DERMOSCOPY
IMAGE ANALYSIS

Digital Imaging and Computer Vision Series

Series Editor

Rastislav Lukac
Foveon, Inc./Sigma Corporation
San Jose, California, U.S.A.

DERMOSCOPY
IMAGE ANALYSIS

Edited by
M. Emre Celebi
Louisiana State University, Shreveport, USA

Teresa Mendonça
University of Porto, Portugal

Jorge S. Marques
Instituto Superior Tecnico, Lisboa, Portugal

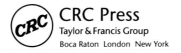

CRC Press
Taylor & Francis Group
Boca Raton London New York

CRC Press is an imprint of the
Taylor & Francis Group, an **informa** business

CRC Press
Taylor & Francis Group
6000 Broken Sound Parkway NW, Suite 300
Boca Raton, FL 33487-2742

First issued in paperback 2017

© 2016 by Taylor & Francis Group, LLC
CRC Press is an imprint of Taylor & Francis Group, an Informa business

No claim to original U.S. Government works

ISBN-13: 978-1-4822-5326-9 (hbk)
ISBN-13: 978-1-138-89287-3 (pbk)

Library of Congress Cataloging-in-Publication Data

Dermoscopy image analysis / edited by M. Emre Celebi, Teresa Mendonca, and Jorge S. Marques.
  p. ; cm. -- (Digital imaging and computer vision)
  Includes bibliographical references and index.
  ISBN 978-1-4822-5326-9 (hardcover : alk. paper)
  I. Celebi, M. Emre, editor. II. Mendonca, Teresa, editor. III. Marques, Jorge S., editor.
IV. Series: Digital imaging and computer vision series.
  [DNLM: 1. Skin Neoplasms--diagnosis. 2. Dermoscopy--methods. 3. Image Interpretation, Computer-Assisted--methods. WR 500]

RC280.S5
616.99'477075--dc23   2015021724

Visit the Taylor & Francis Web site at
http://www.taylorandfrancis.com

and the CRC Press Web site at
http://www.crcpress.com

Contents

Preface

Malignant melanoma is one of the most rapidly increasing cancers in the world. Invasive melanoma alone has an estimated incidence of 73,870 and an estimated total of 9940 deaths in the United States in 2015 [1]. Early diagnosis is particularly important since melanoma can be cured with a simple excision if detected early.

In the past, the primary form of diagnosis for melanoma has been unaided clinical examination. In recent years, dermoscopy has proved valuable in visualizing the morphological structures in pigmented lesions. However, it has also been shown that dermoscopy is difficult to learn and subjective. Therefore, the development of automated image analysis techniques for dermoscopy images has gained importance.

The goal of this book is to summarize the state of the art in the computerized analysis of dermoscopy images and provide future directions for this exciting subfield of medical image analysis. The intended audience includes researchers and practicing clinicians, who are increasingly using digital analytic tools.

The book opens with two chapters on preprocessing. In "Toward a Robust Analysis of Dermoscopy Images Acquired under Different Conditions," Barata et al. investigate the influence of color normalization on classification accuracy. The authors investigate three color constancy algorithms, namely, gray world, max-RGB, and shades of gray, and demonstrate significant gains in sensitivity and specificity on a heterogeneous set of images. In "A Bioinspired Color Representation for Dermoscopy Image Analysis," Madooei and Drew propose a new color space that highlights the distribution of underlying melanin and hemoglobin color pigments. The advantage of this new color representation, in addition to its biological underpinnings, lies in its attenuation of the effects of confounding factors such as light color, intensity falloff, shading, and camera characteristics. The authors demonstrate that the new color space leads to more accurate classification and border detection results.

The book continues with two chapters on border detection (segmentation). In "Where's the Lesion? Variability in Human and Automated Segmentation of Dermoscopy Images of Melanocytic Skin Lesions," Bogo et al. examine the extent of agreement among dermatologist-drawn borders and that among dermatologist-drawn borders and automatically determined ones. The authors conclude that state-of-the-art border detection algorithms can achieve a level of agreement that is only slightly lower than the level of agreement among experienced dermatologists themselves. In "A State-of-the-Art Survey on Lesion Border Detection in Dermoscopy Images," Celebi et al. present a comprehensive overview of 50 published border detection methods. The authors review preprocessing, segmentation, and postprocessing aspects of these methods and discuss performance evaluation issues. They also propose guidelines for future studies in automated border detection.

The book continues with four chapters on feature extraction. In "Comparison of Image Processing Techniques for Reticular Pattern Recognition in Melanoma Detection," García Arroyo and García Zapirain present an in-depth overview of the state of the art in the extraction of pigment networks from dermoscopy images. The authors give a detailed explanation of 20 selected methods and then compare them with respect to various criteria, including the number and diagnostic distribution of the images used for validation and the numerical results obtained in terms of sensitivity, specificity, and accuracy. In "Global Pattern Classification in Dermoscopic Images," Sáez et al. present an overview of six methods for extracting the global patterns (namely, reticular, globular, cobblestone, homogeneous, starburst, parallel, multicomponent, and lacunar patterns) as defined in the pattern analysis diagnostic scheme. The authors first illustrate each pattern and then describe the automated methods designed for extracting these patterns. The chapter concludes with a critical discussion of global pattern extraction. In "Streak Detection in Dermoscopic Color Images Using Localized Radial Flux of Principal Intensity Curvature," Mirzaalian et al. present an automated method for detecting streaks based on the concept of quaternion tubularness and nonlinear support vector machine classification. The authors demonstrate the performance of their feature extraction method on 99 images from the EDRA atlas. Finally, in "Dermoscopy Image Assessment Based on Perceptible Color Regions," Lee et al. present a method for detecting perceptually significant colors in dermoscopy images. The authors first partition the image into 27 color regions by dividing each of the red, green, and blue channels into three levels of brightness using a multithresholding algorithm. They then extract various color features from these regions. The classification performance of these features is demonstrated on 150 images obtained from the Korea University Guro Hospital.

The book continues with four chapters on classification. In "Improved Skin Lesion Diagnostics for General Practice by Computer-Aided Diagnostics," Møllersen et al. present a computer-aided diagnosis (CAD) system for melanomas that features an inexpensive acquisition tool, clinically meaningful features, and interpretable classification feedback. The authors evaluate their system on 206 images acquired at two sites. In "Accurate and Scalable System for Automatic Detection of Malignant Melanoma," Abedini et al. present a comprehensive literature review on CAD systems for melanomas. The authors then propose a highly scalable CAD system implemented in the MapReduce framework and demonstrate its performance on approximately 3000 images obtained from two sources. In "Early Detection of Melanoma in Dermoscopy of Skin Lesion Images by a Computer Vision–Based System," Zare and Toossi present a novel CAD system for melanomas that involves hair detection/removal based on edge detection, thresholding, and inpainting;

border detection using region-based active contours; extraction of various low-level features; feature selection using the t-test; and classification using a neural network classifier. The authors demonstrate the performance of their system on 322 images obtained from two dermoscopy atlases. Finally, in "From Dermoscopy to Mobile Teledermatology," Rosado et al. discuss telemedicine aspects of dermatology. The authors first present an overview of dermatological image databases. They then discuss the challenges involved in the preprocessing of clinical skin lesion images acquired with mobile devices and describe a patient-oriented system for analyzing such images. Finally, they conclude with a comparative review of smart phone-adaptable dermoscopes.

A chapter titled "PH^2: A Public Database for the Analysis of Dermoscopic Images" by Mendonça et al. completes the book. The authors present a publicly available database of dermoscopy images, which contains 200 high-quality images along with their medical annotations. This database can be used as ground truth in various dermoscopy image analysis tasks, including preprocessing, border detection, feature extraction, and classification. The authors also describe some of their projects that made use of this database.

As editors, we hope that this book on computerized analysis of dermoscopy images will demonstrate the significant progress that has occurred in this field in recent years. We also hope that the developments reported in this book will motivate further research in this exciting field.

REFERENCE

1. R. L. Siegel, K. D. Miller, and A. Jemal, "Cancer Statistics, 2015," *CA: A Cancer Journal for Clinicians*, vol. 65, no. 1, pp. 5–29, 2015.

M. Emre Celebi
Louisiana State University
Shreveport, Louisiana

Teresa F. Mendonça
Universidade do Porto
Porto, Portugal

Jorge S. Marques
Instituto Superior Técnico
Lisbon, Portugal

MATLAB® is a registered trademark of The MathWorks, Inc. For product information, please contact:

The MathWorks, Inc.
3 Apple Hill Drive
Natick, MA 01760-2098 USA
Tel: 508 647 7000
Fax: 508-647-7001
E-mail: info@mathworks.com
Web: www.mathworks.com

Editors

M. Emre Celebi earned a BSc in computer engineering at the Middle East Technical University, Ankara, Turkey, in 2002. He earned MSc and PhD degrees in computer science and engineering at the University of Texas at Arlington, Arlington, Texas, in 2003 and 2006, respectively. He is currently an associate professor and the founding director of the Image Processing and Analysis Laboratory in the Department of Computer Science at the Louisiana State University in Shreveport.

Dr. Celebi has actively pursued research in the field of image processing and analysis, with an emphasis on medical image analysis and color image processing. He has worked on several projects funded by the U.S. National Science Foundation (NSF) and National Institutes of Health (NIH) and published more than 120 articles in reputable journals and conference proceedings. His recent research is funded by grants from the NSF.

Dr. Celebi is an editorial board member of 5 international journals and reviewer for more than 90 international journals, and he has served on the program committee of more than 100 international conferences. He has been invited to speak at several colloquia, workshops, and conferences, is the organizer of several workshops, and is the editor of several journal special issues and books. He is a senior member of the Institute of Electrical and Electronics Engineers and SPIE.

Teresa F. Mendonça earned mathematics and PhD degrees at the University of Porto, Portugal, in 1980 and 1993, respectively. Currently she is an assistant professor with the Mathematics Department, Faculty of Sciences, University of Porto, and a researcher at the Institute for Systems and Robotics–Porto. Her research interests are in the areas of identification, modeling, and control applied to the biomedical field. In recent years, she has been involved in projects for modeling and control in anesthesia and in medical image analysis.

Jorge S. Marques earned EE, PhD, and aggregation degrees at the Technical University of Lisbon, Portugal, in 1981, 1990, and 2002, respectively. Currently he is an associate professor with the Electrical and Computer Engineering Department, Instituto Superior Técnico, Lisbon, Portugal, and a researcher at the Institute for Systems and Robotics, Portugal. He was the co-chairman of the IAPR Conference IbPRIA 2005, president of the Portuguese Association for Pattern Recognition (2001–2003), and associate editor of the *Statistics and Computing Journal*, Springer. His research interests are in the areas of statistical image processing, medical image analysis, and pattern recognition.

Contributors

Mani Abedini
IBM Research Australia
Melbourne, Australia

Begoña Acha
Department of Signal Theory and
    Communications
University of Seville
Seville, Spain

Jose Luis García Arroyo
Deustotech-LIFE Unit (eVIDA)
University of Deusto
Bilbao, Spain

Catarina Barata
Institute for Systems and Robotics
Instituto Superior Técnico
Universidade de Lisboa
Lisbon, Portugal

Federica Bogo
Dipartimento di Ingegneria
    dell'Informazione
Università degli Studi di Padova
Padova, Italy

and

Perceiving Systems Department
Max Planck Institute for Intelligent
    Systems
Tuebingen, Germany

Rui Castro
Fraunhofer Portugal AICOS
Porto, Portugal

M. Emre Celebi
Department of Computer Science
Louisiana State University
Shreveport, Louisiana

Qiang Chen
IBM Research Australia
Melbourne, Australia

Noel C. F. Codella
IBM T. J. Watson Research Center
Yorktown Heights, New York

Mark S. Drew
School of Computing Science
Simon Fraser University
British Columbia, Canada

Pedro M. Ferreira
Faculdade de Engenharia
Universidade do Porto
Porto, Portugal

Anna Belloni Fortina
Unità di Dermatologia
Dipartimento di Pediatria
Università degli Studi di Padova
Padova, Italy

Rahil Garnavi
IBM Research Australia
Melbourne, Australia

Fred Godtliebsen
Department of Mathematics and
    Statistics
University of Tromsø
Tromsø, Norway

Ghassan Hamarneh
Medical Image Analysis Lab
Simon Fraser University
British Columbia, Canada

Kristian Hindberg
Department of Mathematics and
    Statistics
University of Tromsø
Tromsø, Norway

Hitoshi Iyatomi
Department of Applied Informatics
Hosei University
Tokyo, Japan

Jaeyoung Kim
Research Institute for Skin Image
College of Medicine
Korea University
Seoul, Korea

Gunwoo Lee
Research Institute for Skin Image
College of Medicine
Korea University
Seoul, Korea

Onseok Lee
Department of Radiological Science
Gimcheon University
Gimcheon, Korea

Tim K. Lee
Photomedicine Institute
Department of Dermatology and
    Skin Science
University of British Columbia and
    Vancouver Coastal Health
    Research Institute
and
Cancer Control Research Program
British Columbia Cancer Agency
British Columbia, Canada

Ali Madooei
School of Computing Science
Simon Fraser University
British Columbia, Canada

André R. S. Marçal
Faculdade de Ciências
Universidade do Porto
Porto, Portugal

Jorge S. Marques
Institute for Systems and Robotics
Instituto Superior Técnico
Universidade de Lisboa
Lisbon, Portugal

Teresa F. Mendonça
Research Center for Systems and
    Technologies
Faculdade de Ciências
Universidade do Porto
Porto, Portugal

Hengameh Mirzaalian
Medical Image Analysis Lab
Simon Fraser University
British Columbia, Canada

Kajsa Møllersen
Norwegian Centre for Integrated
    Care and Telemedicine
University Hospital of North Norway
Tromsø, Norway

Jongsub Moon
Neural Network Laboratory
Korea University
Seoul, Korea

Chilhwan Oh
Department of Dermatology
Guro Hospital
College of Medicine
Korea University
Seoul, Korea

Francesco Peruch
Dipartimento di Ingegneria
  dell'Informazione
Università degli Studi di Padova
Padova, Italy

Enoch Peserico
Dipartimento di Ingegneria
  dell'Informazione
Università degli Studi di Padova
Padova, Italy

Joana Rocha
Hospital Pedro Hispano
Matosinhos, Portugal

Luís Rosado
Fraunhofer Portugal AICOS
Porto, Portugal

Jorge Rozeira
Hospital Pedro Hispano
Matosinhos, Portugal

Aurora Sáez
Department of Signal Theory and
  Communications
University of Seville
Seville, Spain

Gerald Schaefer
Department of Computer Science
Loughborough University
Loughborough, United Kingdom

Thomas R. Schopf
Norwegian Centre for Integrated
  Care and Telemedicine
University Hospital of North Norway
Tromsø, Norway

Carmen Serrano
Department of Signal Theory and
  Communications
University of Seville
Seville, Spain

Kouhei Shimizu
Department of Applied Informatics
Hosei University
Tokyo, Japan

Stein Olav Skrøvseth
Norwegian Centre for Integrated
  Care and Telemedicine
University Hospital of North Norway
Tromsø, Norway

Xingzhi Sun
IBM Research Australia
Melbourne, Australia

João Manuel R. S. Tavares
Instituto de Engenharia Mecânica e
  Gestão Industrial
Departamento de Engenharia
  Mecânica
Faculdade de Engenharia
Universidade do Porto
Porto, Portugal

**Mohammad Taghi Bahreyni
  Toossi**
Medical Physics Research Center
Medical Physics Department
Faculty of Medicine
Mashhad University of Medical
  Sciences
Mashhad, Iran

Maria João M. Vasconcelos
Fraunhofer Portugal AICOS
Porto, Portugal

Quan Wen
School of Computer Science and
    Engineering
University of Electronic Science and
    Technology of China
Chengdu, People's Republic of China

Begoña García Zapirain
Deustotech-LIFE Unit (eVIDA)
University of Deusto
Bilbao, Spain

Hoda Zare
Medical Physics Research Center
Medical Physics Department
Faculty of Medicine

and

Radiologic Technology Department
Faculty of Paramedical Sciences
Mashhad University of Medical
    Sciences
Mashhad, Iran

Huiyu Zhou
School of Electronics, Electrical
    Engineering and Computer
    Science
Queen's University Belfast
Belfast, United Kingdom

Maciel Zortea
Department of Mathematics and
    Statistics
University of Tromsø
Tromsø, Norway

1 Toward a Robust Analysis of Dermoscopy Images Acquired under Different Conditions

Catarina Barata
Instituto Superior Técnico
Lisbon, Portugal

M. Emre Celebi
Louisiana State University
Shreveport, Louisiana

Jorge S. Marques
Instituto Superior Técnico
Lisbon, Portugal

CONTENTS

1.1 INTRODUCTION

Dermoscopy images can be acquired using different devices and illumination conditions. A typical example is teledermoscopy, where the images are acquired at different clinical units and sent to a main hospital to be diagnosed [1]. In each clinical unit, the equipment may be different, and the illumination conditions are different as well. It is well known that both factors can significantly alter the colors of dermoscopy images. Figure 1.1 exemplifies this problem. These images were selected from the EDRA dataset [2] that contains images from three different hospitals.

The human brain is capable of dealing with color variability caused by different acquisition setups. However, computer systems cannot cope with such changes. Thus, this is an aspect that must be taken into account while developing a computer-aided diagnosis (CAD) system, since these kinds of changes strongly influence the commonly used color features (e.g., color histograms). This makes the system less robust and more prone to errors when dealing with multisource images. However, most of the CAD systems proposed in literature do not incorporate a strategy to deal with this problem. A notable exception is the Internet-based system proposed by Iyatomi et al. [3], which includes a color normalization step based on the HSV color space [4].

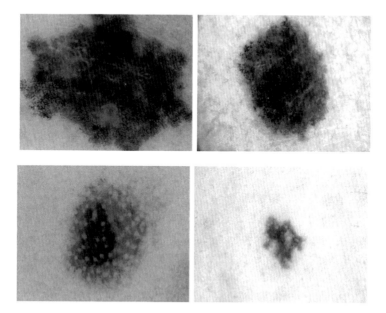

FIGURE 1.1 Different lesions from the EDRA dataset. (Reprinted with permission from Argenziano, G. et al., *Dermoscopy: A Tutorial*, EDRA Medical Publishing and New Media, Milan, Italy, 2002.)

Color normalization is a problem that has been addressed many times in image processing and computer vision. One of approaches used is called color constancy, where the color of the light source is estimated and used to normalize the images. Different color constancy algorithms have been proposed. However, some of these algorithms require knowledge about the acquisition setup. This information is not available for most dermoscopy images. Therefore, we are interested in using a color constancy algorithm that can normalize the images, without needing information about the acquisition system. In this work, we use the shades of gray algorithm [5], which normalizes the colors using only low-level image features. This algorithm not only is fast and easy to implement, but also can achieve performances similar to those of more complex algorithms that use color calibration and training [6].

In this chapter, we show that shades of gray can be used to improve the performance of two different CAD systems, and make them more robust to heterogeneous datasets. The first is a classification system based on the bag-of-features (BoF) model [7, 8]. In this case, we show that the performance of the system significantly improves with color constancy when it is applied to a dataset of images from multiple sources. In the second case, we show that color constancy can improve the detection of colors in dermoscopy images using the algorithm proposed in [9].

The remainder of this chapter is organized as follows: Section 1.2 provides an overview of the proposed calibration methods for dermoscopy images. The information about color constancy and the algorithm used is provided in Section 1.3. Sections 1.4 and 1.5 describe the two CAD systems considered in this chapter and present experimental results for each of them, with and without color constancy. Finally, Section 1.6 concludes the chapter.

1.2 RELATED WORK

Different research groups have proposed color normalization strategies to deal with dermoscopy images. Most of the approaches are hardware based [10–13]. These approaches calibrate images by determining a set of internal camera parameters (e.g., camera offset, color gain, and aperture) as well as a transformation matrix that is used to convert the images to a device-independent color space.

Haeghen et al. [10] were among the first to propose a calibration model of this type. Their calibration procedure consists of converting the images from an unknown RGB color space, which depends on the acquisition system, to the device-invariant sRGB space. Calibration is performed in a set of sequential steps. First, they start by sequentially determining the specific parameters of the acquisition system, namely, the camera offset, the frame grabber, the camera aperture, and the color gains of the camera. By knowing these four parameters, it is possible to maximize the dynamic range and resolution of the system. Then, they use the 24 GretagMacbeth ColorChecker (GMCC) patches to compute the parameters of the transformation matrix. This task is performed in two different stages. First, using a spectrophotometer, they acquire the commission internationale de l'éclairage (CIE) L*a*b* values of each patch after their conversion to sRGB. This allows them to determine the real values of the transformation RGB to sRGB. Next, they have to compute the specific transformation matrix of the imaging system. This task is accomplished by acquiring the 24 GMCC patches using the imaging system. With these two sets of values, it is possible to obtain a set of linear equations that can be used to estimate the components of the transformation matrix.

Grana et al.'s calibration model [11] starts with the correction of border and illumination defects. The former is applied to remove the black pixels associated with the frame of the image or with the black ring of the dermatoscope. The latter consists of a filtering step, whose purpose is to correct the regions of the image where the illumination is not uniform. This filtering step is carried out separately for each color channel. Their following step is to compute the gamma value of the camera and correct it in all the images. With this correction, they obtain the RGB values that can be transformed into device-independent XYZ values. To determine the coefficients of the matrix that transforms RGB into XYZ, they follow the same approach as Haeghen et al. [10], using the GMCC patches and XYZ instead of L*a*b*. Finally, they convert the images from XYZ to a new standard color space. Grana et al. state that the sRGB space used by Haeghen et al. [10] is not appropriate for dermoscopy images, since there is less color contrast with this color space. Therefore, Grana et al. propose a new color space to describe the images. To determine the parameters of the conversion matrix from XYZ to the new space, they have used a set of different colors extracted from dermoscopy images.

Wighton et al. [12] proposed a color calibration model for low-cost digital dermatoscopes. Their method not only corrects color and inconsistent illumination, but also deals with chromatic aberrations. First, they start by performing color correction. This task is carried out as in the work of Grana et al. [11]. The following step is lighting calibration. Wighton et al. start by creating an illumination map for each channel of XYZ. This task is performed using the white patch of the GMCC. After acquiring the patch, its XYZ values are compared with the ground truth values obtained with the spectrophotometer. The ratio between the ground truth and the acquired values leads to the correction maps. Finally, they correct the chromatic aberrations.

The main issue with hardware-based calibration methods is that they require the estimation of device parameters as well as conversion matrix. In both cases, we need to have access to the acquisition device in order to be able to work with the GMCC. This is not always possible in multisource systems (e.g., teledermoscopy networks) or when using commercial heterogeneous databases like EDRA [2]. Furthermore, after a period of time, the acquisition system requires recalibration (e.g., [10]), which might be time-consuming and, consequently, overlooked.

To tackle the aforementioned issues, Iyatomi et al. [4] proposed a calibration system that is software based. Their method performs a fully automated color normalization using image content in the HSV color space. Although Iyatomi et al.'s method does not require knowledge about the acquisition setup, it has a training step. In this step, they start by extracting simple HSV color features from a dataset of dermoscopy images. Then, they use these features to build a set of independent normalization filters. In this stage, they include a selection process in which they reject the less relevant filters.

We are interested in exploring a different and somewhat simpler direction based only on image information that does not require knowledge of the acquisition system properties or a training step. Some of the color constancy algorithms require information about the acquisition device, like the well-known Gamut mapping [14], while others include a training step [14–16]. An alternative is to apply a statistical method based on low-level image features to estimate the color of the light source. Among the possible alternatives [6] we have selected shades of gray, since it has been demonstrated that with appropriate parameter values, this method achieves performance similar to that obtained by more complex methods [5, 6, 17]. Furthermore, this method is a generalization of other well-known color constancy methods (gray world [18] and max-RGB [19]) and is easy to implement.

1.3   COLOR CONSTANCY

1.3.1   SHADES OF GRAY

The goal of color constancy methods is to transform the colors of an image I, acquired under an unknown light source, so that they appear identical to colors under a canonical light source [6, 20, 21]. This task is accomplished by performing two separate steps: estimation of the color of the light source in RGB coordinates, $\mathbf{e} = [e_R, e_G, e_B]^T$, and transformation of the image using the estimated illuminant.

Different algorithms have been proposed to estimate the color of the light source [6]. In this work we apply the shades of gray method [5].

For a color image I, each component of the illuminant e_c, $c \in \{R, G, B\}$, is estimated using the Minkowski norm of the cth color channel, as follows:

$$\left(\frac{\int (I_c(\mathbf{x}))^p \mathrm{d}\mathbf{x}}{\int \mathrm{d}\mathbf{x}} \right)^{1/p} = k e_c \quad c \in \{R, G, B\} \tag{1.1}$$

where I_c is the cth color component of image I, $\mathbf{x} = (x, y)$ is the position of each pixel, k is a normalization constant that ensures that $\mathbf{e} = [e_R, e_G, e_B]^T$ has unit length, using the Euclidean norm, and p is the degree of the norm. The value of p can be tuned according to the dataset used as well as according to the type of system. Shades of gray is a generalization of two other color constancy algorithms: gray world [18], when $p = 1$, and max-RGB [19], when $p = \infty$.

After estimating $\mathbf{e}$, the next step transforms the image I. A simple way to model this transformation is the von Kries diagonal model [22]:

$$\begin{pmatrix} I_R^t \\ I_G^t \\ I_B^t \end{pmatrix} = \begin{pmatrix} d_R & 0 & 0 \\ 0 & d_G & 0 \\ 0 & 0 & d_B \end{pmatrix} \begin{pmatrix} I_R^u \\ I_G^u \\ I_B^u \end{pmatrix} \tag{1.2}$$

where $[I_R^u, I_G^u, I_B^u]^T$ is the pixel value acquired under an unknown light source, and $[I_R^t, I_G^t, I_B^t]^T$ is the transformed pixel value as it would appear under the canonical light source, which is assumed to be the perfect white light, that is, $\mathbf{e}^w = (1/\sqrt{3}, 1/\sqrt{3}, 1/\sqrt{3})^T$. The matrix coefficients $\{d_R, d_G, d_B\}$ are related to the estimated illuminant $\mathbf{e}$ as follows:

$$d_c = \frac{1}{e_c}, \quad c \in \{R, G, B\} \tag{1.3}$$

The color constancy method described above is applied to the RGB color space. Nonetheless, it has been shown that color constancy can also be combined with color space conversion, in a sequential way. First, color correction is performed, and then a color space transformation is applied. van de Weijer and Schmid [23] have shown that color constancy can be used to improve object detection and image classification using HSV features. Thus, we include two color spaces in our experiments: RGB and HSV.

1.3.2 GAMMA CORRECTION

Image acquisition systems, such as the ones used to acquire dermoscopy images, transform sRGB values through gamma (γ) correction, leading to what is referred to as nonlinear R'G'B'. In practice, this correction is applied for visualization purposes, since it reduces the dynamic range, that is, increases the low values and decreases the high values, as can be seen in Equation 1.4, where $I_c(\mathbf{x}) \in [0, 1]$ and $c \in \{R, G, B\}$. By adjusting the dynamic range, it is possible to compensate the way humans perceive light and color.

$$I_c'(\mathbf{x}) = \begin{cases} 12.92 I_c(\mathbf{x}) & \text{if } I_c(\mathbf{x}) \le 0.0031308 \\ 1.055 I_c(\mathbf{x})^{1/\gamma} - 0.055 & \text{otherwise} \end{cases} \tag{1.4}$$

The main problem with γ correction is that digital systems store images after this correction is applied. However, the color normalization algorithms are derived for the sRGB values. Thus, before processing the dermoscopy images, it is necessary to undo the γ correction. The transformation of R'G'B' to sRGB is simply performed by inverting Equation 1.4:

$$I_c(\mathbf{x}) = \begin{cases} \frac{I'_c(\mathbf{x})}{12.92} & \text{if } I_c(\mathbf{x}) \leq 0.03928 \\ \left(\frac{I'_c(\mathbf{x})+0.055}{1.055}\right)^\gamma & \text{otherwise} \end{cases} \tag{1.5}$$

where γ is set to the standard value of 2.2 [24]. We have applied Equation 1.5 to all the images before performing color constancy. Nonetheless, for visualization purposes, the images shown in the remaining sections of the chapter have been corrected using Equation 1.4, after color normalization.

1.3.3 GENERAL FRAMEWORK

The block diagram of our experiments is displayed in Figure 1.2. We start by performing gamma correction using Equation 1.5. Then we estimate the color of the lighting source using Equation 1.1 and normalize image colors using Equation 1.2. If we want to use other color space besides RGB, the color space transformation is performed after color normalization (see Figure 1.2). In the color transformation block, the color components of each pixel are changed to the new color coordinates. Finally, we are able to apply one of the CAD systems considered in this work (lesion classification or color detection). Figure 1.3 exemplifies the color normalization process on an image from the EDRA dataset.

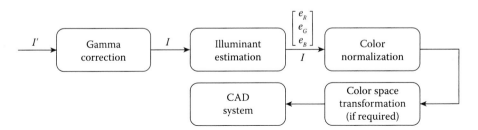

FIGURE 1.2 Color normalization framework.

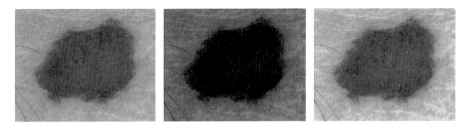

FIGURE 1.3 Example of color normalization: original image (left), gamma correction (middle), and corrected image ($p = 6$). (Reprinted with permission from Argenziano, G. et al., *Dermoscopy: A Tutorial*, EDRA Medical Publishing and New Media, Milan, Italy, 2002.)

1.4   LESION CLASSIFICATION

Different CAD systems have been proposed for the classification of dermoscopy images. Most of these systems extract global image features, which means that they segment the lesion and compute a feature vector that contains information about the whole lesion [3, 25–27]. An alternative to this kind of analysis consists of dividing the lesion into small patches, and separately characterizing each of them using local features. A popular algorithm for this kind of analysis is BoF, which has already been shown to perform well in the classification of dermoscopy images [7, 8] using only color features. The images used in the previous works [7, 8] are selected from the publicly available PH^2 dataset [28] and were acquired at a single hospital, using the same equipment and illumination conditions. Our goal is to extend the BoF system to multiple acquisition sources, as it happens in the case of teledermoscopy, where the images are acquired at multiple facilities and sent to a central dermatology service to be diagnosed.

1.4.1   BoF MODEL

The CAD system used in this chapter is summarized in Figure 1.4. First, the lesion is separated from the surrounding skin. To do so, we have used manual segmentations to prevent classification errors due to incorrect border detection. Segmentations were validated by an expert. Then, we trained and tested a BoF model [29] to obtain a classification rule. The BoF system used in this work is trained as described in [7, 8, 30].

The BoF model performs a description of a lesion using local information (small patches). It starts by separately analyzing different patches of the lesion and then uses them to compute a signature. Then, this signature is used to characterize the lesion and classify it as melanoma or benign. The easiest way to separate the lesion into different sections is to search for salient points located on specific texture regions, such as lines or dots/blobs. In this chapter,

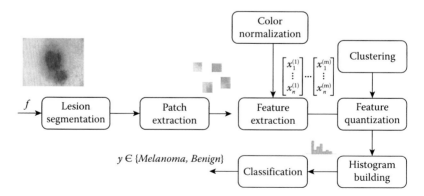

FIGURE 1.4   Block diagram of the classification system.

this task is accomplished using one of the most popular keypoint detectors in literature: the Harris–Laplace detector, which is applied after converting the color image into a grayscale image [31]. This detector performed well in previous studies [7, 8, 30]. After finding the keypoints, it is then possible to extract their support regions, which correspond to square patches centered on the keypoints. We then remove all the patches that are not fully contained in the lesion region and intersect the lesion in less than 50% of its area.

In the next step, we extract a vector of color features from each of the patches. This step is directly related to the theme of this paper since the color calibration step alters the color information of an image and, as a result, the values of the extracted features. Therefore, the features extracted in this step are computed over the normalized images.

Skin lesions have different areas. Moreover, the number of keypoints detected inside each lesion varies. Therefore, an intermediate step in which the patch features are converted into usable information is necessary. The strategy used in BoF is to use all feature vectors of the training set to predict K centroids [29]. This task is carried out using the K-means algorithm. The computed set of centroids is often called a codebook and contains a set of typical features that represent the training data. These centroids are then used to label each patch according to the closest centroid (the one that minimizes the Euclidean distance). It is then possible to represent each lesion by counting the number of times each centroid is selected. This information is stored in a histogram and considered the signature of the lesion.

During the training phase, histograms of the training set as well as the lesion labels (melanoma/benign) are used to train a support vector machine (SVM) classifier with the χ^2 kernel:

$$K_{\chi^2}(\mathbf{x}, \mathbf{y}) = e^{-\rho d_{\chi^2}(\mathbf{x},\mathbf{y})} \tag{1.6}$$

where $\mathbf{x}$ and $\mathbf{y}$ are image histograms, ρ is a width parameter, and

$$d_{\chi^2}(\mathbf{x}, \mathbf{y}) = \sum_i \frac{(x_i - y_i)^2}{x_i + y_i} \tag{1.7}$$

To classify unseen images, we use the set of centroids computed during the training phase to label the patches and compute the lesion histograms. Then, we apply the SVM classifier to label each lesion as melanoma or benign.

In this work, we use one-dimensional (1-D) RGB and HSV histograms to describe the patches. We select the former because color constancy algorithms are performed on the RGB color space. Thus, the influence of color normalization should be more evident in RGB features. We also use HSV to show that color constancy can be combined with color space transformations, as proposed in [23]. Furthermore, both color spaces achieved very good classification results in previous works [7, 8]. In the following section, we evaluate the BoF classifier with and without color constancy.

1.4.2 EXPERIMENTAL RESULTS

The experiments were conducted on a multisource dataset of 482 images (50% melanomas and 50% benign), randomly selected from the EDRA dataset [2]. EDRA contains images from three university hospitals: University Federico II of Naples (Italy), University of Graz (Austria), and University of Florence (Italy), which makes this dataset particularly challenging for classification systems that use color features.

To assess the influence of the color calibration methods, we have trained two BoF systems for each color space. The first was trained using nonnormalized images and the other using the color-corrected images. To evaluate the performance of each system, we compute three metrics: sensitivity (SE), specificity (SP), and accuracy (ACC). SE corresponds to the percentage of melanomas that are correctly classified, and SP is the percentage of correctly classified benign lesions. All metrics are computed using a stratified ten fold cross-validation scheme. We have tried different values of $p \in \{2, 10\}$ in Equation 1.1 as well as the two special instances of the color constancy algorithm: gray world ($p = 1$) and max-RGB ($p = \infty$).

Table 1.1 shows the classification results achieved with and without color correction. These results were obtained with $p = 6$. It can be seen that, as expected, the color constancy method significantly improves the classification results with 1-D RGB histograms. In this case, the ACC of the system is improved by 14%. In the case of HSV, the BoF model without color correction performs better than the corresponding RGB one. Nonetheless, it is still possible to improve the performance of HSV by using color normalization.

Figures 1.5 and 1.6 show some examples of color-normalized images, using different values of p (Equation 1.1), including the two special instances of shades of gray: gray world ($p = 1$) and max-RGB ($p = \infty$). It is clear that shades of gray corrects the colors of the images, making them look more similar. Please note that as the value of p increases, the images look less grayish and achieve a more natural coloration. In some cases of $p = \infty$, the normalized image is very similar to the original one. Furthermore, it is possible to correct

---

TABLE 1.1

Classification Results for the EDRA Dataset without and with Color Correction

Color Space	Color Constancy	Sensitivity	Specificity	Accuracy
RGB	None	71.0%	55.2%	63.1%
	Shades of gray	79.7%	76.0%	77.8%
HSV	None	73.8%	76.8%	75.3%
	Shades of gray	73.9%	80.1%	77.0%

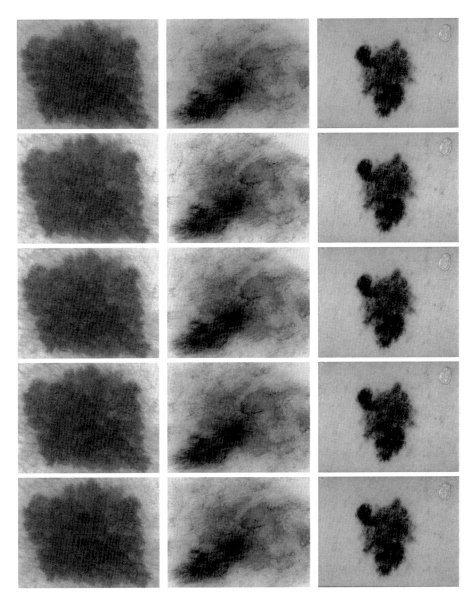

FIGURE 1.5 (See color insert.) Examples of color normalization using different values of p melanomas. From top row to bottom: original image, $p = 1$, $p = 3$, $p = 6$, and $p = \infty$. (Reprinted with permission from Argenziano, G. et al., *Dermoscopy: A Tutorial*, EDRA Medical Publishing and New Media, Milan, Italy, 2002.)

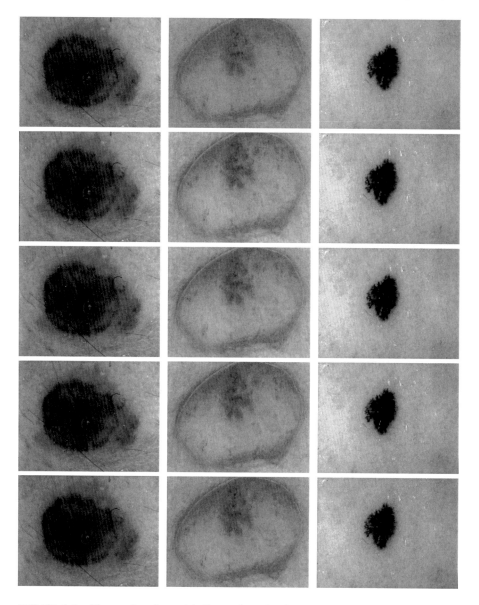

FIGURE 1.6 (See color insert.) Examples of color normalization using different values of p benign. From top row to bottom: original image, $p = 1$, $p = 3$, $p = 6$, and $p = \infty$. (Reprinted with permission from Argenziano, G. et al., *Dermoscopy: A Tutorial*, EDRA Medical Publishing and New Media, Milan, Italy, 2002.)

color channel saturations. In some of the examples, the red channel of the acquisition camera is clearly saturated, making the image look reddish. Color normalization also allows a better visualization of the colors of the lesion, enhances the contrast inside the lesion, and in some cases, even improves the contrast between the lesion and the surrounding skin.

1.5 COLOR DETECTION

The classification model used is not fully clinically oriented, despite performing a local analysis of the lesion based on the detection of relevant textures. In recent years, there has been a growing interest in the development of clinically oriented CAD systems. These systems analyze and diagnose the lesions in a way similar to that of dermatologists, by detecting relevant dermoscopic characteristics [32–35].

One of the more relevant dermoscopic characteristics is color. Dermatologists can either count the number of colors in the lesion (ABCD rule [36] and Menzies' score [37]) or search for relevant color structures (7-point checklist [38]). Both approaches have been investigated, and CAD systems have been proposed that perform the former [9, 32, 39, 40] or the latter [33, 41, 42]. All of the previous systems require the extraction of color features. As we have shown in the Section 1.4, color features are significantly influenced by the acquisition setup. Thus, it is important to study the role of color normalization in the color detection problem.

In this section, we investigate the importance of color normalization using the color detection algorithm proposed in [9]. This algorithm uses Gaussian mixture models to describe a set of five relevant dermoscopy colors (blue–gray, black, white, dark brown, and light brown).

Figure 1.7 shows the block diagram of the system. In the preprocessing, artifacts such as hairs are removed using the algorithm proposed in [34], and the lesions are manually segmented. The training of the color models and color detection process will be described next.

1.5.1 LEARNING COLOR MIXTURE MODELS

The ABCD rule of dermoscopy considers a set of six colors that may be present in a skin lesion (white, red, light brown, dark brown, blue–gray, and black) [2]. During a routine examination, the medical doctor should determine how many colors are visible in the lesion. This operation has been recently tackled representing each color by a Gaussian mixture learned from examples [9]. In [9], the authors compute a model for five of the six possible colors: white, light brown, dark brown, blue–gray, and black. This leads to a color palette of five Gaussian mixtures. This approach was possible because it uses a set of medically annotated images from the PH^2 dataset (see [28] for more details). In this work, we use the same training set, which consists of 29 dermoscopy images. For each image, the different color regions were manually segmented

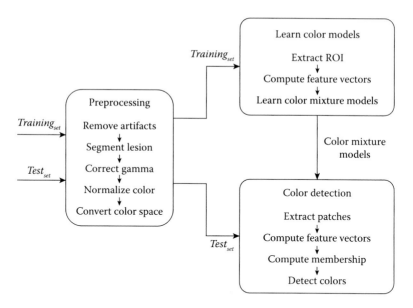

FIGURE 1.7 Block diagram of the color detection system.

and labeled by an expert dermatologist (see an example for each color in Figure 1.8). This resulted in 17 examples of both dark brown and light brown, 6 examples of blue–gray, and 4 examples of both black and white. The red color is not present in this dataset and was not considered.

Features are extracted from the training set in the following way. A set of round patches, with a 5-pixel radius, is randomly selected from each region. Since there are considerably more examples of dark brown and light brown than of the remaining colors, the number of patches extracted from each of the corresponding regions depends on the color. Therefore, we selected 250 patches from each light brown and dark brown region, 350 patches from each blue–gray region, and 500 patches from each white and black region. The final step computes a feature vector to characterize each patch, which is its mean color. As in [9], we compute the color features in the HSV space.

Each skin color $c = 1, \ldots, 5$ is represented by a Gaussian mixture model:

$$p(\mathbf{y}|c, \theta^c) = \sum_{m=1}^{k_c} \alpha_m^c \, p(\mathbf{y}|c, \theta_m^c) \tag{1.8}$$

where k_c is the number of components of the cth color mixture, $\alpha_1^c \ldots \alpha_k^c$ are the mixing probabilities ($\alpha_m^c \geq 0$ and $\sum_{m=1}^{k_c} \alpha_m^c = 1$), and θ_m^c is the set of parameters that defines the mth component of the cth Gaussian mixture. In our work, $\mathbf{y}$ is a 3-D feature vector associated with each patch, and

$$p(\mathbf{y}|c, \theta_m^c) = \frac{(2\pi)^{-(d/2)}}{\sqrt{|R_m^c|}} \exp\left\{ -\frac{1}{2}(\mathbf{y} - \mu_m^c)^T (R_m^c)^{-1} (\mathbf{y} - \mu_m^c) \right\} \tag{1.9}$$

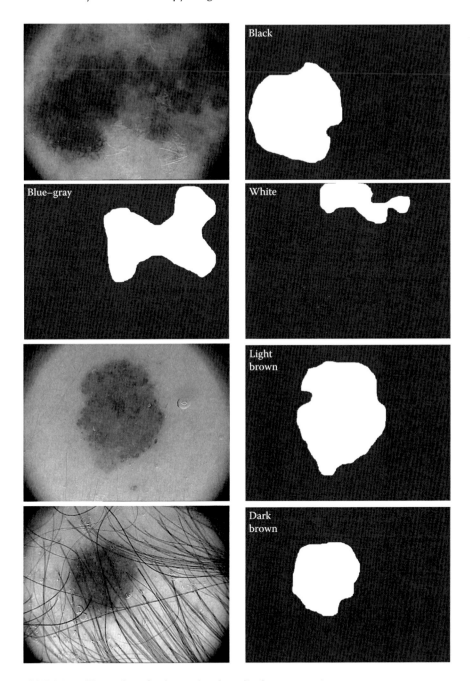

FIGURE 1.8 Examples of color regions' medical segmentations.

where $\theta_m^c = (\mu_m^c, R_m^c, \alpha_m^c)$. Thus, the parameters to be estimated when learning a mixture are the mean and covariance of each component (μ_m^c, R_m^c) and the corresponding mixing probabilities α_m^c. The parameters of each mixture are estimated using the algorithm proposed by Figueiredo and Jain [43] that also estimates the model complexity, that is, the number of Gaussians needed to represent the data.

1.5.2 COLOR IDENTIFICATION

The color identification approach proposed in [9] is a hierarchical decision scheme with two steps: patch labeling and lesion labeling.

First, the lesion is sampled into small patches of size 12×12 using a regular grid. For each patch, its mean color $\mathbf{y}$ is computed and its membership to each color model is determined using a Bayesian law:

$$p(c|\mathbf{y}) = \frac{p(\mathbf{y}|c, \widehat{\theta}^c)p(c)}{p(\mathbf{y}|\widehat{\theta})} \tag{1.10}$$

where $\widehat{\theta}^c = (\widehat{\mu}^c, \widehat{R}^c, \widehat{\alpha}^c)$, $\widehat{\theta} = (\widehat{\theta}^1, \dots, \widehat{\theta}^5)$, and $p(c) = 1/5$ are set to be equal for all colors, and

$$p(\mathbf{y}|\widehat{\theta}) = \sum_{c=1}^{5} p(\mathbf{y}|c, \widehat{\theta}^c)p(c) \tag{1.11}$$

By selecting the model with the highest degree of membership, it is possible to segment the different color regions. The described steps correspond to the patch labeling process. In order to label the lesion and count the number of colors, the area of each color region is compared with a threshold.

1.5.3 EXPERIMENTAL RESULTS

To assess the influence of color constancy on the color detection problem, we trained two different sets of color models, using 29 images from the PH^2 dataset, with medical segmentations of colors. In the first case, we trained the models without performing the color normalization step, while in the second case, we train the models with a color correction step, where we correct the RGB images. We have empirically determined that $p = 3$ (see Equation 1.11) is a suitable value.

To test the color detection systems, we used two datasets: one with 123 images from the PH^2 dataset (different from the training examples) and the other with 340 images from EDRA. Please note the mismatch between training and test sources in the second case. For each of these images there is a medical ground truth annotation (color label) stating whether each color is present or absent. The computed statistics are the SE, the average percentage of correctly identified colors; SP, the average percentage of correctly nonidentified colors, and ACC.

Table 1.2 shows the performances obtained with the two tested frameworks. These results show that the system performance is significantly improved when the color constancy algorithm is applied. This conclusion is valid for both datasets. We stress that in the case of the EDRA dataset, the models were trained with 29 images from the PH^2 dataset. This shows that color normalization improves the robustness of the proposed method, making it more suitable to deal with images acquired under different conditions.

Figures 1.9 and 1.10 show examples of color detection without and with color normalization. Similarly to what was observed in Section 1.4, color normalization makes the images look more similar and improves the color contrast

TABLE 1.2

Color Detection Results for the Single- and Multisource Datasets

Dataset	Color Constancy	Sensitivity	Specificity	Balanced Accuracy
PH^2	None	79.7%	73.9%	76.8%
	Shades of gray	91.7%	74.5%	81.7%
EDRA	None	75.5%	55.5%	65.7%
	Shades of gray	80.5%	69.7%	75.1%

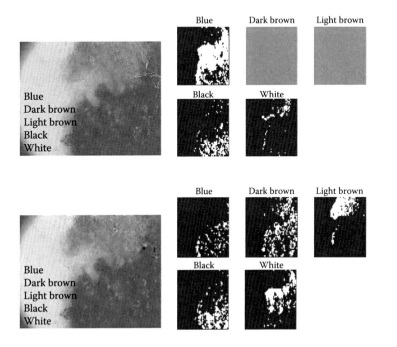

FIGURE 1.9 Example of color detection without and with color constancy.

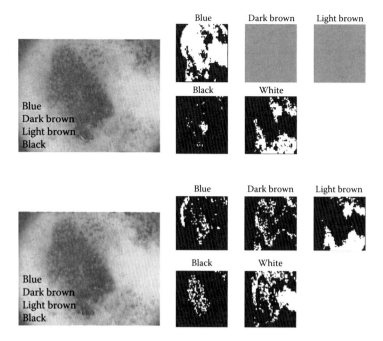

FIGURE 1.10 Example of color detection without and with color constancy.

inside the lesion. Observing these examples, it is clear that color normalization has an important role in improving color discrimination. After applying color correction, the algorithm is capable of identifying the presence of all the colors, which did not happen before. In Figure 1.10, the algorithm incorrectly identifies the skin color as white. This incorrect detection is understandable, since the algorithm does not have a model for the color of the skin.

1.6 CONCLUSIONS

A color-based CAD system for the analysis of dermoscopy images must be able to cope with multisource images, acquired using different setups and illumination conditions. This work studies the use of color constancy algorithms in two important tasks: melanoma detection and color detection and counting. To apply color constancy, we have selected the shades of gray method. We have also tested gray world and max-RGB, since these methods are particular cases of shades of gray for $p = 1$ and $p = \infty$, respectively. Nonetheless, we have determined that other values of p are more suitable for our applications.

In the lesion classification problem, we have shown that color constancy improves the performance of a BoF model in the classification of multi-source images. When we use RGB color features after color correction, the performance of the system is increased by 14%. We have also shown that color constancy improves the performance of HSV features.

The color detection problem is another challenging task. We have investigated the performance of a recently proposed color detection algorithm [9] with and without color normalization and observed significant improvements even when the images come from a single source. Color correction seems to enhance color discrimination.

In this work, we have represented color using RGB and HSV color spaces and showed that color constancy significantly improves the performance of the tested systems in both cases.

ACKNOWLEDGMENTS

This work was partially funded with grant SFRH/BD/84658/2012 and by Fundação para a Ciência e Tecnologia (FCT) projects PTDC/SAU-BEB/103471/2008 and FCT [UID/EEA/50009/2013].

We would like to thank Prof. Teresa Mendonça and Pedro Ferreira from Faculdade de Ciências, Universidade do Porto, and Dr. Jorge Rozeira and Dr. Joana Rocha from Hospital Pedro Hispano for providing the annotated PH^2 dataset. We would also like to thank Prof. Mário Figueiredo from the Institute of Telecommunications, Instituto Superior Técnico, for his contribution to the color detection algorithm.

REFERENCES

1. C. Massone, A. Brunasso, R. Hofmann-Wellenhof, A. Gulia, and H. Soyer, Teledermoscopy: Education, discussion forums, teleconsulting and mobile teledermoscopy, *Giornale italiano di dermatologia e venereologia*, vol. 145, no. 1, pp. 127–132, 2010.
2. G. Argenziano, H. P. Soyer, V. De Giorgi, D. Piccolo, P. Carli, M. Delfino, A. Ferrari, V. Hofmann-Wellenhog, D. Massi, G. Mazzocchetti, M. Scalvenzi, and I. H. Wolf, *Interactive Atlas of Dermoscopy*, EDRA Medical Publishing and New Media, Milan, Italy, 2000.
3. H. Iyatomi, H. Oka, M. E. Celebi, M. Hashimoto, M. Hagiwara, M. Tanaka, and K. Ogawa, An improved Internet-based melanoma screening system with dermatologist-like tumor area extraction algorithm, *Computerized Medical Imaging and Graphics*, vol. 32, pp. 566–579, 2008.
4. H. Iyatomi, M. E. Celebi, G. Schaefer, and M. Tanaka, Automated color calibration method for dermoscopy images, *Computerized Medical Imaging and Graphics*, vol. 35, pp. 89–98, 2011.
5. G. Finlayson and E. Trezzi, Shades of gray and colour constancy, in *IS&T/SID 12th Color Imaging Conference*, pp. 37–41, 2004.
6. A. Gijsenij, T. Gevers, and J. van de Weijer, Computational color constancy: Survey and experiments, *IEEE Transactions on Image Processing*, vol. 20, no. 9, pp. 2475–2489, 2011.
7. C. Barata, M. Ruela, T. Mendonça, and J. S. Marques, A bag-of-features approach for the classification of melanomas in dermoscopy images: The role of color and

texture descriptors, in *Computer Vision Techniques for the Diagnosis of Skin Cancer* (J. Scharcanski and M. E. Celebi, eds.), pp. 49–69, Springer, Berlin, 2014.

8. C. Barata, M. Ruela, M. Francisco, T. Mendonça, and J. S. Marques, Two systems for the detection of melanomas in dermoscopy images using texture and color features, *IEEE Systems Journal*, vol. 8, no. 3, pp. 965–979, 2014.

9. C. Barata, M. A. T. Figueiredo, M. E. Celebi, and J. S. Marques, Color identification in dermoscopy images using Gaussian mixture models, in *IEEE International Conference on Acoustics, Speech, and Signal Processing*, Florence, Italy, pp. 3611–3615, 2014.

10. Y. V. Haeghen, J. M. A. D. Naeyaert, and I. Lemahieu, An imaging system with calibrated color image acquisition for use in dermatology, *IEEE Transactions on Medical Imaging*, vol. 19, no. 7, pp. 722–730, 2000.

11. C. Grana, G. Pellacani, and S. Seidanari, Pratical color calibration for dermoscopy applied to a digital epiluminescence microscope, *Skin Research and Technology*, vol. 11, pp. 242–247, 2005.

12. P. Wighton, T. K. Lee, H. Lui, D. McLean, and M. S. Atkins, 'Chromatic aberration correction: An enhancement to the calibration of low-cost digital dermoscopes, *Skin Research and Technology*, vol. 17, pp. 339–347, 2011.

13. J. Quintana, R. Garcia, and L. Neumann, A novel method for color correction in epiluminescence microscopy, *Computerized Medical Imaging and Graphics*, vol. 35, pp. 646–652, 2011.

14. D. Forsyth, A novel algorithm for color constancy, *International Journal of Computer Vision*, vol. 5, no. 1, pp. 5–36, 1990.

15. G. Finlayson, S. Hordley, and P. Hubel, Color by correlation: A simple, unifying framework for color constancy, *IEEE Transactions on Pattern Analysis and Machine Intelligence*, vol. 23, no. 11, pp. 1209–1221, 2001.

16. J. van de Weijer, C. Schmid, and J. Verbeek, Using high-level visual information for color constancy, in *IEEE International Conference on Computer Vision*, Rio de Janeiro, Brasil, pp. 8–11, 2007.

17. J. van de Weijer, T. Gevers, and A. Gijsenij, Edge-based color constancy, *IEEE Transactions on Image Processing*, vol. 16, no. 9, pp. 2207–2214, 2007.

18. G. Buchsbaum, A spatial processor model for object colour perception, *Journal of the Franklin Institute*, vol. 210, pp. 1–26, 1980.

19. E. Land, The retinex theory of color vision, *Scientific American*, vol. 237, pp. 108–128, 1977.

20. S. Shafer, Using color to separate reflection components, *Color Research and Application*, vol. 10, no. 4, pp. 210–218, 1985.

21. G. Klinker, S. Shafer, and T. Kanade, A physical approach to color image understanding, *International Journal of Computer Vision*, vol. 4, no. 1, pp. 7–38, 1990.

22. J. von Kries, Influence of adaptation on the effects produced by luminous stimuli, *Sources of Color Vision*, pp. 109–119, 1970.

23. J. van de Weijer and C. Schmid, Coloring local feature extraction, in *European Conference on Computer Vision*, Graz, Austria, pp. 246–268, 2006.

24. C. Poynton, *Digital Video and HD: Algorithms and Interfaces.* Morgan Kaufmann, Burlington, MA, 2012.

25. H. Ganster, P. Pinz, R. Rohrer, E. Wildling, M. Binder, and H. Kittler, Automated melanoma recognition, *IEEE Transactions on Medical Imaging*, vol. 20, no. 3, pp. 233–239, 2001.

26. M. E. Celebi, H. Kingravi, B. Uddin, H. Iyatomi, Y. Aslandogan, W. Stoecker, and R. Moss, A methodological approach to the classification of dermoscopy images, *Computerized Medical Imaging and Graphics*, vol. 31, pp. 362–373, 2007.

27. Q. Abbas, M. E. Celebi, I. F. Garcia, and W. Ahmad, Melanoma recognition framework based on expert definition of ABCD for dermoscopic images, *Skin Research and Technology*, vol. 19, pp. e93–e102, 2013.

28. T. Mendonca, P. M. Ferreira, J. S. Marques, A. R. S. Marcal, and J. Rozeira, PH2: A dermoscopic image database for research and benchmarking, in *35th Annual International Conference of the IEEE Engineering in Medicine and Biology Society (EMBC)*, Osaka, Japan, pp. 5437–5440, 2013.

29. J. Sivic and A. Zisserman, Video Google: A text retrieval approach to object matching in videos, in *9th IEEE International Conference on Computer Vision*, Nice, France, pp. 1470–1477, 2003.

30. C. Barata, J. S. Marques, and J. Rozeira, The role of keypoint sampling on the classification of melanomas in dermoscopy images using bag-of-features, in *Iberian Conference on Pattern Recognition and Image Analysis*, Madeira, Portugal, pp. 715–723, 2013.

31. K. Mikolajczyk and C. Schmid, Scale and affine invariant interest point detectors, *International Journal of Computer Vision*, vol. 60, no. 1, pp. 63–86, 2004.

32. S. Seidenari, G. Pellacani, and C. Grana, Computer description of colours in dermoscopic melanocytic lesion images reproducing clinical assessment, *British Journal of Dermatology*, vol. 149, no. 3, pp. 523–529, 2003.

33. M. E. Celebi, H. Iyatomi, W. V. Stoecker, R. H. Moss, H. S. Rabinovitz, G. Argenziano, and H. P. Soyer, Automatic detection of blue-white veil and related structures in dermoscopy images, *Computerized Medical Imaging and Graphics*, vol. 32, pp. 670–677, 2008.

34. C. Barata, J. S. Marques, and J. Rozeira, A system for the detection of pigment network in dermoscopy images using directional filters, *IEEE Transactions on Biomedical Engineering*, vol. 10, pp. 2744–2754, 2012.

35. M. Sadeghi, T. Lee, H. Lui, D. McLean, and S. Atkins, Detection and analysis of irregular streaks in dermoscopic images of skin lesions, *IEEE Transactions on Medical Imaging*, vol. 32, pp. 849–861, 2013.

36. W. Stolz, A. Riemann, and A. B. Cognetta, ABCD rule of dermatoscopy: A new practical method for early recognition of malignant melanoma, *European Journal of Dermatology*, vol. 4, pp. 521–527, 1994.

37. S. Menzies, C. Ingvar, K. Crotty, and W. H. McCarthy, Frequency and morphologic characteristics of invasive melanomas lacking specific surface microscopic features, *Archives of Dermatology*, vol. 132, pp. 1178–1182, 1996.

38. G. Argenziano, G. Fabbrocini, P. Carli, V. De Giorgi, E. Sammarco, and E. Delfino, Epiluminescence microscopy for the diagnosis of doubtful melanocytic skin lesions: Comparison of the ABCD rule of dermatoscopy and a new 7-point checklist based on pattern analysis, *Archives of Dermatology*, vol. 134, pp. 1563–1570, 1998.

39. A. R. S. Marcal, T. Mendonca, C. S. P. Silva, M. A. Pereira, and J. Rozeira, Evaluation of the Menzies method potential for automatic dermoscopic image analysis, in *Computational Modelling of Objects Represented in Images— CompImage 2012*, pp. 103–108, 2012.

40. M. E. Celebi and A. Zornberg, Automated quantification of clinically significant colors in dermoscopy images and its application to skin lesion classification, *IEEE Systems Journal*, vol. 8, no. 3, pp. 980–984, 2014.

41. G. Di Leo, G. Fabbrocini, A. Paolillo, O. Rescigno, and P. Sommella, Towards an automatic diagnosis system for skin lesions: Estimation of blue-whitish veil and regression structures, in *6th International IEEE Multiconference on Systems, Signals and Devices*, Djerba, Tunisia, pp. 1–6, 2009.

42. A. Madooei, M. S. Drew, M. Sadeghi, and M. S. Atkins, Automatic detection of blue-white veil by discrete colour matching in dermoscopy images, in *Medical Image Computing and Computer-Assisted Intervention—MICCAI 2013*, pp. 453–460, Springer, Nagoya, Japan, 2013.

43. M. A. T. Figueiredo and A. K. Jain, Unsupervised learning of finite mixture models, *IEEE Transactions on Pattern Analysis and Machine Intelligence*, vol. 24, no. 3, pp. 381–396, 2002.

2 A Bioinspired Color Representation for Dermoscopy Image Analysis

Ali Madooei
Simon Fraser University
Vancouver, Canada

Mark S. Drew
Simon Fraser University
Vancouver, Canada

CONTENTS

2.1   INTRODUCTION

In this chapter, we investigate the use of color features representing biological properties of skin with application to dermoscopy image analysis. As a case study, we focus on two applications: segmentation and classification. The main contribution is a new color-space representation that is used, as a feature space, in supervised learning to achieve excellent melanoma versus benign skin lesion classification. This is a step toward building a more reliable computer-aided diagnosis system for skin cancers.

The proposed color space is aimed at understanding the underlying biological factors that are involved in human skin coloration, that is, melanin and hemoglobin. These two chromophores strongly absorb light in the visible spectrum and thus are major contributors to skin color and pigmentation. This motivates the hypothesis that, through analysis of skin color, one may extract information about the underlying melanin and hemoglobin content.

Few studies have investigated the use of color features representing biological properties of skin lesions. Among these, a notable study is the work of Claridge et al. [1]. These authors have figured prominently, with emphasis on the use of intermediate multispectral modeling to generate images disambiguating dermal and epidermal melanin, thickness of collagen, and blood [1]. This type of analysis is interesting, as it offers the possibility of obtaining information about skin physiology and composition in a noninvasive manner. Such information may potentially be useful for diagnosis of skin diseases. However, the method in [1] (and other similar techniques, such as skin spectroscopy) requires specific optical instruments. It would be economically and computationally beneficial if this information could be extracted from conventional clinical images. In particular, the melanin and hemoglobin content of skin images can aid analysis of skin pigmentation, erythema, inflammation, and hemodynamics.

This study focuses on using conventional dermatological images such as dermoscopy images. In other words, we aim at utilizing only red, green, blue (RGB) color and not considering multispectral image modeling. The closest research to our work is the seminal study by Tsumura et al. [2, 3] who employed independent component analysis (ICA) of skin images for extracting melanin and hemoglobin information. While Tsumura et al.'s goal was to develop a computationally efficient model of skin appearance for image synthesis, we employ the extracted information as a feature space for supervised classification of class melanoma versus class benign.

We develop a model of skin coloration based on physics and biology of human skin, which is shown to be compatible with the ICA data model. This model utilizes Tsumura's work and combines it with another stream of work proposed by Finlayson et al. [4]. The latter is an image analysis approach that is devised to find an intrinsic reflectivity image, that is, an image that is invariant to lighting and lighting-related factors such as shading.

The proposed skin coloration model succeeds in largely removing confounding factors in the imagery system, such as (1) the effects of the particular camera characteristics for the camera system used in forming RGB images, (2) the color of the light used in the imagery system, (3) shading induced by imaging non-flat skin surfaces, and (4) light intensity, removing the effect of light intensity falloff toward the edges of the skin lesion image. In the context of a blind source separation of the underlying color (here embodied in the ICA algorithm), we arrive at intrinsic melanin and hemoglobin images.

In addition, we put forward an empirical solution to determine which separated component (after applying ICA) corresponds to melanin distribution and which one corresponds to hemoglobin distribution. This issue has not been addressed by Tsumura et al. or any others to date. It is an important consideration, because ICA delivers underlying source answers without an inherent ordering, and for a fully automated system, it is crucial to establish which component is which.

In the lesion classification task, a set of simple statistical measures calculated from the channels of the proposed color space are used as color and texture features, in supervised learning, to achieve excellent melanoma versus benign classification. Moreover, in the lesion segmentation task, based on simple gray-level thresholding, the geometric mean (geo-mean) of RGB color, one component in our new color space, is found to substantially improve the accuracy of segmentation, with results outperforming the current state of the art.

The rest of this chapter is organized as follows. Section 2.2 is devoted to explaining the theory behind the methods employed here. It provides a detailed description of the contributions of this study. Section 2.3 presents experimental results where the significance of the contributions is analyzed and discussed. The chapter concludes with Section 2.4, with an outline of proposals for future work.

2.2 METHOD

As theoretical underpinnings, we begin with a brief overview of independent component analysis (ICA). This is followed by theoretical considerations aimed at developing a model of skin coloration by incorporating optics of human skin into a color image formation model.

2.2.1 INDEPENDENT COMPONENT ANALYSIS

Independent component analysis is a powerful computational method that has been successfully used in many application domains, but more specifically for signal processing aimed at solving the blind source separation (BSS) problem. It essentially defines a generative model of the observed data as linear mixtures of some underlying (hidden) factors that are assumed to be statistically independent. Because of its importance, we briefly recapitulate ICA here.

As a motivating example, consider the classic BSS example: the cocktail party problem. This is a situation where there are a number of people speaking simultaneously at a party. Assume that there are several microphones recording an overlapping combination of the speakers' voices. These microphones are at different locations, so each records a mixture of original source signals with slightly different weights (because each microphone is at a different distance from each of the speakers). The problem is to separate the original speech signals using these microphone recordings.

To formalize this problem, further assume there are n speakers and m microphones $(n \leq m)$. Each microphone records a signal; let us call it observed signal and denote it by $x_i(t)$, which is a weighted sum of the speech signals denoted by $s_j(t)$, where the weights depend on the distances* between microphone i and speaker j. Putting this into mathematical notation, we have

$$x_i(t) = \sum_j a_{ij} s_j(t) \ \text{ for } \ i = 1 \ldots m \ \text{ and } \ j = 1 \ldots n \qquad (2.1)$$

Note that the weight coefficients a_{ij} are assumed to be *unknown*, as well as the speech signals $s_j(t)$, since the basic problem is that we cannot record them directly; instead, what is recorded is a set of microphone measurements $x_i(t)$. To further generalize the problem, we drop the time index (t) and consider each signal as a random variable. Then, the matrix–vector form of the aforementioned is

$$\mathbf{x} = \mathbf{As} \qquad (2.2)$$

where $\mathbf{x}$ is a random vector of observations $(x_1, x_2, \ldots, x_m)$, $\mathbf{s}$ is a random vector containing the source components $(s_1, s_2, \ldots, s_n)$, and the matrix $\mathbf{A}$ contains the weight coefficients a_{ij}. Equation 2.2 is, in fact, a general representation of the BSS problem. Here, *blind* means that we know very little, if anything, about the original source signals and the mixing process, and our goal is to recover these quantities using minimum assumptions. The solution to the BSS problem is usually formulated as

$$\mathbf{s} \simeq \mathbf{Wx} \qquad (2.3)$$

---

* For simplicity, we omit time delay between microphones, echo, amplitude difference, and other extra factors.

where $\mathbf{W} = \mathbf{A}^+$ (where $^+$ denotes pseudoinverse; in case $\mathbf{A}$ is square and invertible, $\mathbf{A}^+$ equals $\mathbf{A}^{-1}$). In this notation, $\mathbf{W}$ is often referred to as the *unmixing* or *separating* matrix and $\mathbf{A}$ as the *mixing* matrix.

Since both $\mathbf{A}$ and $\mathbf{s}$ are unknown, the BSS problem is underdetermined; additional assumptions are necessary to solve it. Depending on what additional assumptions are considered, various methods apply. ICA is one; other popular approaches are factor analysis [5], principal component analysis (PCA) [6], sparse component analysis [7], nonnegative matrix factorization (NMF) [8], and others.

For an ICA solution, the additional assumptions are that source components are mutually statistically independent and have non-Gaussian distributions.* ICA can then be formally defined as finding a linear transformation matrix $\mathbf{W}$ in Equation 2.3, where the data model is given by Equation 2.2, and ICA model assumptions are met.

For two random variables, independence intuitively means that knowing the value of one would not convey any information for the value of the second one. More formally, statistical independence is defined in terms of probability densities. Two or more random variables $(x_1, x_2, x_3, \ldots)$ are mutually independent if their joint probability density may be factorized as the product of their marginal densities, that is,

$$p(x_1, x_2, x_3, \ldots) = \prod_i p(x_i) \tag{2.4}$$

Although this definition is fairly intuitive, it does not lend itself easily to forming a computational procedure for finding independent components from their mixtures. Fortunately, there are analytically tractable ways to approach this problem under certain assumptions. One such approach is based on the principle of maximizing non-Gaussianity of sources, motivated by the central limit theorem (CLT). Here, we omit theoretical discussions (these can be found in [9, 10]). However, a short overview is illuminating: the CLT says, quite generally, that the sum of a sufficiently large number of mutually independent random variables (each with finite mean and variance) tends toward a normal (Gaussian) distribution. As a result, a sum of any number of independent random variables has a distribution that is closer to Gaussian than any of the original random variables. The implication of this observation can be used to form a new assumption for ICA solution: if statistically independent signals can be extracted from signal mixtures, then these extracted signals must be from a non-Gaussian distribution. To understand why, let us analyze the solution to the BSS problem by attempting to estimate one independent component.

---

* The assumptions of independence and that the components are non-Gaussian are complementary to one another.

From Equation 2.3, each estimated source component can be obtained by an inner product of the observed data with the corresponding row of $\mathbf{W}$, denoted by $\mathbf{w}_j$:

$$\hat{s}_j = \mathbf{w}_j^T x \text{ where } \mathbf{w}_j = (w_{j1}, w_{j2}, \ldots, w_{jm})^T$$

This simply states that the estimated sources can be written as a linear combination of the observed data. We move forward from this by making a change of variables and introducing a variable $\mathbf{z}$ as follows: $\hat{s}_j = \mathbf{w}_j^T \mathbf{x} = \mathbf{w}_j^T(\mathbf{As}) = (\mathbf{w}_j^T \mathbf{A})\mathbf{s} = \mathbf{z}^T\mathbf{s}$. Thus, the variable $\mathbf{z} = \mathbf{A}^T\mathbf{w}_j$ is a weight vector that gives one estimated component as a linear combination of (actual) source components. It is obvious that the estimated component $\hat{s}_j$ is equal to actual source component s_j only if all elements of $\mathbf{z}$ are zero except the jth element ($z_j = 1$). This would hold true if $\mathbf{w}_j$ were one of the rows of the inverse of $\mathbf{A}$. However, in practice, we cannot determine such a $\mathbf{w}_j$ exactly because we have no knowledge of matrix $\mathbf{A}$. Now let us assume that $\mathbf{z}$ has more than one nonzero element. Since the sum of two or more independent random variables is more Gaussian than the original variables, $\hat{s}_j$ is more Gaussian than any of the elements of $\mathbf{s}$, including the actual s_j. Note that as more elements of $\mathbf{z}$ are nonzero, the more the distribution of $\hat{s}_j$ tends to Gaussian; conversely, as more elements of $\mathbf{z}$ are zero, $\hat{s}_j$ becomes less Gaussian, and it is least Gaussian when $\mathbf{z}$ has in fact only one nonzero element (i.e., when $\hat{s}_j$ is equal to s_j).

The above observation leads to the following principle in ICA estimation: if the $\mathbf{w}_j$ vector is determined such that it maximizes the non-Gaussianity of $\mathbf{w}_j^T\mathbf{x}$, then such a vector would correspond (in the transformed coordinate system) to a $\mathbf{z}$ that is sparse and, ideally, has only one nonzero element. This means that $\mathbf{w}_j^T\mathbf{x} = \mathbf{z}^T\mathbf{s}$ equals one of the independent components.

The property of non-Gaussianity can be measured using higher-order statistics (e.g., kurtosis) or information theory (e.g., negentropy) [11]. Having a quantitative measure of non-Gaussianity allows us to employ methods such as gradient descent or expectation maximization (EM) to estimate $\mathbf{w}_j$ in an iterative scheme (see [11] for popular algorithms).

Here we make use of a fast and fixed-point algorithm, referred to as FastICA [12], which employs an approximation of negentropy to measure non-Gaussianity.* In this approximation, the negentropy of a random variable $J(\mathbf{y})$ is estimated as

$$J(y) \propto E\{G(\mathbf{y})\} - E\{G(\mathbf{v})\} \tag{2.5}$$

where $E\{\}$ denotes the expected value of a random variable, $G()$ denotes any nonquadratic function such as $G(\mathbf{u}) = \log\cosh(\mathbf{u})$ [11], and $\mathbf{v}$ is a (standardized) Gaussian random variable. Note that in Equation 2.5, both $\mathbf{y}$ and $\mathbf{v}$ are assumed to be of zero mean and unit variance.

---

* A MATLAB® implementation of the FastICA algorithm available online [13] is used for the experiments reported in this chapter.

The basic fixed-point iteration in the FastICA algorithm minimizes a generic cost function $E\{G(\mathbf{w}_j^T \tilde{\mathbf{x}})\}$, where $\tilde{\mathbf{x}}$ is the observed $\mathbf{x}$ after being centered and "whitened," meaning applying a matrix transform such that $E\{\tilde{\mathbf{x}}\tilde{\mathbf{x}}^T\} = \mathbf{I}$. The resulting $\mathbf{w}_j$ is a direction, that is, a unit vector, which maximizes the non-Gaussianity of $\mathbf{w}_j^T \tilde{\mathbf{x}}$. At each iteration, $\mathbf{w}_j$ is updated according to the following rule (which would of course be followed by the normalization of $\mathbf{w}_j$):

$$\mathbf{w}_j \leftarrow E\{\tilde{\mathbf{x}}g(\mathbf{w}_j^T \tilde{\mathbf{x}})\} - E\{g'(\mathbf{w}_j^T \tilde{\mathbf{x}})\}\mathbf{w}_j \qquad (2.6)$$

where g is the derivative of G, and g' is the derivative of g — in [11]; a robust choice of these is given as $g(\mathbf{u}) = \tanh(\mathbf{u})$ and $g'(\mathbf{u}) = 1 - \tanh^2(\mathbf{u})$. The algorithm usually converges in a small number of steps. Now, a complete solution to ICA needs to find all $\mathbf{w}_j$ vectors, that is, estimation of $\mathbf{W}$ in Equation 2.3. A possible solution can be formulated as shown in Algorithm 2.1.

Algorithm 2.1: FastICA

1: Center the data: $\hat{\mathbf{x}} = \mathbf{x} - E\{\mathbf{x}\}$
2: Apply a whitening matrix $\mathbf{M}$ to $\hat{\mathbf{x}}$ such as $\tilde{\mathbf{x}} = \mathbf{M}\hat{\mathbf{x}}$
3: **for** j in 1 to n **do**
4:    $\mathbf{w}_j \leftarrow$ random vector of length m
5:    **while** $\mathbf{w}_j$ changes **do**
6:        $\mathbf{w}_j \leftarrow E\{\tilde{\mathbf{x}}g(\mathbf{w}_j^T \tilde{\mathbf{x}})\} - E\{g'(\mathbf{w}_j^T \tilde{\mathbf{x}})\}\mathbf{w}_j$
7:        $\mathbf{w}_j \leftarrow \mathbf{w}_j / \|\mathbf{w}_j\|$
8:    **end while**
9: **end for**

Note the whitening process in step 2 of Algorithm 2.1: whitening the data involves linearly transforming the data so that the new components are uncorrelated and have unit variance. This can be done using eigenvalue decomposition of the covariance matrix of the data: $E\{\mathbf{x}\mathbf{x}^T\} = \mathbf{U}\mathbf{D}\mathbf{U}^T$, where $\mathbf{U}$ is the matrix of eigenvectors and $\mathbf{D}$ is the diagonal matrix of eigenvalues. Once eigenvalue decomposition is done, the whitened data are

$$\tilde{\mathbf{x}} = \mathbf{U}\mathbf{D}^{-1/2}\mathbf{U}^T\mathbf{x} = \mathbf{M}\mathbf{x} \qquad (2.7)$$

where $\mathbf{M} = \mathbf{U}\mathbf{D}^{-1/2}\mathbf{U}^T$ is the whitening matrix. Note that $E\{\tilde{\mathbf{x}}\tilde{\mathbf{x}}^T\} = \mathbf{I}$.

In the ICA data model, rows of matrix $\mathbf{W}$ (i.e., $\mathbf{w}_j$) are called ICA *filter* vectors. We filter the observed data with the corresponding row of $\mathbf{W}$, once they are estimated, to obtain each component source vector: $s_j = \mathbf{w}_j^T \mathbf{x}$. Rows of matrix $\mathbf{W}$ correspond to columns of matrix $\mathbf{A}$ (denoted by $\mathbf{a}_j$), which are also known as ICA *basis* vectors. They span the ICA space: the observed data are given as a linear mixtures of $\mathbf{a}_j$, where the coefficient of each vector is given by the corresponding independent component s_j, that is, $\mathbf{x} = \sum_{j=1}^{n} s_j \mathbf{a}_j$.

By selecting a subset of ICA basis vectors, one can transform the observed data into a subspace of selected independent components. This has clear application in data representation and dimension reduction.

In this study, we intend to apply independent component analysis to images of skin lesions. The color of skin is the result of interaction of light with its internal structure. In order to extract and retain information regarding the interior structure, a mathematical bio-optical model of human skin is needed. This model has to be compatible with the ICA data model, if the intention is to reveal this information by independent component analysis. In what follows, we will briefly overview a color image formation, as well as describe optics of human skin, with a focus on the light–skin interaction. The two will come together to form a model of skin coloration, as described in Section 2.2.4.

2.2.2 COLOR IMAGE FORMATION

A digital image is created when the light reflected from the scene passes through the lens or microlens of a camera and hits the sensor array at pixel positions. The sensor elements are light sensitive; they transform the photons conveyed by the reflected light (scene radiance) to electrical charge, creating electric current proportional to the intensity of the incoming radiance. This electric current is then converted into numerical values by analog-to-digital (A/D) conversion, producing the intensity (a.k.a. pixel, gray-level) values of the digital image. This process can be mathematically formalized as

$$R_k(x, y) = \int_\lambda C(x, y, \lambda) Q_k(\lambda) d\lambda \tag{2.8}$$

where $R_k(x, y)$ is the pixel value registered by the kth sensor with sensitivity function $Q_k(\lambda)$, at position (x, y). The $C(x, y, \lambda)$ factor represents the scene radiance. A detailed computational model of C could be very complex since the interaction of light/matter and reflectance can be involved and intricate, especially when considering factors such as interreflection and specularities. For computer vision applications, to simplify matters, it is common to assume a simple model of scene radiance based solely on the information given by the surface albedo:

$$R_k(x, y) = \int_\lambda E(x, y, \lambda) S(x, y, \lambda) Q_k(\lambda) d\lambda \tag{2.9}$$

where $E(x, y, \lambda)$ is the illuminant spectral power distribution, and in the reflective case, the surface spectral reflectance function is $S(x, y, \lambda)$. This basic model is shown in Figure 2.1.

To further simplify the formulation, we can approximate camera sensors as narrowband, or they can be made narrowband via a spectral sharpening operation [14]. In this approximation, sensor curve $Q_k(\lambda)$ is simply assumed to be a delta function: $Q_k(\lambda) = q_k \delta(\lambda - \lambda_k)$, where specific wavelengths λ_k

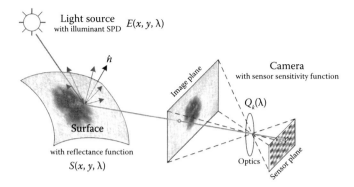

FIGURE 2.1   A simplified model of photometric image formation.

and sensor-curve heights q_k are properties of the camera used. Therefore, Equation 2.9 can be written as

$$R_k(x,y) = E(x,y,\lambda_k)S(x,y,\lambda_k)q_k \qquad (2.10)$$

Conventional cameras are trichromatic, that is, have three different sensors ($k = 1 \cdots 3$), which respond distinctly to different wavelengths across the visible spectrum $\omega = 400$–$700\,\text{nm}$. When a trichromatic camera captures an image, the light reflected from the scene is converted into a discrete triple of values, usually RGB color values, based on the model described above:

$$\begin{bmatrix} R(x,y) \\ G(x,y) \\ B(x,y) \end{bmatrix} = \begin{bmatrix} E(x,y,\lambda_R)S(x,y,\lambda_R)q_R \\ E(x,y,\lambda_G)S(x,y,\lambda_G)q_G \\ E(x,y,\lambda_B)S(x,y,\lambda_B)q_B \end{bmatrix} \qquad (2.11)$$

This simple model can be used for dermoscopy images as well. A dermoscope can be seen as a conventional RGB camera equipped with optical magnification and cross-polarized lighting to allow enhanced visualization of skin morphological characteristics.

2.2.3   LIGHT–SKIN INTERACTION

Human skin is a multilayered structure. The manner in which skin reflects and transmits light of different colors, or wavelengths, is determined by the inherent optical properties of the skin layers [15].

We consider a simplified skin tissue model composed of three layers from the top: epidermis, dermis, and subcutis (Figure 2.2). The optical properties of epidermis and dermis depend mainly on the light scattering and absorption properties of melanin and hemoglobin, respectively, whereas the subcutis mainly contains fat cells that are assumed to diffuse all visible light [16].

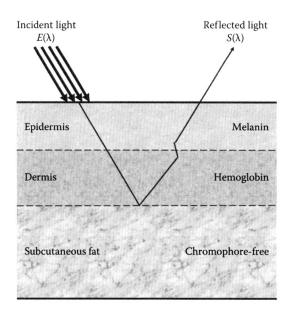

FIGURE 2.2 A simplified model of light–skin interaction.

By adapting a simple Lambert–Beer type of law for radiance from the multilayer skin tissue similar to that in [17], the spectral reflection of skin can be given by*

$$S(x, y, \lambda) = \exp\{-\rho_m(x, y)\alpha_m(\lambda)l_m(\lambda) - \rho_h(x, y)\alpha_h(\lambda)l_h(\lambda) - \zeta(\lambda)\} \quad (2.12)$$

where $\rho_{m,h}$ are densities of melanin and hemoglobin, respectively (cm^{-3}), and are assumed to be independent of each other. The cross-sectional areas for scattering absorption of melanin and hemoglobin are denoted $\alpha_{m,h}$ (cm^2), and $l_{m,h}$ are the mean path lengths for photons in the epidermis and dermis layers, which are used as the depth of the medium in this modified Lambert–Beer law. The term ζ encapsulates scattering loss and any other factors that contribute to skin appearance, such as absorbency of other chromophores (e.g., β-carotene) and thickness of the subcutis.

2.2.4 SKIN COLORATION MODEL

In this section we develop a model of skin coloration. To this end, Equation 2.10 can be expanded as

$$R_k(x, y) = \omega(x, y)E(x, y, \lambda_k)$$
$$\times \exp\{-\rho_m(x, y)\alpha_m(\lambda)l_m(\lambda) - \rho_h(x, y)\alpha_h(\lambda)l_h(\lambda) - \zeta(\lambda)\}q_k$$
$$(2.13)$$

---

* Here, for simplicity, specular reflection and interreflection inside each layer are ignored.

Note that we included the term $\omega(x,y)$, which denotes shape-induced shading variation (e.g., Lambertian shading is surface normal dotted into the light direction, although we do not necessarily assume Lambertian surfaces here).

Moreover, in keeping with [4], we adopt a simple model for the illuminant: we assume the light can be written as a Planckian radiator (in Wien's approximation):

$$E(x,y,\lambda,T) \simeq I(x,y)k_1\lambda^{-5}\exp\left(\frac{-k_2}{T\lambda}\right) \tag{2.14}$$

where k_1 and k_2 are constants, T is the correlated color temperature characterizing the light spectrum, and I is the lighting intensity at pixel (x,y), allowing for a possible roll-off in intensity toward the periphery of the skin image. The light temperature T is assumed constant across the image (but is, in general, unknown).

By substituting Equation 2.14 into Equation 2.13 and taking the logarithm, we arrive at a linear model that captures the relationship between the color of skin and the underlying composition of its color pigments:

$$\log R_k(x,y) = -\rho_m(x,y)\sigma_m(\lambda_k) - \rho_h(x,y)\sigma_h(\lambda_k) - \varsigma(\lambda_k)$$
$$+ \log(k_1 I(x,y)\omega(x,y)) + \left[\log\left(\frac{1}{\lambda_k^5}\right) - \frac{k_2 q_k}{\lambda_k T}\right] \tag{2.15}$$

where we have lumped terms:

$$\sigma_m(\lambda_k) = \alpha_m(\lambda_k)l_m(\lambda_k)$$
$$\sigma_h(\lambda_k) = \alpha_h(\lambda_k)l_h(\lambda_k)$$

Further, for notational convenience, denote

$$u_k = \log(1/\lambda_k^5)$$
$$e_k = -k_2 q_k/\lambda_k$$
$$m_k = \sigma_m(\lambda_k)$$
$$h_k = \sigma_h(\lambda_k)$$
$$\varsigma_k = \varsigma(\lambda_k)$$
$$c(x,y) = \log(k_1 I(x,y)\omega(x,y))$$

giving the skin coloration model as

$$\log R_k(x,y) = -\rho_m(x,y)m_k - \rho_h(x,y)h_k - \varsigma_k + c(x,y) + u_k - e_k\left(\frac{1}{T}\right) \tag{2.16}$$

Now let us move forward by making the observation that the same type of chromaticity analysis as appears in [4] can be brought to bear here for the skin coloration model (Equation 2.16). Chromaticity is color without intensity, for example, an L_1 norm–based chromaticity is $\{r, g, b\} = \{R, G, B\}/(R+G+B)$. Here, suppose we instead form a band ratio chromaticity by dividing by one color channel R_p, for example, green for $p = 2$. (In practice, we shall instead follow [4] and divide by the geometric mean color, $\mu = \sqrt[3]{R \cdot G \cdot B}$, so as not to favor one particular color channel, but dividing by R_p is clearer in exposition.) Notice that dividing removes the term $c(x, y)$ (in Equation 2.16); that is, it removes the effect of shading ω and light intensity field I.

We further define a log-chromaticity $\chi(x, y)$ as the log of the ratio of color component R_k divided by R_p:

$$\chi_k(x, y) = \log \left(\frac{R_k(x, y)}{R_p(x, y)} \right) \tag{2.17}$$

$$= -\rho_m(x, y)(m_k - m_p) - \rho_h(x, y)(h_k - h_p) + w_k - (e_k - e_p) \left(\frac{1}{T} \right)$$

with $w_k \equiv (u_k - u_p) - (\zeta_k - \zeta_p)$. The import of this equation is that if we were to vary the lighting (in this simplified model), then the chromaticity χ would follow a straight line as temperature T changes. In fact, we also have that this linear behavior is also obeyed by the mean $\bar{\chi}$ over the image of this new chromaticity quantity:

$$\bar{\chi}_k = -\bar{\rho}_m(m_k - m_p) - \bar{\rho}_h(h_k - h_p) + w_k - (e_k - e_p) \left(\frac{1}{T} \right) \tag{2.18}$$

Now notice that we can remove all terms in the camera-offset term w_k and the illuminant color term T by subtracting the mean from χ. Let χ^0 be the mean-subtracted vector:

$$\chi_k^0(x, y) = \chi_k(x, y) - \bar{\chi}_k \tag{2.19}$$
$$= -(\rho_m(x, y) - \bar{\rho}_m)(m_k - m_p) - (\rho_h(x, y) - \bar{\rho}_h)(h_k - h_p)$$

Equation 2.19 is then a model of skin coloration that depends only on melanin m and hemoglobin h. If we apply the assumption that m and h terms can be disambiguated using ICA, then from the new feature χ^0, we can extract the melanin and hemoglobin content in skin images (where the vectors $(m_k - m_p)$ and $(h_k - h_p)$ are considered constant vectors in each image). The camera characteristic still persists to some degree through the dependence of m_k and h_k on λ_k, a camera-specific set of wavelengths. Nonetheless, the removal of w_k has in large measure removed the influence of the camera; moreover, the ICA process is applied independently to each image, from different cameras, and the good results obtained justify the suitability of this approach.

The two new image features, $\rho_m^0(x, y) = (\rho_m(x, y) - \bar{\rho}_m)$ and $\rho_h^0(x, y) = (\rho_h(x, y) - \bar{\rho}_h)$, represent the spatial distribution of melanin and hemoglobin content in the image. As an example, consider Figure 2.3a showing a melanoma lesion, and the ρ_m^0 and ρ_h^0 components in (b) and (c). In computer vision,

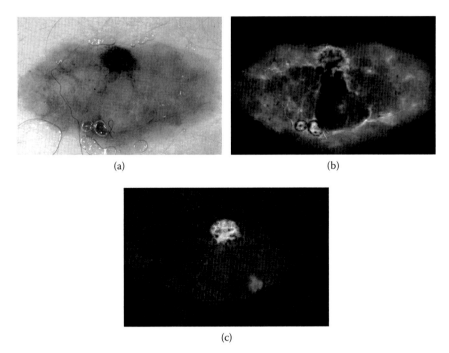

(a)   (b)

(c)

FIGURE 2.3   Separation of melanin and hemoglobin content. Here, the separation is the result of ICA on the proposed model for skin coloration. (a) Input image. (b) Melanin component. (c) Hemoglobin component. (Reprinted with permission from Argenziano, G. et al., *Dermoscopy: A Tutorial*, EDRA Medical Publishing and New Media, Milan, Italy, 2002.)

images with lighting removed are denoted intrinsic images, and thus our two new features are indeed intrinsic.

2.2.4.1   Geometric Mean Chromaticity

As mentioned before, in order to not rely on any particular color channel when forming the chromaticity image, we divide not by R_p, but by the geometric mean $\mu(x, y)$ at each pixel, for which the invariance properties above persist:

$$\psi_k(x, y) \equiv \log\left[\frac{R_k(x, y)}{\mu(x, y)}\right]$$

Then ψ is a 3-vector; it is orthogonal to $(1, 1, 1)$. Therefore, instead of 3-vectors, one can easily treat these as 2-vector values, lying in the plane orthogonal to $(1, 1, 1)$: if the 3×3 projector onto that two-dimensional (2-D) subspace is $\mathbf{V}$, then the singular value decomposition is $\mathbf{V} = \mathbf{U}\mathbf{U}^T$, where $\mathbf{U}$ is a 3×2 matrix. Thus, to find the skin data plane, we project the log-chromaticity image data onto 2-D vectors ϕ in the plane coordinate system via $\mathbf{U}^T$ (but N.B. [2] used PCA to find the skin plane):

$$\phi = \mathbf{U}^T \psi \tag{2.20}$$

where ϕ is 2-D. The mean subtraction step from above still holds in projected color, and therefore we here propose carrying out ICA in the plane $\phi - \bar{\phi}$:

$$\text{Feature: } \eta = \text{ICA}(\phi - \bar{\phi}) \tag{2.21}$$

2.2.4.2 Summary

In short, by running ICA on $(\phi - \bar{\phi})$, that is, the mean-subtracted 2-D projected data of log-chromaticity of skin color vectors, we can obtain η, which we assume corresponds to distributions of underlying melanin and hemoglobin contents in an image of a skin lesion. This procedure is summarized in Algorithm 2.2. The corresponding ICA data model is

$$\phi = \mathbf{A}\eta \tag{2.22}$$

where, for notational convenience, we simplify by denoting $\phi \equiv \phi - \bar{\phi}$.

Algorithm 2.2: Independent Component Analysis of Skin Lesion Images

1: Load an image of skin lesion.
2: Assume the intensity values at pixel (x, y) are represented by the function $R_k(x, y)$, where k indexes R,G,B channels.
3: Obtain the band ratio 3-vector chromaticity $c_k(x, y) = R_k(x, y)/\mu(x, y)$, where $\mu(x, y) = (\prod_{k=1}^{3} R_k)^{\frac{1}{3}}$, the geometric mean at each pixel.
4: Take the log of the (geo-mean) chromaticity: $\psi_k(x, y) \equiv \log c_k(x, y)$.
5: Reshape $\psi_k(x, y)$ into a $N \times K$ matrix ψ, where N is the number of pixels and $K = 3$ for R,G,B.
6: Project the log-chromaticity image data (ψ) onto the 2-D plane orthogonal to $(1, 1, 1)$: $\phi = \mathbf{U}^T \psi$, where $\mathbf{U}$ is any 3×2 transformation matrix onto that 2-D subspace.
7: Run ICA on the 2-D plane $(\phi - \bar{\phi})$ to find independent components (source) data η (and separating matrix $\mathbf{W}$).

Equation 2.22 is similar to the ICA data model (Equation 2.2), although, here, η and ϕ are both $N \times 2$ matrices (where N is the number of pixels) as opposed to $\mathbf{x}$ and $\mathbf{s}$ (in Equation 2.2), which are both (random) vectors. This is not a problem since the ICA data model can be easily extended to a matrix notation where the observed data are a collection of k random vectors $\mathbf{x}_k$, collected into a $m \times k$ matrix $\mathbf{X}$, with a corresponding $n \times k$ matrix collection of sources, $\mathbf{S}$, giving $\mathbf{X} = \mathbf{AS}$, where $\mathbf{A}$ is still the same matrix as in Equation 2.2. Accordingly, the ICA solution can be given by $\mathbf{S} = \mathbf{WX}$. In Equation 2.22, $k = 2$, $m = n =$ number of pixels, independent components are $\boldsymbol{\eta}_1$ and $\boldsymbol{\eta}_2$, and observed data are $\boldsymbol{\phi}_1$ and $\boldsymbol{\phi}_2$. The corresponding ICA solution model is

$$\boldsymbol{\eta} = \mathbf{W}\boldsymbol{\phi} \tag{2.23}$$

As discussed, ICA estimates the separating matrix $\mathbf{W}$ such that $\boldsymbol{\eta}_1$ and $\boldsymbol{\eta}_2$ are maximally statistically independent. Since the input (observed) data are an image (i.e., the skin lesion image), we take each $\boldsymbol{\eta}_j$ vector and reshape it as a 2-D signal, that is, a (monochromatic) image $\eta_j(x, y)$. The output images $\eta_j(x, y)$ are expected to show the spatial distribution of underlying melanin and hemoglobin contents of the input image (Figure 2.3).

2.2.5 ICA AMBIGUITIES

So far we have discussed independent component analysis in general and when applied to dermoscopy images. We continue in this section with an important question: To what degree can $\mathbf{W} = \mathbf{A}^{-1}$ be recovered?

In Equation 2.3, once the independent components are estimated, they can be scaled, negated, and permuted with permutation matrix $\mathbf{P}$ and scaling matrix $\mathbf{S}$ such that new components remain independent: $\mathbf{s}' = \mathbf{SPs} = \mathbf{SPWx}$. So any matrix $\mathbf{W}' = \mathbf{SPW}$ is also a valid separating matrix within the ICA framework. This is often referred to as the inherent *ambiguity* in the ICA model [18]. That is, "independent sources can only be recovered up to *scale*, *sign* and *permutation*" [19]. Without any prior knowledge about the sources ($\mathbf{s}$) and the mixing matrix ($\mathbf{A}$), it is impossible to avoid these ambiguities.

In what follows, we shall discuss the effect of these ambiguities on the proposed skin coloration model, as well as strategies to alleviate those effects.

2.2.5.1 Permutation Ambiguity

ICA solutions do not provide information regarding the order of the independent components; that is, all permutations of the separated sources are equally valid [18]. Let us change $\mathbf{s}$ to $\mathbf{s}' = \mathbf{Ps}$, where $\mathbf{P}$ is a permutation matrix. The elements of $\mathbf{s}'$ are the original independent variables s_j, but in another order. Further, we can change $\mathbf{A}$ to $\mathbf{A}' = \mathbf{AP}^{-1}$ and rewrite the ICA data model as $\mathbf{x} = \mathbf{A}'\mathbf{s}' = \mathbf{AP}^{-1}\mathbf{Ps} = \mathbf{As}$. Hence, the permutation ambiguity is inherent to the ICA model.

In this study, however, it is of interest to correspond each independent component to either melanin or hemoglobin content. Unfortunately, this is a difficult task, even with user intervention; there is usually little visual evidence for indication of each component.

Tsumura et al. [3] proposed active biophysical tests to, for example, use biological response to methyl nicotinate (applied to a human subject arm) for indication and validation of a hemoglobin component. Such indication strategies are difficult, limited, and most importantly, impractical in our study.

As suggested above, distinction of the melanin and hemoglobin components is a difficult task. Notwithstanding the difficulties, in some skin lesion images there are visual cues that would increase the confidence for indication of each component, for example, the presence of blood or vessels in the image or inflammation around the lesion, all expected to show up in the hemoglobin image (see Figure 2.4 for a few examples).

In a set of experiments, we have carefully selected 116 images (out of 944) that contained some of the aforementioned visual cues. Following Algorithm 2.2, we have manually labeled the outcome of ICA to melanin and hemoglobin. Then, the following observations were made.

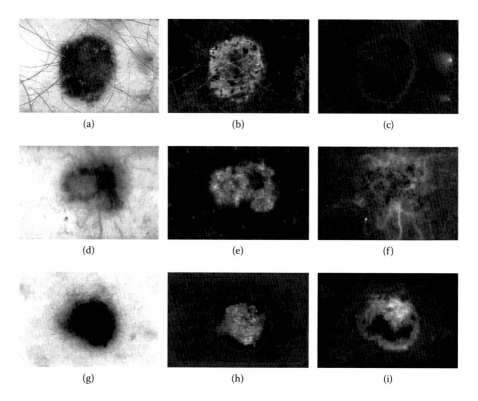

FIGURE 2.4 Indication of melanin and hemoglobin components from visual cues. In some skin lesion images, there are visual cues that could aid us in corresponding each independent component to distribution of either melanin (b, e, h) or hemoglobin. For example, the presence of blood (a) Clark's nevus, vessels (d) melanoma, or inflammation around the lesion (g) Clark's nevus, is expected to show up in the hemoglobin image (c, f, i). (Reprinted with permission from Argenziano, G. et al., *Dermoscopy: A Tutorial*, EDRA Medical Publishing and New Media, Milan, Italy, 2002.)

2.2.5.2 Observation 1

The two types of ICA basis vector are clustered. As shown in Figure 2.5, basis vectors in the same class (melanin or hemoglobin) are seen to cluster, indicating that *intraclass* distances are smaller than *interclass* distances. Thus, a classifier could be trained to discriminate between the two classes. For example, a k-nearest-neighborhood (k-NN) classifier would be able to decide if a new instance belongs to the melanin or hemoglobin class based on a distance function and nearest-neighbor procedure.

We formulate a probabilistic framework of the k-NN procedure. Given a new instance of ICA basis vector ($\mathbf{a}_j$), we consider ($k = 10$) nearest neighbors to this vector in the *training* set (i.e., 464 manually labeled vectors from 116

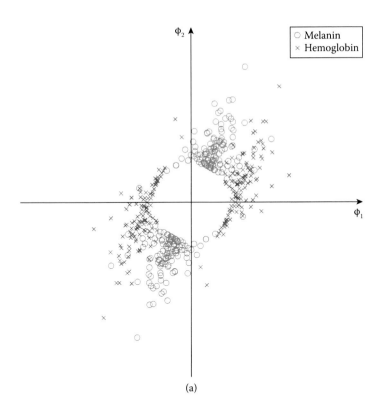

(a)

FIGURE 2.5 ICA basis vectors corresponding to each component are closer together. ICA basis vectors of 116 images are labeled manually and plotted as 2-D points in observation space. To obviate the sign ambiguity, we have kept both possible signs of each vector; hence, there are 2×116 points shown in each class (symmetric with respect to the origin), making a total of 464 samples.

selected images—refer to the caption of Figure 2.5 for details) and define the following probability:

$$P(\mathbf{a}_j : M) = \sum_{k=1}^{10} t_k w_k \tag{2.24}$$

where M indicates melanin component, and t_k is the target value of each nearest neighbor, set to 1 if the label of nearest neighbor is M and 0 otherwise. In Equation 2.24, w_k is the weight coefficient to control and adjust the effect of the k-NN procedure; that is, more weight is given to closer neighbors. Here, the weights are predefined and fixed: (N.B. $\sum w_k = 1$)

$$w_k = \{0.19 \ 0.17 \ 0.15 \ 0.13 \ 0.11 \ 0.09 \ 0.07 \ 0.05 \ 0.03 \ 0.01\}; \quad k = 1 \cdots 10$$

Also, it is clear that since a component corresponds to either melanin (M) or hemoglobin (H), the following is true:

$$P(\mathbf{a}_j : H) = 1 - P(\mathbf{a}_j : M) \tag{2.25}$$

Finally, as M and H components are independent, their joint probability is the product of their marginals:

$$P(\mathbf{a}_1 : M, \ \mathbf{a}_2 : H) = P(\mathbf{a}_1 : M) \times P(\mathbf{a}_2 : H)$$
$$P(\mathbf{a}_1 : H, \ \mathbf{a}_2 : M) = P(\mathbf{a}_1 : H) \times P(\mathbf{a}_2 : M) \tag{2.26}$$

Therefore, Equation 2.26 could be used to indicate which order of independent components is more likely the correct one.

2.2.5.3 Observation 2

For many images, the hemoglobin component and the a* channel of CIE L*a*b* color space are similar. This is not surprising since studies [20, 21] showed high correlation between the skin's erythema index (redness) and a* channel map. The hemoglobin component, in a sense, embodies a similar meaning, that is, redness of skin.

In Figure 2.6, the CIE L*a*b* channels for two examples from Figure 2.4 are illustrated. Notice the hemoglobin component and a* channel are very similar. The similarity between the b* channel and melanin component is noticeable too. Therefore, similarity to a* and b* channels of CIE L*a*b* could be used as an indicator of hemoglobin and melanin distribution, respectively.

In order to measure the similarity of $\eta_j(x, y)$ images to a* or b* channels, computing the 2-D correlation coefficient between them would suffice, since the images are of the same size without any affine distortion.

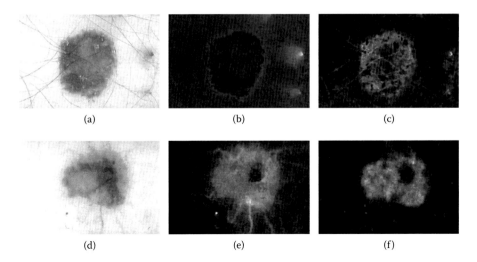

FIGURE 2.6 CIE L*a*b* channels of sample images from Figure 2.4. (a, b, c) are, respectively, the L*, a*, and b* channels of image (a) in Figure 2.4. Similarly, (d, e, f) are the L*, a*, and b* channels of image (b) in Figure 2.4. Notice the similarity between melanin and hemoglobin images in Figure 2.4 (respectively) to the b* and a* channel maps here.

The 2-D correlation coefficient, $\mathfrak{r}$, is calculated by the following equation, where A and B are two monochromatic images both of size $m \times n$:

$$\mathfrak{r}(A, B) = \frac{\sum_m \sum_n (A_{mn} - \bar{A})(B_{mn} - \bar{B})}{\sqrt{\left(\sum_m \sum_n (A_{mn} - \bar{A})^2\right)\left(\sum_m \sum_n (B_{mn} - \bar{B})^2\right)}} \qquad (2.27)$$

Thus, one can measure which component is more similar to which channel of CIE L*a*b*. A fair comparison should take into account the similarity of each component to both channels. Hence, we define the following probabilities as a measure for likeliness of each component corresponding to each channel, that is, corresponding to melanin or hemoglobin contents:

$$\mathcal{P}(\boldsymbol{\eta}_j : \mathrm{M}) = \frac{|\mathfrak{r}(\boldsymbol{\eta}_j, \mathrm{b}^*)|}{|\mathfrak{r}(\boldsymbol{\eta}_j, \mathrm{a}^*)| + |\mathfrak{r}(\boldsymbol{\eta}_j, \mathrm{b}^*)|}$$

$$\mathcal{P}(\boldsymbol{\eta}_j : \mathrm{H}) = \frac{|\mathfrak{r}(\boldsymbol{\eta}_j, \mathrm{a}^*)|}{|\mathfrak{r}(\boldsymbol{\eta}_j, \mathrm{a}^*)| + |\mathfrak{r}(\boldsymbol{\eta}_j, \mathrm{b}^*)|} \qquad (2.28)$$

Notice that $\mathcal{P}(\boldsymbol{\eta}_j : \mathrm{H}) = 1 - \mathcal{P}(\boldsymbol{\eta}_j : \mathrm{M})$. Also, as mentioned before, since M and H components are independent, their joint probability is the product of their marginals:

$$\mathcal{P}(\boldsymbol{\eta}_1 : \mathrm{M}, \ \boldsymbol{\eta}_2 : \mathrm{H}) = \mathcal{P}(\boldsymbol{\eta}_1 : \mathrm{M}) \times \mathcal{P}(\boldsymbol{\eta}_2 : \mathrm{H})$$

$$\mathcal{P}(\boldsymbol{\eta}_1 : \mathrm{H}, \ \boldsymbol{\eta}_2 : \mathrm{M}) = \mathcal{P}(\boldsymbol{\eta}_1 : \mathrm{H}) \times \mathcal{P}(\boldsymbol{\eta}_2 : \mathrm{M}) \qquad (2.29)$$

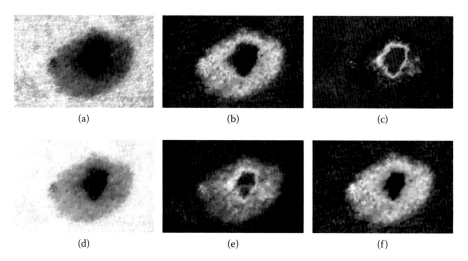

FIGURE 2.7 ICA outcome is different from CIE L*a*b* color-space conversion. (a) Combined nevus. (b) Melanin. (c) Hemoglobin. (d) L. (e) a*. (f) b*. (Reprinted with permission from Argenziano, G. et al., *Dermoscopy: A Tutorial,* EDRA Medical Publishing and New Media, Milan, Italy, 2002.)

Similar to Equation 2.26, the above equation can also be used to indicate which ordering of independent components is more likely the correct one.

An extracted component more likely corresponds, for example, to melanin distribution if both probabilities of $\mathcal{P}(\mathbf{a}_j : M)$ and $\mathcal{P}(\mathbf{\eta}_j : M)$ are high. Thus, in order to indicate the order of estimated components, it is best to consider both aforementioned observations. In other words, we need a measure that combines both Equations 2.26 and 2.29. We assume here (for simplicity) that the aforementioned observations are independent of each other (although in reality they are not) and define the following probabilities:

$$
\begin{aligned}
\mathcal{P}(\mathrm{IC}_1{:}\mathrm{M},\ \mathrm{IC}_2{:}\mathrm{H}) &= \mathcal{P}(\mathbf{a}_1 : \mathrm{M}\ ,\ \mathbf{a}_2 : \mathrm{H}) \times \mathcal{P}(\mathbf{\eta}_1 : \mathrm{M}\ ,\ \mathbf{\eta}_2 : \mathrm{H}) \\
\mathcal{P}(\mathrm{IC}_1{:}\mathrm{H},\ \mathrm{IC}_2{:}\mathrm{M}) &= \mathcal{P}(\mathbf{a}_1 : \mathrm{H}\ ,\ \mathbf{a}_2 : \mathrm{M}) \times \mathcal{P}(\mathbf{\eta}_1 : \mathrm{H}\ ,\ \mathbf{\eta}_2 : \mathrm{M})
\end{aligned}
\tag{2.30}
$$

Here, if $\mathcal{P}(\mathrm{IC}_1{:}\mathrm{M}\ ,\ \mathrm{IC}_2{:}\mathrm{H}) \geq \mathcal{P}(\mathrm{IC}_1{:}\mathrm{H},\ \mathrm{IC}_2{:}\mathrm{M})$, then the first extracted independent component (IC_1) corresponds to melanin distribution and the second estimated IC is hemoglobin (and vice versa).

As a final note on this section, the outcome of the image analysis proposed here is different in general from results simply using CIE L*a*b* values. For instance, Figure 2.7 shows an example where, for example, the hemoglobin image is not similar to the a* channel.

2.2.5.4   Scaling and Sign Ambiguity

Since both **A** and **s** in Equation 2.2 are unknown, any scalar multiplier in one of the sources s_j could always be canceled by dividing the corresponding column $\mathbf{a}_j$ of $\mathbf{A}$ by the same scalar; therefore, we cannot determine the true variance of source signals, hence the ambiguity in scale (and magnitude). Fortunately, for many applications, this ambiguity is not significant (e.g., scaling a speaker's speech affects only the volume of his speech).

In ICA solution methods, the matrix $\mathbf{W}$ is often estimated such that each independent component has unit variance (i.e., $E\{s_j^2\} = 1$). Since s_j is a random variable, the assumption of having unit variance can be made without loss of generality.

The above strategy is also employed in the FastICA algorithm. Therefore, the outcome of Equation 2.21, that is, $\boldsymbol{\eta}_1$ and $\boldsymbol{\eta}_2$, will have unit variance. Since the image data do not usually have unit variance, we *L2-normalize* the ICA filters (i.e., scale each row of $\mathbf{W}$ to be of unit Euclidean length) so the estimated source data $\boldsymbol{\eta}$ has the same variance as the observed data $\boldsymbol{\phi}$ (equality results from the additivity of variances: $\sum var(\boldsymbol{\eta}_j) = \sum var(\boldsymbol{\phi}_i)$).

Either adapting $\mathbf{W}$ such that s_j would have unit variance or L2-normalizing rows of $\mathbf{W}$ so $\sum var(\boldsymbol{\eta}_j) = \sum var(\boldsymbol{\phi}_i)$ will still leave the ambiguity of the **sign**: the sign of sources cannot be determined. This ambiguity can be ignored in many applications (e.g., a sound signal, S, is identical to $-S$ when played on a speaker). In general, the sources can be multiplied by -1 without affecting the ICA model and the estimation [18].

Here too, the sign ambiguity is unimportant, although there is one concern: if we take each source vector $\boldsymbol{\eta}_j$ and reshape it as a 2-D signal, that is, a (monochromatic) image $\eta_j(x, y)$, the unknown sign might cause some inconsistencies in, for example, visualization. For instance, in Figure 2.8, one has to consider either images (a, d) or images (b, c) as independent components. In other words, either the darker or brighter areas should be taken as regions corresponding to the content of a component (melanin/hemoglobin) in an image.

To address this problem, we propose to always choose the sign such that brighter pixels would represent higher content of each component [i.e., images (c, d) in Figure 2.8]. Besides maintaining consistency in visualization, by normalizing $\eta_j(x, y)$ values to $[0, 1]$, the output image could be considered a spatial probability distribution map of each component (where brighter pixels depict higher likelihood).

While this proposal is advantageous, it requires user intervention. For each input, the user has to identify the correct two images from among the four possible outcomes. For large image datasets, this will obviously be a tedious task. In order to eliminate user intervention and automate this process, we will make use of the following observations.

2.2.5.5 Observation 3

Figure 2.9 shows the intensity histogram of the four images illustrated in Figure 2.8. Notice that the histograms of desired outcomes (b, c) are skewed to the left, with their highest peak (first mode) on the darker side of the red bar. This means that most of the pixels in the desired image are dark

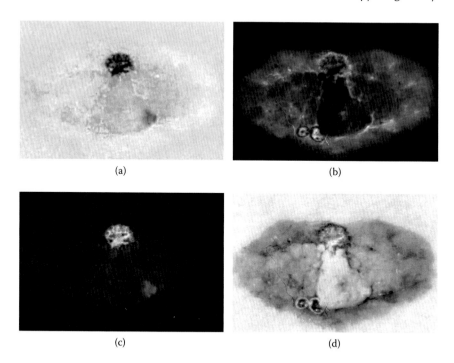

FIGURE 2.8 Illustration of the sign ambiguity. (a) $\eta_1(x,y)$. (b) $\eta_2(x,y)$. (c) $-\eta_1(x,y)$. (d) $-\eta_2(x,y)$. (a, b) Outcomes of FastICA. (c, d) are *complement* (negative) images of (a, b), representing four different possible outcomes due to the ambiguity in sign. Note that all images are normalized between $[0,1]$.

(with intensity value <0.5), which can be observed in Figure 2.8 as well. This observation is admissible because (1) the melanin and hemoglobin contents are expected to be higher in the lesion areas and (2) the lesion is often smaller than the background (healthy skin).

In conclusion, the bin index of peak(s) of the intensity histogram of $\eta_j(x,y)$ can be used as an indicator for determining the correct sign. Pertinent to this strategy, we will describe a computational procedure. Before we proceed to that, however, we would like to emphasize that the sign of an independent component will be canceled out in the inverse-matrix operation to, for example, reconstruct chromaticity images (for example, in back-projecting estimated sources to 2-D log-chromaticity space, i.e., $\hat{\phi} = \mathbf{A}\hat{\eta}$).

If we take $-\hat{\eta}_j$, instead of any $\hat{\eta}_j$, the sign of corresponding ICA basis should change to $-\mathbf{a}_j$ too (because $-\hat{\eta}_j = (-\hat{\mathbf{w}}_j) \times \phi_i$), and multiplying them together, we get the same answer for $\hat{\phi}_i = \mathbf{a}_j \times \hat{\eta}_j$ regardless of the sign.

2.2.5.6 Observation 4

The correlation coefficient ($\mathbf{r}$) between the correct $\eta_j(x,y)$ image and corresponding channel of CIE L*a*b* is usually positive (by "correct," it is meant

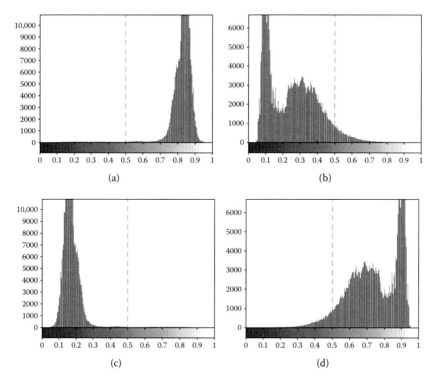

FIGURE 2.9 Intensity histograms of $\eta_j(x, y)$ images from Figure 2.8. (a) hist$\langle\eta_1(x, y)\rangle$. (b) hist$\langle\eta_2(x, y)\rangle$. (c) hist$\langle-\eta_1(x, y)\rangle$. (d) hist$\langle-\eta_2(x, y)\rangle$.

that the sign of that component is the desired one, and by "corresponding," it is meant the channel that has higher correlation with the component). For example, Figure 2.8b is highly correlated to the b* channel. The correlation coefficient is $\tau = 0.955$, whereas its complement (negative) image (i.e., Figure 2.8c) has correlation $\tau = -0.955$.

We will use this observation with the previous one in a unified voting scheme to decide the correct sign of an estimated independent component as follows.

The *first vote* is based on an intensity histogram of $\pm\eta_j(x, y)$ images. If the highest peak (first mode) of the histogram is in the bright side of the red bar (its bin index is >0.6), then the first vote goes to changing the sign of that component. For example, the bin index of the highest peak of Figure 2.9a is 0.8, which indicates correctly that our desired output should be the complement (negative) of this image (i.e., Figure 2.8c).

The *second vote* is based on the observation that intensity histograms of desired images are skewed to the left. This means most of the pixels in the image are dark. If more than half of the values of each $\pm\eta_j(x, y)$, when normalized to $[0, 1]$, are greater than 0.5, then the second vote goes to changing the sign of that component. For example, in Figure 2.8a, almost 98% of pixel values are greater than 0.5, which correctly indicates its sign has to be changed.

Finally, the *third vote* is based on the sign of the correlation coefficient (τ) between the component and its corresponding channel of CIE L*a*b*. If $\tau < 0$, the third vote goes to changing the sign of that component.

The sign of a component will only change if the majority of votes are in favor of the change.

2.2.5.7 Proposed Recovery Algorithm

To summarize, Algorithm 2.3 describes the proposed strategy taken here to deal with ICA ambiguities. For maintaining consistency in the implementation, Algorithm 2.3 is implemented to always output the melanin component as $\eta_1(x, y)$ and hemoglobin as $\eta_2(x, y)$.

Algorithm 2.3: Recovery from ICA Ambiguities

1: Load an image of skin lesion.
2: Run Algorithm 2.2 to estimate the separating matrix $\mathbf{W}$.
3: L2-normalize rows of $\mathbf{W}$, i.e., ICA filters.
4: Compute ICA basis: $\mathbf{A} = \mathbf{W}^+$, where $^+$ indicates Moore–Penrose pseudoinverse.
5: Compute independent components: $\boldsymbol{\eta} = \mathbf{W}\boldsymbol{\phi}$.
6: Reshape each estimated $\boldsymbol{\eta}_j$ to a 2-D signal, i.e., a (monochromatic) image $\eta_j(x, y)$.
7: First decide on the order of independent components as outlined in Section 2.2.5.1.
8: Then decide on the correct sign of independent components as outlined in Section 2.2.5.4.

2.2.6 PROPOSED COLOR-SPACE FORMULATION

In the previous sections, we have defined a model for skin coloration based on bio-optical properties of human skin. This model has been shown to be compatible with the ICA data model. Therefore, the ICA solution was used to disambiguate melanin and hemoglobin content in dermoscopy image content. As a result of the image analysis employed here, the extracted melanin and hemoglobin components are free of lighting artifacts. In fact, we have discarded the luminance (intensity) part of the input image. However, image intensities do carry a great deal of useful information [22]. For example, many texture extraction methods use only the intensity information. It is therefore of interest to somehow include intensity information in the model proposed here. For that purpose, we can go on to include the grayscale geometric mean image (Figure 2.10f) information, μ, together with extracted components,

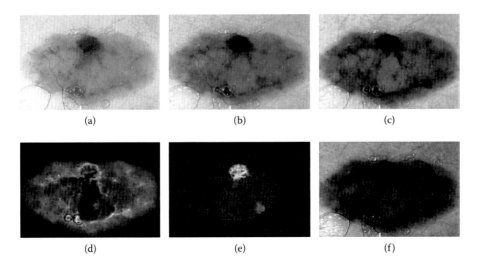

FIGURE 2.10 RGB color space vs. MHG color space. Melanin, hemoglobin, and geometric mean (MHG) is the proposed color space. (a) $R_r(x,y)$. (b) $R_g(x,y)$. (c) $R_b(x,y)$. (d) $\eta_m(x,y)$. (e) $\eta_h(x,y)$. (f) $\mu(x,y)$.

that is, use a color-space separation $\{\eta_1, \eta_2, \mu\}$. We denote this color space as *MHG*, standing for melanin, hemoglobin, and geometric mean. In Figure 2.10, the color channels R,G,B are illustrated together with color channels of the proposed M,H,G.

As will be shown in Section 2.3, MHG as a feature space yields excellent results for classification of melanoma versus benign skin lesions. Moreover, in the lesion segmentation task, μ will be shown to improve the precision and sensitivity of segmentation.

2.3 EXPERIMENTS AND RESULTS

We started this chapter by suggesting that the use of color features representing biological underpinnings of skin may benefit image analysis of skin lesions. In this section, we experimentally test that hypothesis. As a case study, we perform supervised classification of melanoma versus benign skin lesions.

Melanoma, the most severe and potentially fatal form of skin cancer, is among the cancers in the world with a rising incidence and high mortality rate [23]. Early detection of melanoma is crucial because it drastically changes the patient's prognosis for greater survival. If it is detected and excised early, particularly when the cancer is still localized in the top layer of the skin (the epidermis), the patient's survival rate is about 90%–97% at 10 years [24, 25].*

---

* The 5- and 10-year survival rates refer to the percentage of patients who live at least this long after their cancer is diagnosed. Of course, many people live much longer than 5 or 10 years (and many are cured).

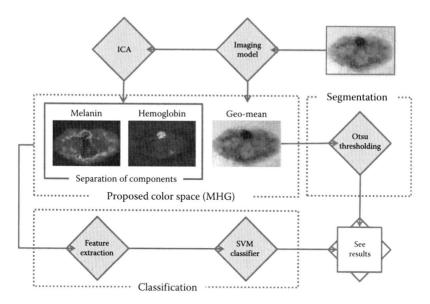

FIGURE 2.11 Schematic representation of proposed method for dermoscopy image analysis.

Unfortunately, if the diagnosis is made at a more advanced stage, when the cancer has penetrated and invaded the lower layer, the dermis, the survival rate drops to 10%–15% at 5 years [26], and progressively worsens with the depth of invasion. Melanoma, once it becomes invasive, may progress to the subcutaneous (under-the-skin) tissues and spread to other organs in the body (i.e., metastasize). At a metastatic stage, melanoma is almost always a fatal disease.

The current practice for early screening of pigmented skin lesions involves visual assessment by a health care professional. Clinical diagnosis of melanoma is, however, difficult even for experienced dermatologists [27, 28]. The problem is that *in vivo* diagnosis of malignant melanoma is highly subjective and uncertain, especially for clinically equivocal pigmented lesions [27]. Even with advanced clinical visualization and imaging tools, the accuracy of experts' diagnosis is estimated to be about 75%–85% [29]. Therefore, there is an increasing demand for computer-aided diagnostic systems to catch early melanomas,* in particular through automatic analysis of dermoscopic images. The latter typically involves successive steps of preprocessing [33–37], segmentation [38–40], feature extraction [40–50], and classification [51–55]. Here, we will go through this pipeline where color-space conversion to our proposed color representation is considered a preprocessing step. A schematic representation of our proposed system is given in Figure 2.11.

---

* There exists extensive literature on skin lesion image analysis: space does not allow a review, and the interested reader is referred to [30–32].

2.3.1   LESION SEGMENTATION

Lesion segmentation involves isolating skin lesions from normal skin surrounding it. It is important for two reasons: Firstly, the lesion boundary provides important information for accurate diagnosis. For example, border asymmetry or irregularity can signal malignancy. Secondly, it is a common practice to perform the feature extraction for the lesion area only, masking the healthy skin surrounding it. Therefore, representativeness of image features depends on the accuracy of the segmentation.

Automatic segmentation of skin lesion images is a challenging task for several reasons, including low contrast between the lesion and its background, the presence of artifacts, and so forth [41].

Throughout this study, it was found empirically that the G channel of the proposed MHG color space, that is, the geometric mean of R,G,B space (μ), intensifies the contrast between the lesion and the normal skin. This is a desired effect for segmentation methods based on gray-level thresholding, as explained in [56]. This effect is illustrated in Figure 2.12, where the G channel of MHG space is compared to L of CIE L*a*b*.

For automatic segmentation of lesions, we simply apply Otsu's method [57] for selecting a gray-level threshold. The Otsu method assumes that the image contains two classes (regions) of pixels (e.g., foreground [lesion] and background [healthy skin]). It then calculates (automatically) the optimum threshold value that separates those two classes such that their overlap is minimum. The overlap here is defined as the within-class variance (aka intraclass variance), that is, a weighted sum of variances of the two classes:

$$\sigma_{within}^2(t) = w_1(t)\sigma_1^2(t) + w_2(t)\sigma_2^2(t)$$

where $w_i(t)$ are the probabilities of the two classes separated by the threshold t and calculated from the image histogram as $w_1(t) = \sum_{i=0}^{t} p(i)$ and $w_2(t) = \sum_{i=t}^{n} p(i)$. The σ_i^2 are the variances of these classes.

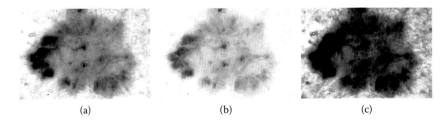

| (a) | (b) | (c) |

FIGURE 2.12 Grayscale image for segmentation. The geometric mean grayscale (c) highlights the lesion from its surroundings. (a) Input. (b) L of CIE L*a*b*. (c) G of MHG.

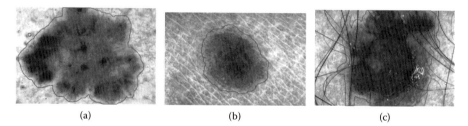

| (a) | (b) | (c) |

FIGURE 2.13 (a–c) Sample dermoscopy images with segmentation output.

Otsu shows [57] that minimizing the within-class variance is the same as maximizing the between-class (interclass) variance, while the former is faster to compute:

$$\sigma_{between}^2(t) = \sigma^2 - \sigma_{within}^2(t)$$
$$= w_1(t)[\mu_1(t) - \mu]^2 + w_2(t)[\mu_1(t) - \mu)]^2$$
$$= w_1(t)w_2(t)[\mu_1(t) - \mu_2(t)]^2$$

The μ_i are the mean of each class, $\mu = w_1(t)\mu_1(t) + w_2(t)\mu_2(t)$ is the total mean, and σ^2 is the total variance. Therefore, we can iteratively compute $\sigma_{between}^2(t)$ for each potential threshold $t \in [0,1]$. The desired threshold corresponds to the $\max_t \sigma_b^2(t)$. This iterative process can be implemented using recurrence relations, which yield efficient implementation [58].

Figure 2.13 shows the result of segmentation, using the proposed method (as summarized in Algorithm 2.4), on three sample images. Note that in our method it is assumed that the lesion is darker than its surrounding. For best results, small (and narrow) segmented regions—which usually correspond to hair and other dark-colored artifacts, such as ruler markings—are removed.

Algorithm 2.4: Proposed Segmentation Method

1: Load an image of a skin lesion.
2: Compute $\mu(x,y) = (\prod_{k=1}^{3} R_k)^{\frac{1}{3}}$, the geometric mean at each pixel.
3: Increase the contrast and smooth $\mu(x,y)$.
4: Create a binary image (mask) of $\mu(x,y)$ by applying Otsu's method.
5: Using morphological image processing:
    5.1: Remove the small regions.
    5.2: Expand and smooth the lesion boundaries.

2.3.2 COLOR/TEXTURE FEATURES

Color plays a substantial role in diagnosis of melanoma. In clinical examination of pigmented lesions, physicians take color variegation as a major sign that signals a possible malignancy. This is encapsulated in the ubiquitous ABCD list [59] and 7-point checklist [60], which are two commonly used clinical approaches for detecting cutaneous melanoma.

Consequently, in computerized analysis of skin lesions, analysis of lesion coloration has been undertaken by many researchers (e.g. [41, 61–63]). For that matter, a common approach is to extract statistical parameters from color channels as color features. Typically, basic statistical measures such as mean and standard deviation are computed (e.g., [55]). Similarly, here we generate mean, standard deviation, the ratio of these (which is the same as the signal-to-noise ratio), variance, skewness, kurtosis, and entropy of each channel as color features:

$$\text{mean: } \bar{x} = \frac{1}{n} \sum_{i=1}^{n} x_i$$

$$\text{std} = \sqrt{\text{var}}$$

$$\text{snr} = \bar{x}/\text{std}$$

$$\text{var} = \frac{1}{n-1} \sum_{i=1}^{n} (x_i - \bar{x})^2$$

$$\text{skew} = \frac{1}{n \times \text{std}^3} \sum_{i=1}^{n} (x_i - \bar{x})^3$$

$$\text{kurt} = \frac{1}{n \times \text{std}^4} \sum_{i=1}^{n} (x_i - \bar{x})^4$$

$$\text{entropy} = -\sum (p(x_i) \times \log_2 p(x_i))$$

Note that in calculation of these features, each color channel is treated as a random vector $\mathbf{x} = (x_1, \ldots, x_n)^T$.

The mean, variance, skewness, and kurtosis are *moments* of a distribution. They provide information about the appearance (shape) of a distribution (e.g., the location and variability of a set of numbers). Note as well that we adopt the standard deviation (which is of course closely related to variance) as the measure to describe dispersion of a distribution. The signal-to-noise ratio (SNR) is a measure that is more commonly used in signal processing to describe the quality of a signal compared to the level of background noise. SNR is also used in image processing as an image feature, and there it is defined as the ratio of the mean pixel values to the standard deviation [64]. Entropy is a statistical measure of randomness that can also be used to characterize the distribution of the pixel values. In the above formulation, $p(x_i)$ is the probability mass function (i.e., normalized histogram counts) of pixel values x_i.

Each of the above-mentioned statistical measures is a scalar, calculated separately for each color channel. Thus, the color feature used is a 21-D vector.

We append texture features onto the color-feature vector set out above, in a fashion similar to the approach used in [65, 66]. Four of the classical statistical texture measures of [67] (contrast, correlation, homogeneity, and energy) are derived from the gray-level co-occurrence matrix (GLCM) of each channel. This is an additional 12-D texture feature vector; thus, we arrive at a 33-D feature vector (11-D for each channel, concatenated into one vector for each image). This process is shown schematically in Figure 2.14.

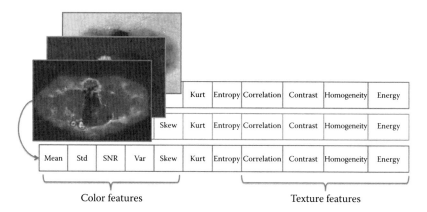

FIGURE 2.14 Feature extraction.

The GLCM is formed by calculating how often a pixel with gray-level (intensity) value i occurs in relation to a pixel with the value j. Consider the input image I; the position operator P is defined as a matrix P_{ij} that counts the number of times a pixel with gray-level i occurs at a certain position from a pixel with gray-level j. The following is an example where P counts horizontal adjacent pixels. Suppose I consists of only four gray-levels, $0, \ldots, 3$. Below, the number of times 0 is followed immediately by 0 horizontally in I is twice; therefore, $P(0,0)$ has the value 2.

$$
I = \begin{matrix} 0 & 0 & 1 & 1 \\ 0 & 0 & 1 & 1 \\ 0 & 2 & 2 & 2 \\ 2 & 2 & 3 & 3 \end{matrix} \quad \Rightarrow \quad P = \begin{array}{c|cccc} i,j & 0 & 1 & 2 & 3 \\ \hline 0 & 2 & 2 & 1 & 0 \\ 1 & 0 & 2 & 0 & 0 \\ 2 & 0 & 0 & 3 & 1 \\ 3 & 0 & 0 & 0 & 1 \end{array}
$$

In general, if the offset being examined is $\Delta x, \Delta y$, then if I is of size $N \times M$, P is given by

$$
P_{\Delta x, \Delta y} = \sum_{p=1} q = 1 \begin{cases} 1 & \text{if } I(p,q) = i \text{ and } I(p + \Delta y, q + \Delta x) = j \\ 0 & \text{otherwise} \end{cases}
$$

If I has Q quantized gray levels, then P is a $Q \times Q$ matrix.

The GLCM is defined by normalizing P (by the total number of pixels) such that each element $\hat{P}(i,j)$ is between $[0,1]$. We can obtain various useful descriptors from $\hat{P}$, by measuring various statistical properties, including the following:

$$
\text{contrast: } \sum_{i,j} |i - j|^2 \, \hat{P}(i,j)
$$

$$
\text{correlation: } \sum_{i,j} \frac{(i - \mu_i)(j - \mu_j)\hat{P}(i,j)}{\sigma_i \sigma_j}
$$

$$\text{energy: } \sum_{i,j} \hat{P}(i,j)^2$$

$$\text{homogeneity: } \sum_{i,j} \frac{\hat{P}(i,j)}{1+|i-j|}$$

Interested readers can refer to [67] for detailed information.

2.3.3 CLASSIFICATION

In this study, the support vector machine (SVM) is used for skin lesion classification. SVM is based on statistical learning theory, and it is considered to be a supervised learning method. Given a set of two-class input data in an N-dimensional space, SVM finds a separating hyperplane that maximizes the distance (margin) between the two class samples.

Although several machine learning methods have been applied to the skin lesion classification task (see [68] for a survey), the use of SVMs has been predominant [28, 55, 68–72]. Here we provide a brief overview of the theory behind SVM. For a more detailed discussion, interested readers are referred to [73].

Consider the simple case of binary linear classification, where the training set is given as $(\mathbf{x}_1, y_1)$, $(\mathbf{x}_2, y_2)$, ..., $(\mathbf{x}_m, y_m)$, class labels are $y \in \{-1, +1\}$, and each feature vector is of length N: $\mathbf{x} \in \mathbb{R}^N$. Assuming there exists a linear function $f(\mathbf{x}) = \mathbf{w}^T \mathbf{x} + b$ such that for the positive class $(y_i = 1)$, $f(\mathbf{x}_i) > 0$, and for the negative class $(y_i = -1)$, $f(\mathbf{x}_i) < 0$, a separating hyperplane can be found by solving $\mathbf{w}^T \mathbf{x} + b = 0$. In other words, new data points $\mathbf{x}$ are classified according to the sign of $f(\mathbf{x})$.

There are many possible choices of $\mathbf{w}$ and b. The SVM algorithm defines the optimal separating hyperplane as the one that is maximally far from any data point. For that matter, SVM attempts to maximize the classifier's margin, that is, the (smallest) distance between the decision boundary and the separating hyperplane.

The SVM as described here was first introduced by Boser et al. [74]. This model was modified by Cortes and Vapnik [75] to account for mislabeled examples (aka the soft margin method), which is still the standard formulation of this model:

$$\arg\min_{\mathbf{w},b,\xi} \frac{1}{2}\mathbf{w}^T\mathbf{w} + C\sum_{i=1}^{m}\xi_i$$
$$\text{subject to} \quad y_i(\mathbf{w}^T\mathbf{x}_i + b) \geq 1 - \xi_i \tag{2.31}$$
$$\xi_i \geq 0, \quad i = 1\ldots m$$

where ξ_i is a *slack variable*, which allows x_i to not exactly meet the margin requirements at a cost $C\xi_i$. The parameter $C > 0$ controls the trade-off between the slack variable penalty and the margin.

2.3.4 RESULTS

2.3.4.1 Segmentation Results

The proposed segmentation method is tested on a dataset of images used by Wighton et al. [39]. The dataset consists of 100 challenging and 20 easy-to-segment images. An image is considered challenging if any of the following conditions are true: "1) the contrast between the skin and lesion is low, 2) there is significant occlusion by either oil or hair, 3) the entire lesion is not visible, 4) the lesion contains variegated colors or 5) the lesion border is not clearly defined" [39].

Wighton et al. presented a modified random walker (MRW) segmentation where seed points were set automatically based on a lesion probability map (LPM). The LPM was created through a supervised learning algorithm using color and texture properties.

Table 2.1 shows the results for the proposed method (Otsu on G) compared to the results in [39]. While the proposed method uses a much simpler algorithm and does not require learning, it achieves comparable results. It is worth mentioning that [39] also applied Otsu's method, but on their lesion probability maps. Their result for this approach is included in Table 2.1 under "Otsu on LPM," with results not nearly as good as ours.

We also compare the results of using the proposed method with those in Khakabi et al. [38]. They proposed "a novel tree structure based representation

---

TABLE 2.1

Results of Segmentation Using Proposed Method vs. Those Reported in [39]

Img. Set	Method	Precision	Recall	F-Score
Simple	MRW on LPM	0.96	0.95	0.95
	Otsu on LPM	**0.99**	0.86	0.91
	Otsu on G	0.95	**0.98**	**0.96**
Challenging	MRW on LPM	0.83	0.90	0.85
	Otsu on LPM	0.88	0.68	0.71
	Otsu on G	**0.88**	**0.91**	**0.88**
Entire	MRW on LPM	0.87	0.92	0.88
	Otsu on LPM	**0.91**	0.74	0.78
	Otsu on G	0.90	**0.92**	**0.90**

Note: Comparing the proposed segmentation method to the modified random walker (MRW) algorithm with Otsu's thresholding, applied to lesion probability map (LPM) [39]. Note that the proposed method (Otsu on G) consistently produces higher f-score, notwithstanding its simplicity and speed.

TABLE 2.2

Results of Segmentation Using Proposed Method vs. Those Reported in [38]

Method	Sensitivity	Specificity
Otsu on G	**0.92**	0.91
Multilayer tree [38]	0.89	0.90
G-Log/LDA [49]	0.88	0.88
KPP [76]	0.71	0.79
DTEA [77]	0.64	**0.99**
SRM [78]	0.77	0.95
JSEG [79]	0.678	**0.99**
FSN [54]	0.81	0.93

Note: Comparing our segmentation method to the multilevel feature extraction method [38] and the output of six other methods reported in [38]. Note that the proposed method (Otsu on G) has the highest sensitivity, whereas its specificity is comparable to other methods.

of the lesion growth pattern by matching every pixel sub-cluster with a node in the tree structure" [38]. This multilayer tree is employed to extract sets of features, which are then used, in a supervised learning framework, to segment lesions. Khakabi et al. tested their method on the same dataset used by Wighton et al. [39] and herein for lesion segmentation. They reported sensitivity and specificity of their segmentation results, comparing with six other skin lesion segmentation methods. See Table 2.2 and references therein.

In another test on 944 test images, the proposed method achieved a precision of 0.86, recall of 0.95, and f-score of 0.88 (with standard deviation 0.19, 0.08, and 0.15, respectively) compared to expert segmentations. Note that results here are averaged over all images.

2.3.4.2 Classification Results

We applied linear SVM to a set of 486 images taken from [80], with two classes consisting of melanoma versus all benign lesions (congenital, compound, dermal, Clark, Spitz, and blue nevus; dermatofibroma; and seborrheic keratosis).

Table 2.3 results are averaged over ten fold cross-validation. The classifier achieves an f-score of 88.2% and area under the curve (AUC) of 0.93, an excellent performance. The receiver operator curve (ROC) and precision–recall (PR) curve of the overall classification is provided in Figure 2.15.

In a ten fold cross-validation procedure, the data are randomly partitioned into 10 complementary subsets of equal size. At each round of cross-validation, the classifier is trained on nine subsets, whereas a single subset is retained as validation (testing) data. Usually, results are averaged over the rounds to form a single estimation (although they can be otherwise combined too).

TABLE 2.3

Results of Classifying the Dataset Using the Proposed Color-Space MHG

Class	n	Precision	Recall	F-Score	AUC
Melanoma	121	0.804	0.711	0.754	
Benign	365	0.908	0.942	0.925	0.93
Weighted avr.	486	0.882	0.885	0.882	

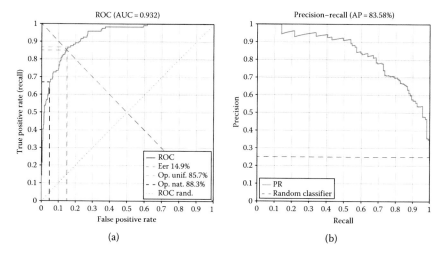

(a)   (b)

FIGURE 2.15 Graphs representing goodness of fit of the classifier. The graphs are based on the SVM classifier that generated the results presented in Table 2.3. Note that SVM (in general) is a decision machine and so does not provide posterior probabilities. The curves here are generated by ranking the decision values. (a) ROC curve. (b) PR curve.

2.3.4.3 Discussion

The significance of using the proposed color space is illustrated in Table 2.4, where the results of classifying the dataset using different color spaces are presented. It can be seen that by using MHG (the proposed color space), the classifier's discriminatory power (AUC) is substantially boosted, while its performance (f-score) is also improved. The latter improvement is marginal for overall classification, yet considerable for the positive class (melanoma), showing that MHG is particularly effective for melanoma lesions. Note that the dataset is unbalanced: a classifier trained on, for example, RGB achieved high scores, yet assigned the benign label to most melanoma instances. Using the proposed color space, on the other hand, produced equally high and steady results for both classes, improving, for example, recall for melanoma cases by

TABLE 2.4

Results of Classifying the Dataset Using Different Color Spaces

Color Space	Class	n	Precision	Recall	F-Score	AUC
MHG	Melanoma	121	0.804	**0.711**	**0.754**	**0.93**
	Benign	365	**0.908**	0.942	0.925	
	Weighted avr.	486	0.882	0.885	**0.883**	
RGB	Melanoma	121	**0.875**	0.636	0.737	0.803
	Benign	365	0.889	0.97	**0.928**	
	Weighted avr.	486	**0.886**	**0.887**	0.88	
HSV	Melanoma	121	0.875	0.579	0.697	0.776
	Benign	365	0.874	**0.973**	0.921	
	Weighted avr.	486	0.875	0.874	0.856	
LAB	Melanoma	121	0.797	0.455	0.579	0.708
	Benign	365	0.842	0.962	0.898	
	Weighted avr.	486	0.831	0.835	0.818	

Note: MHG is the proposed color space. Note that using MHG the AUC is significantly boosted.

TABLE 2.5

Results of Classifying the Dataset Using Different Subsets of Our Feature-Set (Color/Texture) and Different Channels of Our Proposed Color-Space MHG

Description	n	Precision	Recall	F-Score	AUC
Color features only on MHG	486	0.707	0.753	0.696	0.736
Texture features only on MHG		0.88	0.819	0.868	0.817
Color + texture on melanin only		0.696	0.751	0.674	0.697
Color + texture on hemoglobin only		0.798	0.811	0.796	0.862
Color + texture on geo-mean only		0.848	0.854	0.847	0.892
Color + texture on MHG		**0.882**	**0.885**	**0.882**	**0.93**

up to 26%. Since the same feature set and classifier are used, the improvement is the result of using the proposed color space.

On a different note, we would like to point out that obtaining these results by using such a simple feature set is very encouraging. We have shown that even such a simple feature set is sufficient to demonstrate its applicability and highlight the significance of using the proposed color space for the task at hand.

To judge the effect of color versus texture features, and the contribution of different channels of the proposed color-space MHG, consider Table 2.5.

This table shows that (1) texture features have higher impact than color features (2) the three channels of MHG contribute more than each individually; the best results overall stem from combining all the features.

2.3.4.4 Quantification of Melanin and Hemoglobin

In order to verify the validity of the proposed skin coloration model, and the employed blind-source separation approach, we need pathological data

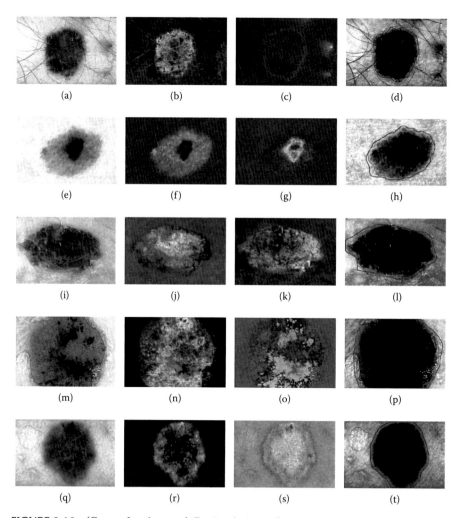

FIGURE 2.16 (See color insert.) Benign lesions. On geo-mean image, the blue border shows expert segmentation, whereas the red border is our segmentation boundary produced by applying Algorithm 2.4. The first column is input image followed by melanin, hemoglobin, and geo-mean channels in the following columns.

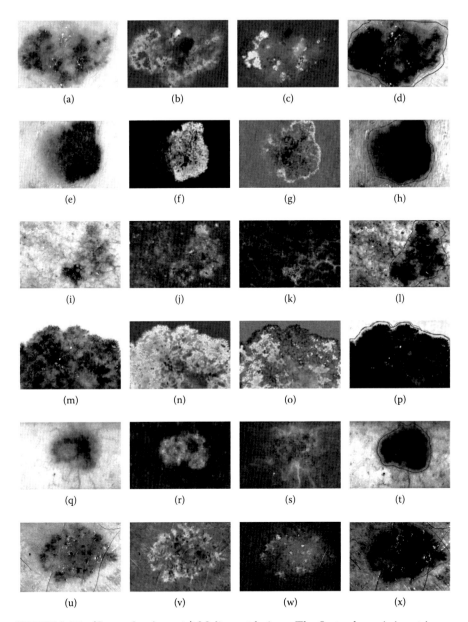

FIGURE 2.17 (See color insert.) Malignant lesions. The first column is input image followed by melanin, hemoglobin, and geo-mean channels in the following columns.

associated with skin images. For our dataset, such information is not available. Thus, we rely on visual assessment: the proposed method seems to succeed in highlighting hyperpigmented spots. Some sample outputs are shown in Figures 2.16 through 2.18.

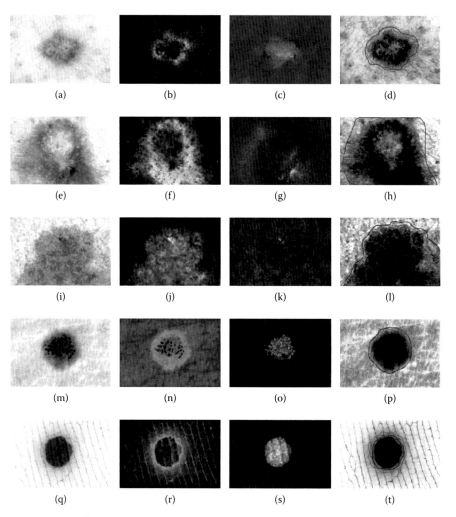

(a)   (b)   (c)   (d)

(e)   (f)   (g)   (h)

(i)   (j)   (k)   (l)

(m)   (n)   (o)   (p)

(q)   (r)   (s)   (t)

FIGURE 2.18 (**See color insert.**) Some more benign lesions. The first column is input image followed by melanin, hemoglobin, and geo-mean channels in the following columns.

2.4 CONCLUSION

We have proposed a new color feature η, which is aimed at apprehending underlying melanin and hemoglobin biological components of dermoscopy images of skin lesions. The advantage of the new feature, in addition to its biological underpinnings, lies in removing the effects of confounding factors such as light color, intensity falloff, shading, and camera characteristics. The new color-feature vectors $\{\eta_1, \eta_2\}$ combined with a geometric mean value, μ, are proposed as a new color-space MHG. In our experiments,

MHG is shown to produce excellent results for classification of melanoma versus benign. Moreover, in the lesion segmentation task, μ is shown to improve accuracy of segmentation. Future work will include (1) exploration of effects and contributions of other color and texture features, combined with those reported here, (2) experimenting with different learning algorithms and strategies, in particular the possibility of multiclass classification, and (3) examination of the extracted melanin and hemoglobin color components as a set of two full-color images, since the equations leading to Equation 2.20 are in fact invertible for each component separately. As 3-D color features, these will support descriptors such as color histograms and correlograms, which may lead to even more improvement.

REFERENCES

1. E. Claridge, S. Cotton, P. Hall, and M. Moncrieff, From colour to tissue histology: Physics-based interpretation of images of pigmented skin lesions, *Medical Image Analysis*, vol. 7, pp. 489–502, 2003.
2. N. Tsumura, H. Haneishi, and Y. Miyake, Independent-component analysis of skin color image, *Journal of the Optical Society of America*, vol. 16, pp. 2169–2176, 1999.
3. N. Tsumura, N. Ojima, K. Sato, M. Shiraishi, H. Shimizu, H. Nabeshima, S. Akazaki, K. Hori, and Y. Miyake, Image-based skin color and texture analysis/synthesis by extracting hemoglobin and melanin information in the skin, *ACM Transactions Graphics*, vol. 22, pp. 770–779, 2003.
4. G. D. Finlayson, M. S. Drew, and C. Lu, Intrinsic images by entropy minimization, in *Proceedings of the 8th European Conference on Computer Vision (ECCV)*, T. Pajdla and J. Matas, Eds., Springer, Berlin, pp. 582–595, 2004.
5. L. Lathauwer, A short introduction to tensor-based methods for factor analysis and blind source separation, in *2011 7th International Symposium on Image and Signal Processing and Analysis (ISPA)*, Bosan, Korea, pp. 558–563, 2011.
6. C. Servire and P. Fabry, Principal component analysis and blind source separation of modulated sources for electro-mechanical systems diagnostic, *Mechanical Systems and Signal Processing*, vol. 19, no. 6, pp. 1293–1311, 2005.
7. Y. Li, A. Cichocki, and S. I. Amari, Sparse component analysis for blind source separation with less sensors than sources, in *Proceedings of Fourth International Symposium on Independent Component Analysis and Blind Source Separation (ICA 2003)*, Nara, Japan, pp. 89–94, 2003.
8. A. Cichocki and R. Zdunek, Multilayer nonnegative matrix factorisation, *Electronics Letters*, vol. 42, no. 16, pp. 947–948, 2006.
9. J. V. Stone, *Independent Component Analysis: A Tutorial Introduction*, MIT Press, Cambridge, MA, 2004.
10. A. Hyvrinen, J. Karhunen, and E. Oja, *Independent Component Analysis*, John Wiley and Sons, New York, 2001.
11. A. Hyvrinen and E. Oja, Independent component analysis: Algorithms and applications, *IEEE Transactions on Neural Networks*, vol. 13, no. 4-5, pp. 411–430, 2000.

12. A. Hyvarinen, Fast and robust fixed-point algorithms for independent component analysis, *IEEE Transactions on Neural Networks*, vol. 10, no. 3, pp. 626–634, 1999.

13. H. Gvert, J. Hurri, J. Srel, and A. Hyvrinen, *FastICA for MATLAB*, version 2.5, http://research.ics.aalto.fi/ica/fastica/, 2005.

14. G. D. Finlayson, M. S. Drew, and B. V. Funt, Spectral sharpening: Sensor transformations for improved color constancy, *Journal of the Optical Society of America*, vol. 11, no. 5, pp. 1553–1563, 1994.

15. R. R. Anderson and J. A. Parrish, The optics of human skin, *Journal of Investigative Dermatology*, vol. 77, no. 1, pp. 13–19, 1981.

16. J. Dawson, D. Barker, D. Ellis, E. Grassam, J. Cotterill, G. Fisher, and J. Feather, A theoretical and experimental study of light absorption and scattering by in vivo skin, *Physics in Medicine and Biology*, vol. 25, no. 4, pp. 695–709, 1980.

17. M. Hiraoka, M. Firbank, M. Essenpreis, M. Cope, S. R. Arrige, P. V. D. Zee, and D. T. Delpy, A Monte Carlo investigation of optical pathlength in inhomogeneous tissue and its application to near-infrared spectroscopy, *Physics in Medicine and Biology*, vol. 38, pp. 1859–1876, 1993.

18. G. R. Naik and D. K. Kumar, An overview of independent component analysis and its applications, *Informatica: An International Journal of Computing and Informatics*, vol. 35, no. 1, pp. 63–81, 2011.

19. J. Hurri, Independent component analysis of image data, Master's thesis, Department of Computer Science and Engineering, Helsinki University of Technology, Espoo, Finland, 1997.

20. H. Takiwaki, Measurement of skin color: Practical application and theoretical considerations, *Journal of Medical Investigation*, vol. 44, no. 3–4, pp. 121–126, 1998.

21. P. Clarys, K. Alewaeters, R. Lambrecht, and A. O. Barel, Skin color measurements: Comparison between three instruments: The Chromameter®, the DermaSpectrometer® and the Mexameter®, *Skin Research and Technology*, vol. 6, no. 4, pp. 230–238, 2000.

22. B. K. P. Horn, Understanding image intensities, *Artificial Intelligence*, vol. 8, no. 2, pp. 201–231, 1977.

23. R. Siegel, J. Ma, Z. Zou, and A. Jemal, Cancer statistics, 2014, *CA: A Cancer Journal for Clinicians*, vol. 64, no. 1, pp. 9–29, 2014.

24. C. M. Balch, S. J. Soong, J. E. Gershenwald, J. F. Thompson, D. S. Reintgen, N. Cascinelli, M. Urist, K. M. McMasters, M. I. Ross, and J. M. Kirkwood, Prognostic factors analysis of 17,600 melanoma patients: Validation of the American Joint Committee on Cancer melanoma staging system, *Journal of Clinical Oncology*, vol. 19, no. 16, pp. 3622–3634, 2001.

25. C. Balch, A. Buzaid, S. Soong, M. Atkins, N. Cascinelli, D. Coit, I. Fleming, J. Gershenwald, A. Houghton Jr., and J. Kirkwood, Final version of the American Joint Committee on Cancer staging system for cutaneous melanoma, *Journal of Clinical Oncology*, vol. 19, no. 16, pp. 3635–3648, 2001.

26. R. Braun, L. French, and J. Saurat, Dermoscopy of pigmented lesions: A valuable tool in the diagnosis of melanoma, *Swiss Medical Weekly*, vol. 134, no. 7/8, pp. 83–90, 2004.

27. R. P. Braun, H. S. Rabinovitz, M. Oliviero, A. W. Kopf, and J. H. Saurat, Dermoscopy of pigmented skin lesions, *Journal of the American Academy of Dermatology*, vol. 52, no. 1, pp. 109–121, 2005.

28. I. Maglogiannis and C. Doukas, Overview of advanced computer vision systems for skin lesions characterization, *IEEE Transactions on Information Technology in Biomedicine*, vol. 13, no. 5, pp. 721–733, 2009.

29. G. Argenziano, H. Soyer, S. Chimenti, R. Talamini, R. Corona, F. Sera, M. Binder, L. Cerroni, G. De Rosa, G. Ferrara et al., Dermoscopy of pigmented skin lesions: Results of a consensus meeting via the Internet, *Journal of the American Academy of Dermatology*, vol. 48, no. 5, pp. 679–693, 2003.

30. J. Scharcanski and M. E. Celebi, *Computer Vision Techniques for the Diagnosis of Skin Cancer*, Springer, Berlin, 2013.

31. K. Korotkov and R. Garcia, Computerized analysis of pigmented skin lesions: A review, *Artificial Intelligence in Medicine*, vol. 56, no. 2, pp. 69–90, 2012.

32. M. E. Celebi, W. V. Stoecker, and R. H. Moss, Advances in skin cancer image analysis, *Computerized Medical Imaging and Graphics*, vol. 35, no. 2, pp. 83–84, 2011.

33. Q. Abbas, I. F. Garcia, M. E. Celebi, and W. Ahmad, A feature-preserving hair removal algorithm for dermoscopy images, *Skin Research and Technology*, vol. 19, no. 1, pp. 27–36, 2013.

34. A. Madooei, M. Drew, M. Sadeghi, and S. Atkins, Automated pre-processing method for dermoscopic images and its application to pigmented skin lesion segmentation, in *Twentieth Color and Imaging Conference: Color Science and Engineering Systems, Technologies, and Applications*, Los Angeles, CA, pp. 158–163, 2012.

35. Q. Abbas, M. E. Celebi, and I. F. Garcia, Hair removal methods: A comparative study for dermoscopy images, *Biomedical Signal Processing and Control*, vol. 6, no. 4, pp. 395–404, 2011.

36. H. Zhou, M. Chen, R. Gass, J. M. Rehg, L. Ferris, J. Ho, and L. Drogowski, Feature-preserving artifact removal from dermoscopy images, in *Proceedings of Medical Imaging 2008: Image Processing*, in SPIE Medical Imaging, vol. 6914, pp. 69141B–69141B-9, 2008.

37. T. Lee, V. Ng, R. Gallagher, A. Coldman, and D. McLean, Dullrazor: A software approach to hair removal from images, *Computers in Biology and Medicine*, vol. 27, no. 6, pp. 533–543, 1997.

38. S. Khakabi, P. Wighton, T. K. Lee, and M. S. Atkins, Multi-level feature extraction for skin lesion segmentation in dermoscopic images, in *Proceedings of Medical Imaging: Computer-Aided Diagnosis*, San Diego, CA, vol. 8315, pp. 83150E–83150E-7, 2012.

39. P. Wighton, M. Sadeghi, T. K. Lee, and M. S. Atkins, A fully automatic random walker segmentation for skin lesions in a supervised setting, in *Proceedings of the 12th International Conference on Medical Image Computing and Computer-Assisted Intervention: Part II*, MICCAI '09, G.-Z. Yang, D. Hawkes, D. Rueckert, A. Noble, and C. Taylor, Eds., Springer, Berlin, pp. 1108–1115, 2009.

40. M. E. Celebi, G. Schaefer, H. Iyatomi, and W. V. Stoecker, Lesion border detection in dermoscopy images, *Computerized Medical Imaging and Graphics*, vol. 33, no. 2, pp. 148–153, 2009.

41. M. E. Celebi and A. Zornberg, Automated quantification of clinically significant colors in dermoscopy images and its application to skin lesion classification, *IEEE Systems Journal*, vol. 8, no. 3, pp. 980–984, 2014.

42. J. L. Garcia Arroyo and B. Garcia Zapirain, Detection of pigment network in dermoscopy images using supervised machine learning and

structural analysis, *Computers in Biology and Medicine*, vol. 44, pp. 144–157, 2014.

43. M. Sadeghi, T. K. Lee, D. McLean, H. Lui, and M. S. Atkins, Detection and analysis of irregular streaks in dermoscopic images of skin lesions, *IEEE Transactions on Medical Imaging*, vol. 32, no. 5, pp. 849–861, 2013.

44. Q. Abbas, M. E. Celebi, C. Serrano, I. Fondon Garcia, and G. Ma, Pattern classification of dermoscopy images: A perceptually uniform model, *Pattern Recognition*, vol. 46, no. 1, pp. 86–97, 2013.

45. A. Madooei, M. S. Drew, M. Sadeghi, and M. S. Atkins, Automatic detection of blue-white veil by discrete colour matching in dermoscopy images, in *Medical Image Computing and Computer-Assisted Intervention—MICCAI 2013*, K. Mori, I. Sakuma, Y. Sato, C. Barillot, and N. Navab, Eds., Springer, Berlin, pp. 453–460, 2013.

46. A. Madooei and M. Drew, A colour palette for automatic detection of blue-white veil, in *21st Color and Imaging Conference: Color Science and Engineering Systems, Technologies, and Applications*, Albuquerque, NM, pp. 200–205, 2013.

47. C. Barata, J. S. Marques, and J. Rozeira, A system for the detection of pigment network in dermoscopy images using directional filters, *IEEE Transactions on Biomedical Engineering*, vol. 59, no. 10, pp. 2744–2754, 2012.

48. M. Sadeghi, M. Razmara, T. K. Lee, and M. S. Atkins, A novel method for detection of pigment network in dermoscopic images using graphs, *Computerized Medical Imaging and Graphics*, vol. 35, no. 2, pp. 137–143, 2011.

49. P. Wighton, T. K. Lee, H. Lui, D. I. McLean, and M. S. Atkins, Generalizing common tasks in automated skin lesion diagnosis, *IEEE Transactions on Information Technology in Biomedicine*, vol. 15, no. 4, pp. 622–629, 2011.

50. M. E. Celebi, H. Iyatomi, W. V. Stoecker, R. H. Moss, H. S. Rabinovitz, G. Argenziano, and H. P. Soyer, Automatic detection of blue-white veil and related structures in dermoscopy images, *Computerized Medical Imaging and Graphics*, vol. 32, no. 8, pp. 670–677, 2008.

51. Q. Abbas, M. E. Celebi, I. F. Garcia, and W. Ahmad, Melanoma recognition framework based on expert definition of ABCD for dermoscopic images, *Skin Research and Technology*, vol. 19, no. 1, pp. 93–102, 2013.

52. A. Madooei, M. S. Drew, M. Sadeghi, and M. S. Atkins, Intrinsic melanin and hemoglobin colour components for skin lesion malignancy detection, in *Medical Image Computing and Computer-Assisted Intervention—MICCAI 2012*, N. Ayache, H. Delingette, P. Golland, and K. Mori, Eds., Springer, Berlin, pp. 315–322, 2012.

53. Q. Abbas, M. E. Celebi, and I. Fondón, Computer-aided pattern classification system for dermoscopy images, *Skin Research and Technology*, vol. 18, no. 3, pp. 278–289, 2012.

54. H. Iyatomi, H. Oka, M. E. Celebi, M. Hashimoto, M. Hagiwara, M. Tanaka, and K. Ogawa, An improved Internet-based melanoma screening system with dermatologist-like tumor area extraction algorithm, *Computerized Medical Imaging and Graphics*, vol. 32, no. 7, pp. 566–579, 2008.

55. M. E. Celebi, H. A. Kingravi, B. Uddin, H. Iyatomi, Y. A. Aslandogan, W. V. Stoecker, and R. H. Moss, A methodological approach to the classification of dermoscopy images, *Computerized Medical Imaging and Graphics*, vol. 31, no. 6, pp. 362–373, 2007.

56. D. D. Gomez, C. Butakoff, B. K. Ersboll, and W. Stoecker, Independent histogram pursuit for segmentation of skin lesions, *IEEE Transactions on Biomedical Engineering*, vol. 55, no. 1, pp. 157–161, 2008.

57. N. Otsu, A threshold selection method from gray-level histograms, *IEEE Transactions on Systems, Man and Cybernetics*, vol. 9, no. 1, pp. 62–66, 1979.

58. M. Sezgin and B. Sankur, Survey over image thresholding techniques and quantitative performance evaluation, *Journal of Electronic Imaging*, vol. 13, no. 1, pp. 146–168, 2004.

59. T. Fitzpatrick, A. Rhodes, A. Sober, and M. Mihm, Primary malignant melanoma of the skin: The call for action to identify persons at risk; to discover precursor lesions; to detect early melanomas, *Pigment Cell*, vol. 9, pp. 110–117, 1988.

60. J. Malvehy, S. Puig, G. Argenziano, A. A. Marghoob, H. P. Soyer, and International Dermoscopy Society board members, Dermoscopy report: Proposal for standardization. Results of a consensus meeting of the International Dermoscopy Society, *Journal of the American Academy of Dermatology*, vol. 57, no. 1, pp. 84–95, 2007.

61. Y. Cheng, R. Swamisai, S. E. Umbaugh, R. H. Moss, W. V. Stoecker, S. Teegala, and S. K. Srinivasan, Skin lesion classification using relative color features, *Skin Research and Technology*, vol. 14, no. 1, pp. 53–64, 2008.

62. R. J. Stanley, W. V. Stoecker, and R. H. Moss, A relative color approach to color discrimination for malignant melanoma detection in dermoscopy images, *Skin Research and Technology*, vol. 13, no. 1, pp. 62–72, 2007.

63. A. Sboner, E. Blanzieri, C. Eccher, P. Bauer, M. Cristofolini, G. Zumiani, and S. Forti, A knowledge based system for early melanoma diagnosis support, in *Proceedings of the 6th IDAMAP Workshop—Intelligent Data Analysis in Medicine and Pharmacology*, London, UK, pp. 30–35, 2001.

64. R. Gonzalez and R. Woods, *Digital Image Processing*, 2nd ed., Upper Saddle River, NJ: Prentice Hall, 2002.

65. B. Shrestha, J. Bishop, K. Kam, X. Chen, R. Moss, W. Stoecker, S. Umbaugh, R. Stanley, M. E. Celebi, A. Marghoob, G. Argenziano, and H. Soyer, Detection of atypical texture features in early malignant melanoma, *Skin Research and Technology*, vol. 16, no. 1, pp. 60–65, 2010.

66. M. Sadeghi, M. Razmara, P. Wighton, T. Lee, and M. Atkins, Modeling the dermoscopic structure pigment network using a clinically inspired feature set, in *Medical Imaging and Augmented Reality*, pp. 467–474, 2010.

67. R. M. Haralick and L. G. Shapiro, *Computer and Robot Vision*, Vol. 1. New York: Addison-Wesley, 1992.

68. S. Dreiseitl, L. Ohno-Machado, H. Kittler, S. Vinterbo, H. Billhardt, and M. Binder, A comparison of machine learning methods for the diagnosis of pigmented skin lesions, *Journal of Biomedical Informatics*, vol. 34, no. 1, pp. 28–36, 2001.

69. X. Yuan, Z. Yang, G. Zouridakis, and N. Mullani, SVM-based texture classification and application to early melanoma detection, in *28th Annual International Conference of the IEEE Engineering in Medicine and Biology Society, EMBS '06*, New York, pp. 4775–4778, 2006.

70. I. Maglogiannis and D. I. Kosmopoulos, Computational vision systems for the detection of malignant melanoma, *Oncology Reports*, vol. 15, pp. 1027–1032, 2006.

71. T. Tommasi, E. La Torre, and B. Caputo, Melanoma recognition using representative and discriminative kernel classifiers, in *Proceedings of the Second ECCV International Conference on Computer Vision Approaches to Medical Image Analysis, CVAMIA '06*, R. R. Beichel and M. Sonka, Eds., Springer, Berlin, pp. 1–12, 2006.

72. M. d'Amico, M. Ferri, and I. Stanganelli, Qualitative asymmetry measure for melanoma detection, in *IEEE International Symposium on Biomedical Imaging: Nano to Macro, 2004*, Arlington, VA, vol. 2, pp. 1155–1158, 2004.

73. N. Cristianini and J. Shawe-Taylor, *An Introduction to Support Vector Machines and Other Kernel-Based Learning Methods*. Cambridge: Cambridge University Press, 2000.

74. B. E. Boser, I. M. Guyon, and V. N. Vapnik, A training algorithm for optimal margin classifiers, in *Proceedings of the 5th Annual ACM Workshop on Computational Learning Theory*, New York, pp. 144–152, 1992.

75. C. Cortes and V. Vapnik, Support-vector networks, *Machine Learning*, vol. 20, no. 3, pp. 273–297, 1995.

76. H. Zhou, M. Chen, L. Zou, R. Gass, L. Ferris, L. Drogowski, and J. M. Rehg, Spatially constrained segmentation of dermoscopy images, in *5th IEEE International Symposium on Biomedical Imaging: From Nano to Macro, ISBI 2008*, Paris, France, pp. 800–803, 2008.

77. M. E. Celebi, Y. A. Aslandogan, W. V. Stoecker, H. Iyatomi, H. Oka, and X. Chen, Unsupervised border detection in dermoscopy images, *Skin Research and Technology*, vol. 13, no. 4, pp. 454–462, 2007.

78. M. E. Celebi, H. Kingravi, H. Iyatomi, Y. Aslandogan, W. Stoecker, R. Moss, J. Malters, J. Grichnik, A. Marghoob, H. Rabinovitz, and S. Menzies, Border detection in dermoscopy images using statistical region merging, *Skin Research and Technology*, vol. 14, no. 3, pp. 347–353, 2008.

79. M. E. Celebi, Q. Wen, S. Hwang, H. Iyatomi, and G. Schaefer, Lesion border detection in dermoscopy images using ensembles of thresholding methods, *Skin Research and Technology*, vol. 19, no. 1, pp. e252–e258, 2013.

80. G. Argenziano, H. Soyer, V. De Giorgio, D. Piccolo, P. Carli, M. Delfino, A. Ferrari, R. Hofmann-Wellenhof, D. Massi, and G. Mazzocchetti, *Interactive Atlas of Dermoscopy*. Milan, Italy: EDRA Medical Publishing and New Media, 2000.

3 Where's the Lesion?
Variability in Human and Automated Segmentation of Dermoscopy Images of Melanocytic Skin Lesions

Federica Bogo
Università degli Studi di Padova
Padova, Italy
and
Max Planck Institute for Intelligent Systems
Tuebingen, Germany

Francesco Peruch
Università degli Studi di Padova
Padova, Italy

Anna Belloni Fortina
Università degli Studi di Padova
Padova, Italy

Enoch Peserico
Università degli Studi di Padova
Padova, Italy

CONTENTS

The first step in the analysis of any dermatoscopic image of a melanocytic lesion is *segmentation*—classification of all points in the image as part of the lesion or simply part of the surrounding nonlesional skin. While segmentation is typically studied in the context of automated analysis of images, it is important to observe that it is a first, necessary step even for human operators who plan to evaluate quantitative features of a lesion such as diameter or asymmetry (for example, in the context of epidemiological studies correlating those features to sun exposure [1–3] or risk of lesion malignancy [4]).

Unfortunately, segmentation of melanocytic lesions is a surprisingly difficult task. The fundamental reason lies in the fact that lesion borders are often fuzzy and there exists no standard operative definition of whether a portion of skin belongs to a lesion or not: dermatologists rely on subjective judgment developed over years of dermatoscopic training. This can lead to appreciable variability in the localization of the precise border of lesions (see Figure 3.1).

Quantifying this variability between dermatologists is crucial for at least two reasons. First, it allows one to estimate the level of noise affecting large, multioperator epidemiological studies. Second, variability between experienced dermatologists effectively provides an upper bound for the segmentation accuracy achievable by dermatologists-in-training or by automated systems.

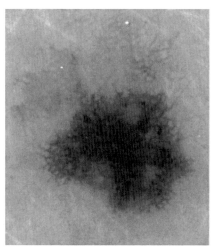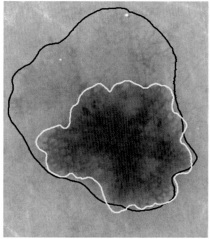

FIGURE 3.1 A dermatoscopically imaged melanocytic lesion (left) and two widely divergent segmentations obtained from two experienced dermatologists (right). (Reprinted from Peruch, F. et al., Simple, fast, accurate melanocytic lesion segmentation in 1-D colour space, in *Proceedings of VISAPP 2013*, pp. 191–200, 2013, Barcelona, Spain. Copyright 2013, with permission from INSTICC/SciTePress.)

For example, if even experienced dermatologists disagree on how to classify 5% of the area of an image, one can never expect to classify "correctly" more than 95% of the area of that image.

This chapter has five sections. Section 3.1 looks at how to formalize the intuitive, but somewhat elusive, notion of disagreement between segmentations of the same lesion. Section 3.2 looks at what disagreement one may expect between different segmentations provided by human dermatologists, providing a survey of the sparse literature on the subject. Section 3.3 very briefly reviews the vast literature on automated segmentation techniques and illustrates one such technique in detail as a representative case study. Section 3.4 compares the segmentations of 60 melanocytic lesions provided by 12 different dermatologists of various degrees of experience and those provided by two variants of the automated technique. In a nutshell, it turns out that state-of-the-art techniques can achieve a level of agreement with the most experienced dermatologists that is only slightly worse than that of other experienced dermatologists, and in fact better than that of dermatologists of little, or even moderate, experience. Finally, Section 3.5 attempts to distill from the results a small set of "take-home messages" for the practitioner of the field.

3.1 COMPARING DIFFERENT SEGMENTATIONS

To formally quantify the intuitive notion of "dissimilarity" or "disagreement" between segmentations, one has to face a number of subtle issues; different approaches to resolve them lead to different definitions. The first and perhaps most crucial issue is that, when comparing two segmentations, their roles are rarely symmetric. Instead, typically one of the two is a reference segmentation (often provided by an experienced dermatologist) used as a ground truth or gold standard against which the other segmentation, the test case, is evaluated.

Most measures of the difference between a reference segmentation and a test case are a function of the number of *true positive* (TP), *true negative* (TN), *false positive* (FP), and *false negative* (FN) pixels—the number of pixels that are judged lesional, respectively, by both the test case and the reference (TP), by neither the test case nor the reference (TN), by the test case but not by the reference (FP), and by the reference but not by the test case (FN). Note that the use of true/false positives/negatives is a classic approach in the evaluation of binary classifiers, not just within the scope of segmentation, and in fact not just in computer science.

Three classic measures in this sense are *precision, recall* or *sensitivity* (also known as *true detection rate*), and *specificity*, each taking values between 0 (the worst case) and 1 (the best case). Precision is the fraction $TP/(TP+FP)$ of pixels classified as lesional by the test case on which test case and reference are in agreement. Recall/sensitivity is the fraction $TP/(TP+FN)$ of pixels classified as lesional by the *reference* on which test case and reference are in agreement. Specificity is the fraction $TN/(TN+FP)$ of pixels classified as *nonlesional* by the reference on which test case and reference are in agreement. Note that a "tight" test case with very few lesional pixels will always have very high precision and specificity (1 if the entire image is classified as non-lesional), while a "lax" test case with very few nonlesional pixels will always have very high recall/sensitivity (1 if the entire image is classified as lesional). For this reason, precision is generally presented alongside recall [6, 7] and specificity alongside sensitivity [8–11], with a good test case having high values in *both* elements of the pair (a test case coinciding with the reference will have precision, recall/sensitivity, and specificity all equal to 1). Alternatively, the average of the two elements of the pair is sometimes presented [8]; or, when some "tightness" parameter controls a trade-off between the two elements, some function of the best achievable value of one element in terms of the other is given—a typical example is the curve of the ratio between sensitivity and 1 minus specificity, also known as the receiver operating characteristic (ROC) curve [9, 10].

Another important set of measures based on true/false positives/negatives is that of *misclassification* or *XOR* measures, all proportional to the number $FP + FN$ of misclassified pixels (the "area of disagreement" between test case and reference, see Figure 3.2). This number is generally divided by the number $TP + FN$ of pixels in the lesion according to the reference segmentation so as to normalize the result for images with different resolutions or for lesions of different size. This is probably the most popular definition of XOR measure, and the most popular measure in the field [5, 12–19].

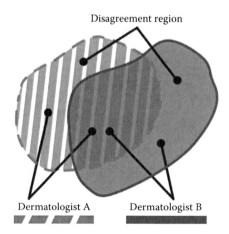

FIGURE 3.2 The XOR measure is proportional to the number $FP + FN$ of misclassified pixels, i.e., the region of disagreement between test case (dermatologist A) and reference (dermatologist B). (Belloni Fortina, A. et al.: Where's the Naevus? Inter-Operator Variability in the Localization of Melanocytic Lesion Border. *Skin Research and Technology*, 2011. 18. 311–315. Copyright Wiley-VCH Verlag GmbH & Co. KGaA. Reproduced with permission.)

TABLE 3.1

Common Measures of Dissimilarity Based on True/False Positives/Negatives

Precision	$\dfrac{TP}{TP + FP}$
Recall/sensitivity	$\dfrac{TP}{TP + FN}$
Specificity	$\dfrac{TN}{TN + FP}$
XOR measure	$\dfrac{FP + FN}{TP + FN}$
Hammoude distance	$\dfrac{FP + FN}{TP + FP + FN}$

Note that this normalization factor is a source of asymmetry: unless reference and test case have exactly the same number of pixels, switching the two yields a different XOR measure. In a few works the normalization factor is instead the number of pixels $TP + FP + FN$ that are lesional according to *either* the reference or the test case (yielding the so-called Hammoude distance) [21, 22] or simply the total number of pixels $TP + FP + TN + FN$ in the entire image [9, 11]; both these normalizations make the error measure symmetric. Table 3.1 summarizes the measures discussed so far.

One measure of dissimilarity not based on true/false positives/negatives that is worth mentioning is the Hausdorff distance between two segmentations of the same lesion [21], equal to the maximum distance of any pixel that is lesional according to either segmentation to the closest pixel that is lesional according to the other segmentation. Informally, the Hausdorff distance attempts to capture the maximum distance between the two lesion borders. One disadvantage of the Hausdorff distance is that it is not invariant to the resolution of the image or the scale of the lesion. A more serious disadvantage is that it fails to distinguish between a test case that diverges from the reference only in a very localized area (for example, because of a spurious hair, see Figure 3.3) and one that diverges all around the border.

We have so far focused on comparisons between *pairs* of segmentations. Given the intrinsic noise affecting the accuracy of any given segmentation, a common strategy is instead to compare the test case not to a single reference, but to an ensemble of references—the idea being that the ensemble provides a more accurate ground truth than any of its constituents in isolation. Once again, this can be done in a number of different ways.

Perhaps the simplest approach is to just compute some measure of pairwise dissimilarity between the test case and *each* reference in the ensemble, and present the set of all results [23]. Much more frequently, the *average* of all results is instead presented [5, 18, 24, 25]. A less common approach is to

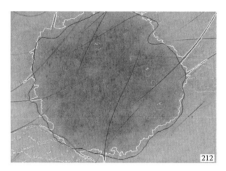

FIGURE 3.3 Melanocytic lesion segmentation performed by a dermatologist (black) and by the technique presented in [5] (white). Automated borders widely diverge from manual ones in localized areas, due to presence of sparse hair.

summarize not the comparison results, but the reference segmentations, into a single segmentation where each pixel is lesional or nonlesional depending on whether it is lesional or nonlesional in the majority of the segmentations of the ensemble [6, 7, 26].

The common problem of all these approaches is that they fail to discriminate between two fundamentally different sources of divergence between a test case and the reference ensemble. If the reference segmentations in the ensemble strongly disagree with each other, then any test case will inevitably sport a high level of disagreement with at least some of the reference segmentations. On the other hand, if the reference segmentations strongly agree with each other, then a test case with a high level of disagreement is a highly suboptimal segmentation that could be drastically improved.

One measure that normalizes the disagreement between a test case and an ensemble of references, adjusting it as a function of the internal disagreement of the ensemble, is the Normalized Probabilistic Random Index (NPRI), first introduced by [27] and proposed for melanocytic lesion segmentation by [28]. NPRI has a complex expression that can be rewritten as a linear rescaling of a function depending solely on the fraction of misclassified pixels in the test case according to each of the reference segmentations [29]. Unfortunately, this dependence is not monotone, so that beyond a certain level of misclassification NPRI will actually improve if classification worsens, yielding counterintuitive results [29] (see Figure 3.4).

A more effective alternative is to present, in addition to the divergence of the test case from the reference ensemble, the average divergence of each element of the ensemble from the others [5, 18, 20]. The latter quantity presents a very clear, immediate lower bound for the divergence achievable by any test case when evaluated against that ensemble. A slight variation (making somewhat less efficient use of the reference ensemble) is to evaluate both the test case and a portion of the ensemble using as ground truth the rest of the ensemble [30, 31].

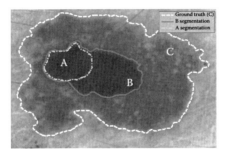

FIGURE 3.4 **(See color insert.)** An example of the counterintuitive behavior of NPRI. Even though segmentation B is in greater agreement than segmentation A with the reference segmentation C, it achieves a lower (i.e., worse) PRI equal to 0.5 (vs. 0.52 of A). NPRI, being simply a linear rescaling of PRI, maintains the anomaly. (Reprinted from *Pattern Recognition Letters*, 31, E. Peserico and A. Silletti, Is (N)PRI suitable for evaluating automated segmentation of skin lesions?, 2464–2467, 2010. Copyright 2010, with permission from Elsevier.)

3.2 VARIABILITY IN HUMAN SEGMENTATIONS

This section reviews the known results on variability in segmentations provided by human dermatologists—a problem that has received relatively little attention so far [32]. A particular focus is on the results of [20], (a portion of) whose dataset is used in Section 3.4 to compare the performance of automated systems with that of human operators.

The first work to study the problem of interoperator variability in melanocytic lesion segmentation is [22]. Interestingly, it is also the only work in the literature that also considers intraoperator variability—having five different dermatologists repeat the segmentation of 25 lesions imaged at 768×512 resolution three times each, at 2-week intervals. The segmentations are drawn on a computer screen as polygons whose vertices are provided by the dermatologists. The authors evaluate the divergence as the Hammoude distance $(FP + FN)/(TP + FP + FN)$ of each of the three pairs of segmentations by each dermatologist, reporting an average divergence of approximately 5% for the "least variable" and of approximately 7% for the "most variable" dermatologist.

Unfortunately, in terms of interoperator variability, the authors adopt a somewhat unorthodox approach that makes it hard to compare their results with others in the literature. They consider a ground truth formed by an ensemble of 21 segmentations: the 15 segmentations provided by the dermatologists and 3 identical segmentations by each of 2 automated algorithms (this triplication is meant to allow each of the automated algorithms the same weight in the ensemble as a human dermatologist). They then report an error probability that coincides with 1 minus the average precision $TP/(TP + FP)$ of each segmentation against the reference ensemble (which includes the test case and in fact includes it three times in the case of automated segmentations). This error is approximately 5% and 6% for the two dermatologists considered above (the other dermatologists are reported to have similar statistics), and 3–4% for the two algorithms considered. Even disregarding the composition of the ensemble note that, as mentioned in Section 3.1, without any recall measure the high precision exhibited by the algorithms is not necessarily indicative of "good" segmentations, but only of "tight" segmentations.

Several other works in the literature, when evaluating the divergence of one or more automated systems from a reference segmentation provided by a human dermatologist, also evaluate the segmentation of a second dermatologist against the same reference as a term of comparison. Using the XOR measure, in [30] and [31] the authors report an average divergence of 8.71% (with a standard deviation of 3.78%) over a group of 70 benign lesions and of 8.13% (with a standard deviation of 3.99%) over a group of 30 melanomas, imaged at various resolutions ranging from 768×512 to 2556×1693. This was markedly less than any of the automated techniques under testing. The authors of [9] instead consider the divergence, from reference segmentations provided by an expert dermatologist over 85 dermatoscopic images at 2000×1334 resolution, of the segmentations provided by a junior dermatologist registrar in his first year of training—again using the XOR measure. The junior dermatologist performed less well than automated algorithms, exhibiting a divergence of at least 10% in more than 80% of the images, at least 15% in more than 50%, and at least 20% in more than 30%. The authors note that junior dermatologists tend to provide segmentations not nearly as tight as those of more experienced dermatologists, an observation confirmed by other studies [18, 20].

The largest study so far on the variability of border localization by different dermatologists, and the only one to consider the impact of dermatologist experience, is [20]. The authors consider a set of 77 dermatoscopic images at 768×512 resolution. Twelve copies of each image were printed in color on 12×18 cm glossy photographic paper, and a copy of each image together with a white marker was given to each of 12 dermatologists. Dermatologists were divided into three cohorts: four *junior*, four *competent*, and four *expert* dermatologists (respectively less than 1 year of dermoscopy training, between 1 and 5 years, and more than 5 years). Each dermatologist was asked to independently draw the border of each lesion with the marker directly on the photographic paper. Each image (with the manually drawn borders) was then scanned and realigned to the same frame of reference. Finally, the contours provided by the markers were extracted and compared by software, identifying for each pixel of each original image the set of dermatologists classifying that pixel as part of the lesion proper or as part of the surrounding nonlesional skin.

The disagreement in each of the $12 \cdot 11 = 132$ distinct (ordered) pairs of dermatologists was evaluated using the XOR measure $(FP + FN)/(TP + FN)$,

TABLE 3.2

Average Disagreement between Pairs of Distinct Dermatologists in Various Experience Groups

Average Disagreement (XOR Measure) of

Expert	Competent	Junior	with
11.90%	14.80%	18.90%	*Expert*
13.58%	14.59%	18.17%	*Competent*
14.91%	15.23%	14.17%	*Junior*

Source: Belloni Fortina, A. et al., *Skin Research and Technology*, 18(3), 311–315, 2011. Copyright 2011.

Note: Measured as the ratio between the disagreement area and the size of the lesion according to the first dermatologist of the pair (XOR measure, $[FP + FN]/[TP + FN]$).

yielding an average disagreement (over all pairs and all images) of 15.28%, with a 90th percentile of over 28%. The average disagreement of dermatologists in each experience cohort with *different* dermatologists in the same and other cohorts is reported in Table 3.2.

Note that *expert* dermatologists appear in greater agreement than merely *competent* ones, which in turn appear in greater agreement than *junior* dermatologists. When validated using one-tailed (nonparametric) permutation tests [33],* these observed differences turned out not to be statistically significant ($p = 0.115$ and $p = 0.286$, respectively). *Expert* dermatologists, however, did turn out to be in significatively ($p = 0.029$) greater agreement than *junior* dermatologists. As in [9], it was also observed that more experienced dermatologists tend to provide tighter segmentations: on average, lesion size according to *expert* dermatologists was only 95.66% of that according to merely *competent* dermatologists, and only 86.87% of that according to *junior* dermatologists. The difference between *expert* and *competent* dermatologists was not statistically significant ($p = 0.129$), but that between *expert* and *junior* dermatologists and that between *competent* and *junior* dermatologists both were ($p = 0.015$ and $p = 0.043$, respectively).

This variability in lesion size evaluation suggested that perhaps divergence between different dermatologists could be more apparent than real, and due at least in part to a systematic bias whereby two dermatologists actually have an identical perception of lesions, but one of the two consistently draws

---

* In a nutshell, when comparing a sample of n_1 more experienced (e.g., *competent*) dermatologists with a sample of n_2 less experienced (e.g., *junior*) dermatologists to test whether greater experience yields a significant positive correlation with some statistic of interest (e.g., interoperator agreement), the p value is the fraction of all possible $(n_1 + n_2/n_1)$ groups of n_1 dermatologists from the two samples associated to an average value of the statistic of interest more extreme than that of the experienced group.

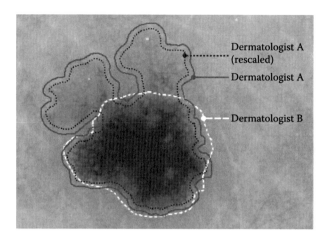

FIGURE 3.5 (See color insert.) Compensation for systematic bias in border drawing, as performed in [20]. All lesions according to dermatologist A are rescaled (in this case tightened) by the same factor, so as to make lesion size identical to that of dermatologist B on average. (Belloni Fortina, A. et al.: Where's the Naevus? Inter-Operator Variability in the Localization of Melanocytic Lesion Border. *Skin Research and Technology*, 2011. 18. 311–315. Copyright Wiley-VCH Verlag GmbH & Co. KGaA. Reproduced with permission.)

a slightly tighter border (e.g., because of greater confidence stemming from greater experience). To address this possibility, when comparing the set of segmentations produced by two dermatologists, the border of all segmentations of the second dermatologist was expanded or reduced by the same scale factor, chosen so as to bring the two dermatologists to the same average lesion size (see Figure 3.5).

This adjustment provided only a minor level of reduction in the divergence between dermatologists; Table 3.3 reproduces the same statistics as Table 3.2 after this size adjustment. Even after rescaling, *expert* dermatologists remained in greater agreement than *competent* ones, which in turn remained in greater agreement than *junior* dermatologists. The difference between *expert* and *junior* dermatologists increased its statistical significance ($p = 0.015$) and, interestingly, the difference between *expert* and *competent* dermatologists also became significative ($p = 0.029$) after rescaling.

3.3 AUTOMATED SEGMENTATION

There is a vast literature on the topic of automated melanocytic lesion segmentation, well beyond the scope of this chapter (see [32, 34, 35] and particularly [36] for surveys). A commonly adopted taxonomy [5, 18, 21, 37] divides the approaches in the literature into three main classes, all three relying to

TABLE 3.3

Average Disagreement between Pairs of Distinct Dermatologists in Various Experience Groups after Lesion Rescaling

Average Disagreement after Rescaling (XOR Measure) of

Expert	Competent	Junior	with
11.03%	13.63%	15.35%	*Expert*
12.74%	13.25%	15.95%	*Competent*
13.03%	14.32%	13.75%	*Junior*

Source: Belloni Fortina, A. et al., *Skin Research and Technology*, 18(3), 311–315, 2011. Copyright 2011.

some extent on some level of preprocessing—typically to remove artifacts such as sparse hair or to calibrate colors.

The first class includes "minimal energy contour" techniques, which try to identify lesion boundaries through the minimization of a well-defined energy function. Commonly used energy functions consider edges and smoothness constraints, or statistical distributions over pixel intensities. A good representative of this class is gradient vector flow (GVF) snakes [31, 38, 39]. The border identification accuracy of techniques in this class typically depends heavily on an initial segmentation estimate, on effective preprocessing (e.g., for hair removal), and on morphological postprocessing [21, 32].

The second class includes "split and merge" techniques. These approaches proceed by either recursively splitting the whole image into pieces based on region statistics or, conversely, merging pixels and regions together in a hierarchical fashion. Representatives of this class include modified JSEG [30], stabilized inverse diffusion equations (SIDE) [14], statistical region merging (SRM) [23], watershed [40]. Performance widely varies depending on a large number of parameters whose values must be carefully tuned [14, 18].

The third class of segmentation techniques for melanocytic lesions discriminates between lesional and nonlesional skin on the image's color histogram to classify each color as lesional or nonlesional. This separation is mapped back onto the original image, from which morphological postprocessing then eliminates small, spurious patches. Simple thresholding techniques like Otsu's method [41] can provide accurate lesion segmentations in some cases, but in general lack robustness [19]; for example, they fail when lesions exhibit variegated coloring or low contrast with respect to the surrounding skin [5, 7]. More sophisticated approaches, such as independent histogram pursuit (IHP) [16], mean shift [8, 42], and fuzzy c-means [18, 42–44], achieve greater robustness—but often at the cost of increased computational loads.

This chapter presents in detail a recent representative of this third class (MEDS [5]) as a case study, because of its high accuracy, low computational load,* and ease of implementation, and because it may yield insight into many of the techniques often used to approach the problem. MEDS proceeds in five stages. The first is optional and simply preprocesses the image to rebalance its colors or automatically remove any hair. The second stage reduces the dimensionality of the color space to one through principal component analysis (PCA) of the color histogram. The third stage applies a blur filter to the resulting image to reduce noise. The fourth stage separates pixels into two clusters through an ad hoc thresholding algorithm that is the heart of the technique and tries to mimic the cognitive process of dermatologists; this effectively partitions the original image into regions corresponding to lesional and non-lesional skin. Finally, the fifth stage morphologically postprocesses the image to remove spurious patches and identify lesional areas of clinical interest.

3.3.1 PREPROCESSING

Hair represents a common obstacle in dermatoscopic analysis of melanocytic lesions [32, 45]; a number of schemes [46–49] have thus been developed to automatically remove it from dermatoscopic images. MEDS is relatively resilient to the presence of hair (see Section 3.4), so it generally can work fairly well even without them. MEDS also works fairly well with any illumination that is reasonably balanced (more specifically, where a white object has red, green, and blue values all between 192 and 255); however, while a cast with a strong red component can significantly worsen the quality of the segmentation, a cast with strong blue, moderate green, and weak red components can marginally improve it. According to [5], the highest accuracy can be achieved when the red, green, and blue (RGB) values of each pixel are multiplied respectively by 0.02, 0.2, and 0.98; the optimality of these parameters, however, could depend on the dataset (and, in particular, on the acquisition system's color calibration). The color balancing can be achieved either physically through the use of appropriate optics or digitally by simply modifying on the fly the RGB values of each pixel the first time it is read from memory—an operation that takes negligible time.

3.3.2 PROJECTION ON 1-D COLOR SPACE

MEDS employs PCA to cluster the colors of the image into two classes, according to their projection on the first principal component of the color histogram.

Consider an m-pixel RGB image. PCA requires the computation of the 3×3 covariance matrix $\mathbf{C}$ as $\mathbf{M}^T\mathbf{M}$, where the ith row $\mathbf{m_i} = \langle r_i g_i b_i \rangle$ of

---

* According to [5] a Java implementation of MEDS segments a 768×512 image in less than 20 ms on a personal computer and in less than 0.5 s on a (2010) Samsung S cell phone, making it well suited for real-time use.

the $m \times 3$ matrix $\mathbf{M}$ represents the three color components of the ith pixel, each component normalized by subtracting the mean value of that color in the image. Effectively, this corresponds to

$$\mathbf{C} = \frac{1}{m} \sum_i \mathbf{m_i}^T \mathbf{m_i} \qquad (3.1)$$

so that $\mathbf{C}$ can be easily computed by "streaming" the image pixel by pixel, subtracting the mean R, G, and B values, computing the six distinct products of the pixel's color components, and adding each of those products to the corresponding product for all other pixels—note that $\mathbf{C}$ is characterized by six elements rather than nine since it is symmetric. The first principal component of $\mathbf{M}$ corresponds to the dominant eigenvector of $\mathbf{C}$. Its computation takes a negligible amount of time, since it only requires extracting the roots of a third-degree polynomial (the characteristic polynomial of $\mathbf{C}$) and inverting a 3×3 matrix. Finally, each row of $\mathbf{M}$ is projected on the principal component; this can be achieved by streaming the image and performing only a few arithmetic operations for each pixel. Thus, the cost of the whole procedure is essentially that of scanning the image from memory three times: once for the average, once for the covariance, and once for the projection.

In challenging cases—for example, when the image contains many artifacts or when only a small fraction of image pixels are lesional—the principal component's direction may vary considerably, resulting in a suboptimal, less discriminative color space. A slightly modified version of MEDS—named MEDS boost—addresses this problem by balancing image colors during pre-processing and then normalizing the mean value of each channel before applying PCA: the red, green, and blue values of each pixel are divided by the mean value of that channel in the image before computing the covariance matrix. The normalization step scales the variance of each channel, ensuring robust PCA and thus accurate segmentations even when the ratio between lesional and nonlesional pixels in the image is very low.

3.3.3   NOISE REDUCTION

After projecting the original image onto the first principal component, MEDS applies a box filter with an $n \times n$ window, where n corresponds roughly to 1.5% of the original image's height. A naive implementation would require $n^2 - 1$ additions plus 1 division for each image pixel. The number of additions can be reduced to 4 by keeping track of the last computed values in a simple, auxiliary data structure; furthermore, each division can be efficiently computed as a multiplication followed by a shift. In this way, filtering the image requires only a single scan and a handful of non-floating-point operations per pixel; this is considerably faster than the fastest median filter implementations, while still providing comparable results in terms of final segmentation accuracy.

3.3.4   COLOR CLUSTERING

Operating on the color histogram $h(\cdot)$ that associates to each color c the number of pixels $h(c)$ of that color, colors (and thus pixels) are separated into two clusters, corresponding respectively to lesional and nonlesional skin. This stage, which is the heart of MEDS and mimics the cognitive process of human dermatologists, can be divided into three main phases. The first phase applies to the histogram a square root operator, followed by a moving-average operator over an $n \times n$ window. The square-root operator enhances smaller values, which is useful when the percentages of lesional and nonlesional tissue differ widely. The averaging smooths out small fluctuations. More precisely, this corresponds to

$$h'(x) = \sqrt{h(x)} \qquad h''(x) = \frac{1}{n} \sum_{y=x-\lfloor n/2 \rfloor}^{x+\lfloor n/2 \rfloor} h'(y) \qquad (3.2)$$

The second phase finds the positions M_ℓ, M_s of two local maxima in $h''(\cdot)$ that can be assumed as color centers of, respectively, lesional and nonlesional skin. Finally, the third phase determines a threshold $F \in [M_\ell, M_s]$ separating the two clusters in the histogram.

The first center M_1 corresponds to the global maximum in $h''(\cdot)$ (see Figure 3.6). Note that M_1 cannot be classified as lesional or nonlesional until the second center is found, since lesion area may be larger or smaller than nonlesional skin area. The second center M_2 is computed as

$$M_2 = \arg\max_x \left(h''(x)(h''(M_1) - h''(m_x)) \right), \ x \neq M_1 \qquad (3.3)$$

where $h''(m_x)$ is the minimum of $h''(\cdot)$ between x and M_1. The two terms $h''(x)$ and $h''(M_1) - h''(m_x)$ in the maximized product favor, in the choice of M_2, a color that is well represented (yielding a high $h''(x)$) and at the same time is sharply separated from M_1 (yielding a high $h''(M_1) - h''(m_x)$). This seems to accurately reflect the cognitive process of dermatologists.

Typically, lesional skin is darker, and therefore corresponds to the lower center:

$$M_\ell = \min(M_1, M_2), \ M_s = \max(M_1, M_2) \qquad (3.4)$$

This assumption is satisfied by almost the totality of melanocytic lesions. The technique could still be easily adapted to work in the extremely rare instances when this is not the case, such as when dealing with amelanotic melanocytic lesions—for example, by assuming that the lesion is entirely contained within the image and does not touch its borders, so that the color of the pixels on the image's borders is that of nonlesional skin.

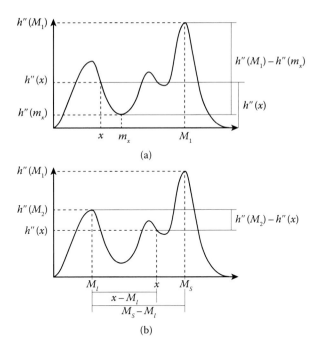

FIGURE 3.6 Partitioning of the color histogram into lesional/nonlesional colors. (Reprinted from Peruch, F. et al., Simple, fast, accurate melanocytic lesion segmentation in 1-D colour space, *Proceedings of VISAPP 2013*, pp. 191–200, 2013, Barcelona, Spain. Copyright 2013, with permission from INSTICC/SciTePress.)

Finally, the threshold between skin and lesion color is set as

$$F = \arg\max_{x} \left(h''(M_2) - h''(x)\right) \left(\frac{x - M_\ell}{M_s - M_\ell}\right)^{\gamma} \tag{3.5}$$

where $\gamma \in \mathbb{R}^+$ is the single tuning parameter of the technique—the smaller γ, the "tighter" the segmentations produced (see Figure 3.7). Informally, the first term in the product favors as threshold a color that is *not* well represented and thus yields a sharp separation between the two clusters. The second term, whose weight grows with γ, favors a color closer to that of nonlesional skin; this reproduces the behavior of human dermatologists, who tend to classify as lesional regions of the image that are slightly darker than the majority of nonlesional skin, even when those regions are considerably lighter than the core of the lesion. Figure 3.7 illustrates how the clustering results vary as γ increases from 0.8 to 1. Note that the fractional exponentiation in Equation 3.5 is carried out at most once for each of the 256 points of the color histogram, incurring an overall computational cost that is virtually negligible.

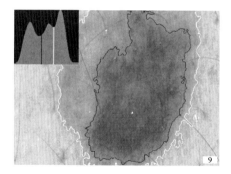

FIGURE 3.7 Identification of the separation point between lesional and nonlesional colors for $\gamma = 1$ (white) and $\gamma = 0.8$ (black). Lower values of γ yield "tighter" segmentations. (Reprinted from Peruch, F. et al., Simple, fast, accurate melanocytic lesion segmentation in 1-D colour space, *Proceedings of VISAPP 2013*, pp. 191–200, 2013, Barcelona, Spain. Copyright 2013, with permission from INSTICC/SciTePress.)

3.3.5 POSTPROCESSING

Mapping the segmentation from color space back onto the original image produces a binary mask, where each pixel is classified as lesional or nonlesional. Two phases of postprocessing follow: first, the image is downsampled in order to easily identify the *boundaries* of each lesional component; then, all boundaries delimiting "too small" connected components are removed. This eliminates artifact patches due to individual pixels slightly darker or lighter than their neighbors and identifies connected components classified as nonlesional but entirely surrounded by lesional pixels—such components usually correspond to air bubbles or lesion regressions and should be classified as lesional.

Denote by $p_{i,j}$ the pixel located at row i and column j in the image, and by $v(p_{i,j})$ its value. Any pixel can be associated to a 4- and an 8-*neighborhood*—informally, the 4 pixels adjacent to it horizontally or vertically and the 8 pixels adjacent to it horizontally, vertically, or diagonally. More formally, for each *internal* (i.e., nonedge and noncorner) pixel $p_{i,j}$ of the image, the following definitions apply:

Definition 3.1
The 4-*neighborhood* of $p_{i,j}$ consists of the 4 pixels $p_{k,l}$ such that $|i - k| + |l - j| = 1$.

Definition 3.2
The 8-*neighborhood* of $p_{i,j}$ consists of the 8 pixels $p_{k,l} \neq p_{i,j}$ such that $|i - k| \leq 1$ and $|l - j| \leq 1$.

In order to deal with pixels located on edges or corners, the image can be simply surrounded with a 1-pixel-wide strip of nonlesional pixels, so that the pixels of the original image correspond to the internal pixels of the expanded image.

In the downsampling phase, the (expanded) image is partitioned into boxes of 3×3 pixels; each pixel in a box takes the value of the central pixel in the box:

$$v(p_{i,j}) \triangleq v(p_{k,l}) \text{ with } k = 3 \left\lfloor \frac{i}{3} \right\rfloor + 1, \ l = 3 \left\lfloor \frac{j}{3} \right\rfloor + 1 \qquad (3.6)$$

Then, *boundary* pixels in the image are identified:

Definition 3.3
A *boundary* pixel is a lesional pixel whose 4-neighborhood contains exactly 3 lesional pixels.

One can then prove the following:

Theorem 3.1
After downsampling, the 8-neighborhood of any boundary pixel contains exactly 2 boundary pixels. ∎

By Theorem 3.1 then, if every boundary pixel is viewed as a vertex of degree 2 connected by an edge to its two adjacent boundary pixels, one can obtain a set of disjoint cycle graphs, corresponding to the boundaries of all (putative lesional) connected components in the image. This makes it extremely easy to "walk" a boundary, starting from any of its pixels, following the edges between adjacent vertices in the corresponding graph.

The last phase of postprocessing computes the area of all connected components of sufficient height. A crucial notion for this phase is that of *d*-row:

Definition 3.4
Consider an image of r rows, numbered from 1 to r starting from the top, and a parameter d $(1 \le d \le r)$. The ith row is a *d*-row if $i \bmod d = 0$.

Only boundary pixels belonging to a *d*-row serve as starting points to follow the corresponding boundary. Every component with height at least d then gets caught, while smaller components may be missed (if no *d*-row intersects them, see Figure 3.8d, but these small components are of no interest. *d*-rows allow considerable speedup as long as d is larger than 5–10, while d values equal to (or smaller than) 5% of the image's height catch all lesions of clinical interest.

The boundary of a connected component allows easy computation of its area: denoting by b_i the ith boundary pixel of the component on a generic row,

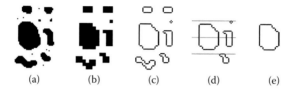

(a)   (b)   (c)   (d)   (e)

FIGURE 3.8   The postprocessing stage. (a) Initial binary mask. (b) Binary mask after downsampling. (c) Boundary pixels. (d) *d*-rows. (e) Single boundary encircling "sufficient" area. (Peruch, F. et al., *IEEE Transactions on Biomedical Engineering*, 61(2), 557–565, 2013. © 2013 IEEE.)

the pixels of the component in that row are those between any two consecutive boundary pixels b_i and b_{i+1} with *odd i*. All boundaries of components with area smaller than one-fifth the area of the largest component are removed: this takes care of both small dark patches in nonlesional skin and small light patches within lesions.

The computational cost of the postprocessing phase is therefore extremely low: it makes a single sequential pass plus a small number of additional accesses to a limited number of pixels.

3.4   VARIABILITY OF HUMANS VERSUS AUTOMATED SYSTEMS

This section compares the divergence, from a reference set of segmentations provided by expert dermatologists, of those provided by dermatologists of differing experience and by two versions of the MEDS technique (see Section 3.3). The comparison has many nuances and a few potential pitfalls.

A FotoFinder digital dermatoscope [50] was used to acquire 60 images of melanocytic lesions at 768×576 resolution (this is a subset of the dataset of [20], highly inhomogeneous in terms of size, color, illumination, and presence of artifacts such as air bubbles or hair). Of each image, 12 copies were printed on 13×18 cm photographic paper. A copy of each image and a marker pen were given to each of 4 *junior*, 4 *senior*, and 4 *expert* dermatologists, having respectively less than 1 year of experience, more than 1 year but no formal dermatoscopic training, and more than 1 year and formal dermatoscopic training. Note that this is a slightly different definition of seniority compared to that of [20] that places greater emphasis on formal training for more experienced dermatologists, reflecting the results of [51]. Each dermatologist was asked to independently draw with the marker the border of each lesion. The results were scanned and realigned to the same frame of reference, and the contours provided by the markers were then extracted and compared—identifying, for each pixel of each original image, the set of dermatologists classifying it as part of the lesion or of the surrounding nonlesional skin. This pen-and-paper approach aimed at maximizing the comfort of dermatologists, thus minimizing the noise in border localization caused by the use of unfamiliar software drawing tools [20].

TABLE 3.4

Disagreement from *Expert* Dermatologists of Automated Techniques and of Dermatologists in Various Experience Groups)

Group	*xor* (avg)	*xor* (std)	*sens* (avg)	*spec* (avg)
Experts	10.39%	6.85%	95.14%	96.77%
Seniors	13.55%	9.51%	95.95%	93.99%
Juniors	17.21%	15.51%	98.40%	91.38%
MEDS boost	11.27%	6.33%	93.34%	96.29%
MEDS	12.35%	7.16%	90.32%	98.15%

Note: XOR measure (average and standard deviation), sensitivity (average) and specificity (average), over the entire 60-image dataset.

The segmentations produced by the 4 *senior* and 4 *junior* dermatologists were evaluated using as ground truth the segmentations produced by the 4 *expert* dermatologists, and the segmentations of each *expert* dermatologist were evaluated using as ground truth the segmentations produced by the remaining 3 *expert* dermatologists. The criteria used were the XOR measure and the pair of sensitivity and specificity (averaged for each test case over the reference segmentations). The same metrics were used to evaluate two versions of MEDS, respectively, with (MEDS boost) or without (MEDS) color preprocessing and PCA normalization. The results are shown in Table 3.4.

The greater the experience of dermatologists providing a segmentation, the smaller the divergence from the reference segmentations provided by *expert* dermatologists—and the smaller the standard deviation of such divergence. The two versions of MEDS achieved a disagreement with *expert* dermatologists between that of other *expert* dermatologists and that of *senior* dermatologists (see Figure 3.9).

Results in Table 3.4 were obtained setting γ (the parameter controlling the "tightness" of the segmentation) equal to 1, a value close, for both MEDS and MEDS boost, to those minimizing average disagreement with *expert* dermatologists on the entire dataset using the XOR measure. Figure 3.10 depicts sensitivity and specificity for different values of γ; Figure 3.11 relates these measures in a single ROC curve. It is important to note that optimizing for a low XOR disagreement may not be quite the same as optimizing for what one may consider the best compromise between sensitivity and specificity. Also, Figure 3.9 suggests that a source of divergence between dermatologists and automated techniques may be that the latter can painstakingly follow even a very jagged and complex border, whereas the former are led to draw a smoother contour even when they can actually *perceive* that the actual border is not as smooth. While automated techniques could be adjusted to remove this discrepancy and thus reduce apparent disagreement [7, 23, 32], it is not obvious that it would lead to actually "better" segmentations.

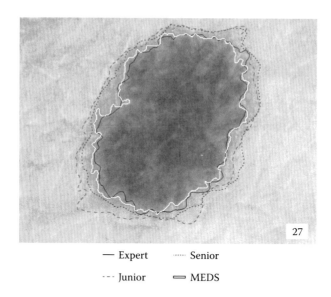

— Expert   ⋯⋯ Senior

‐‐‐ Junior   ⇒ MEDS

FIGURE 3.9 (**See color insert.**) Melanocytic lesion segmentation performed by human dermatologists and MEDS. (Reprinted from Peruch, F. et al., Simple, fast, accurate melanocytic lesion segmentation in 1-D color space, in *Proceedings of VISAPP 2013*, pp. 191–200, 2013, Barcelona, Spain. Copyright 2013, with permission from INSTICC/SciTePress.)

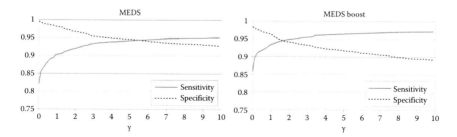

FIGURE 3.10 Sensitivity and specificity of MEDS and MEDS boost, averaged over the entire dataset, as a function of γ.

When working with parametrizable algorithms and relatively small datasets, it is crucial to take steps so as to avoid overfitting the parameters to the data. To this end, 30 trials of random subsampling validation were carried out for both versions of MEDS. In each trial, the 60-lesion dataset was randomly partitioned into a 30-lesion training set and a 30-lesion validation set, measuring average disagreement with *expert* dermatologists on the validation set using the value of γ that minimizes average disagreement on the training set. Figure 3.12 shows the values of γ and of average XOR disagreement for each trial; trials are sorted by increasing disagreement. As for

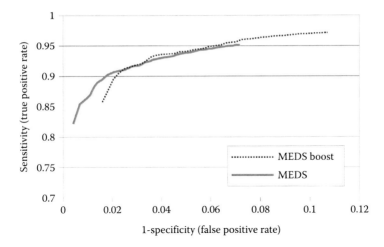

FIGURE 3.11 ROC curve relating sensitivity and specificity of MEDS and MEDS boost, averaged over the entire dataset, as a function of γ.

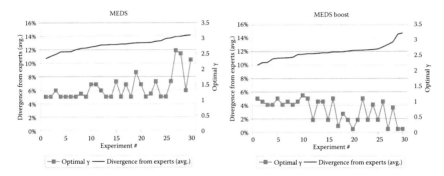

FIGURE 3.12 Disagreement of MEDS (left) and MEDS boost (right) with *expert* dermatologists averaged over 30 random images, using the optimal value of γ obtained for the remaining 30 images, for each of 30 trials sorted by increasing disagreement.

MEDS, in 26 out of 30 trials γ was in the interval $[1, 1.6]$; in the remaining 4 it was in the interval $[1.9, 2.6]$, yielding slightly higher disagreement. Average disagreement per trial ranged from 10.78% to 14.18%—for an overall average of 12.72%. MEDS boost turned out to be slightly less robust, with an optimal value for γ ranging from 0.1 to 1.2; in 17 out of 30 trials, γ was in the interval $[0.9, 1.2]$. Average disagreement per trial ranged from 10.04% to 14.76%, with an overall average of 11.92%.

In the light of cross-validation analysis, results in Table 3.4 appear slightly too optimistic even though MEDS retains a performance somewhere between that of *expert* and *senior* dermatologists. *This highlights the dangers of overfitting, particularly for algorithms with many more parameters than MEDS and when working with even smaller datasets.*

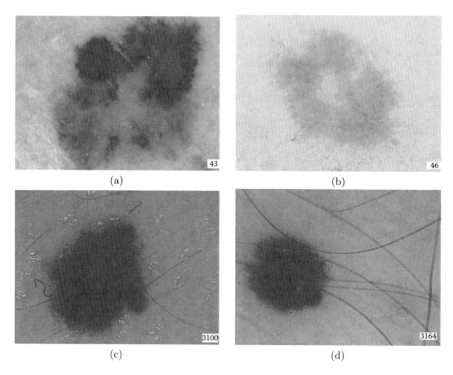

(a)   (b)

(c)   (d)

FIGURE 3.13 Melanocytic lesions exhibiting inhomogeneous pigmentation (a), low color contrast against surrounding skin (b), air bubbles (c), and hair (d). (Peruch, F. et al., *IEEE Transactions on Biomedical Engineering*, 61(2), 557–565, 2013. © 2013 IEEE.)

The variability of the "ideal" γ (and the disagreement achievable with the reference segmentation set) highlights another aspect of crucial importance: some dermatoscopically imaged lesions are considerably harder to segment than others [10, 32]. This can be due to intrinsic properties of the lesion, such as inhomogeneous pigmentation or low color contrast with the surrounding skin (see Figure 3.13a and b), or to artifacts of image acquisition, such as unshaved hair, air bubbles trapped in the antireflective gel, or shadows cast by the dermatoscope (see Figure 3.13c and d). In fact, this variability in difficulty applies not only to automated algorithms but also to human operators. To assess it, four (nondisjoint) subsets of the lesion dataset were identified, containing respectively 33 lesions with inhomogeneous pigmentation, 19 lesions with low color contrast against the surrounding skin, 35 lesions imaged with air bubbles, and 24 lesions imaged with unshaved hair. Tables 3.5 through 3.8 reproduce the results of Table 3.4 for each subset.

Note that the most difficult images, both for MEDS and for dermatologists, are those of lesions with low contrast against the surrounding skin, and at least

TABLE 3.5

Results of Table 3.4 Reported on a Subset of 33 Lesions Exhibiting Inhomogeneous Pigmentation

Group	*xor* (avg)	*xor* (std)	*sens* (avg)	*spec* (avg)
Experts	11.15%	8.86%	94.91%	95.97%
Seniors	13.03%	8.47%	95.72%	93.92%
Juniors	15.63%	13.69%	98.31%	90.51%
MEDS boost	10.25%	5.45%	93.89%	95.43%
MEDS	12.56%	7.82%	90.04%	97.80%

TABLE 3.6

Results of Table 3.4 Reported on a Subset of 19 Lesions Exhibiting Low Color Contrast against the Surrounding Skin

Group	*xor* (avg)	*xor* (std)	*sens* (avg)	*spec* (avg)
Experts	11.12%	3.78%	94.64%	95.40%
Seniors	17.96%	12.19%	95.54%	88.89%
Juniors	18.48%	10.85%	98.15%	86.41%
MEDS boost	13.70%	7.94%	91.32%	95.41%
MEDS	14.25%	7.69%	88.57%	97.37%

TABLE 3.7

Results of Table 3.4 Reported on a Subset of 35 Lesions Imaged with Air Bubbles

Group	*xor* (avg)	*xor* (std)	*sens* (avg)	*spec* (avg)
Experts	11.03%	8.50%	94.94%	96.21%
Seniors	13.26%	8.17%	95.74%	93.94%
Juniors	17.44%	15.93%	98.34%	90.51%
MEDS boost	11.12%	5.52%	93.73%	95.22%
MEDS	12.19%	7.23%	90.93%	97.53%

some (as can be evinced by the higher standard deviation among *experts*) of those with highly inhomogeneous pigmentation. It is important to note that inhomogeneous pigmentation is a common symptom of malignancy, and indeed other works [23, 30, 31] report more variance in the segmentation of malignant lesions than in that of benign ones. Image defects, such as air bubbles or presence of unshaved hair, are instead easily ignored by human and automated techniques alike.

TABLE 3.8

Results of Table 3.4 Reported on a Subset of 24 Lesions Imaged with Unshaved Hair

Group	*xor* (avg)	*xor* (std)	*sens* (avg)	*spec* (avg)
Experts	8.95%	3.83%	95.68%	97.43%
Seniors	12.76%	9.19%	96.30%	94.87%
Juniors	15.18%	8.98%	98.53%	92.85%
MEDS boost	10.07%	3.64%	95.21%	96.70%
MEDS	11.14%	5.04%	92.49%	97.49%

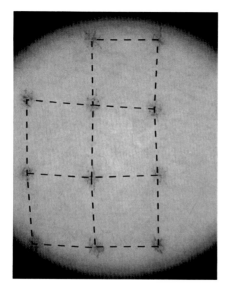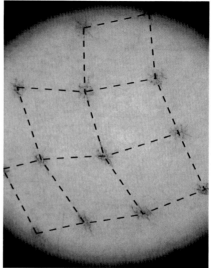

FIGURE 3.14 Deformation caused by dermatoscope pressure on a 4×4 dot grid drawn on the skin.

One last aspect that should be kept in mind is that different images of the same lesion, even taken within few seconds of each other and with the same equipment, zoom, and framing, can present to the viewer considerably "different" lesions: it is difficult to guarantee consistent illumination, while even mild pressure from the dermatoscope can cause significant deformation of the skin (see Figure 3.14). It is interesting to assess how these variations affect segmentation. To assess segmentation robustness in the presence of skin deformations, each image was deformed with a combination of a roto-translation, a perspective distortion, and a barrel distortion, trying to include all possible factors affecting an actual dermatoscopic image (and producing much more dramatic deformations than those observed in practice). The disagreement of the deformed segmentations produced on the *original* images by the automated techniques and by *expert* dermatologists, with the segmentations produced by the automated techniques *directly* on the deformed images, was measured. The average (XOR) disagreement between the segmentations produced by MEDS and MEDS boost on the original and deformed images was 3.17% and 3.09%, respectively (about 1% attributable to rounding in the deformation). The average disagreement with *expert* dermatologists was 13.07% for MEDS and 12.21% for MEDS boost.

As for sensitivity to moderate illumination variations, 27 versions of each image were considered, obtained by independently reducing the red, green, and blue color values by 0%, 12.5%, or 25%. The average (XOR) disagreement of MEDS between versions was 1.00%, and that of MEDS boost 1.55%. The average disagreement from *expert* dermatologists was 12.50% for MEDS and 11.60% for MEDS boost.

3.5 CONCLUSIONS

There is no formal, operative definition of whether a portion of skin belongs to a melanocytic lesion or not. As a result, the only gold standard for accurate border localization is the subjective judgment developed by dermatologists over years of training and practice. The variability in such judgment is inevitably an upper bound for the precision achievable in the task (whether by other dermatologists or by automated systems) and an unavoidable level of background noise for large, multioperator epidemiological studies.

This variability tends to decrease with dermatologist experience and with formal dermatoscopic training, but even with pairs of experienced dermatologists the area of the disagreement region remains of the order of 10% of the size of the lesion (climbing to 15% and beyond for less experienced ones). This should be taken as a very rough figure, for several reasons. One is the presence of several similar, but subtly different, measures of the quantitative disagreement between two segmentations. A much more fundamental reason is that the level of disagreement depends heavily on the characteristics of the lesion: lesions with light, fuzzy pigmentation at low contrast with the surrounding skin, as well as lesions sporting highly inhomogeneous pigmentation, can lead to much higher disagreement.

The segmentations provided by state-of-the-art automated techniques today can almost match those of experienced dermatologists: highly experienced dermatologists disagree with them only slightly more than they disagree with those of other highly experienced dermatologists, and in fact less than they disagree with those of dermatologists of little, or even moderate, experience. This is true even for some very fast techniques that can segment mid-resolution images on portable devices such as smart phones in a fraction of a second, operating in real time. And automated techniques do appear to yield, in comparison to dermatologists, excellent reproducibility of their own segmentations, even in the presence of moderate illumination variations and marked skin deformations.

REFERENCES

1. K. Pettijohn, N. Asdigian, J. Aalborg, J. Morelli, S. Mokrohisky, R. Dellavalle, and L. Crane, Vacations to waterside locations result in nevus development in Colorado children, *Cancer Epidemiology, Biomarkers and Prevention*, vol. 18, no. 2, pp. 454–463, 2009.

2. D. Dobrosavljevic, D. Brasanac, M. Apostolovic, and L. Medenica, Changes in common melanocytic naevi after intense sun exposure: Digital dermoscopic study with a 1-year follow-up, *Clinical and Experimental Dermatology*, vol. 34, no. 6, pp. 672–678, 2009.

3. I. Zalaudek, M. Manzo, I. Savarese, G. Docimo, G. Ferrara, and G. Argenziano, The morphologic universe of melanocytic nevi, *Seminars in Cutaneous Medicine and Surgery*, vol. 28, no. 3, pp. 149–156, 2009.

4. F. Nachbar, W. Stolz, T. Merkle, A. Cognetta, T. Vogt, M. Landthaler, P. Bilek, O. Braun-Falco, and G. Plewig, The ABCD rule of dermatoscopy. High prospective value in the diagnosis of doubtful melanocytic skin lesions, *Journal of the American Academy of Dermatology*, vol. 30, no. 4, pp. 551–559, 1994.

5. F. Peruch, F. Bogo, M. Bonazza, V. Cappelleri, and E. Peserico, Simpler, faster, more accurate melanocytic lesion segmentation through MEDS, *IEEE Transactions on Biomedical Engineering*, vol. 61, no. 2, pp. 557–565, 2013. Available at http://www.ncbi.nlm.nih.gov/pubmed/22092600 (epub year: 2011; issue year: 2012).

6. H. Iyatomi, H. Oka, M. Saito, A. Miyake, M. Kimoto, J. Yamagami, S. Kobayashi et al., Quantitative assessment of tumour extraction from dermoscopy images and evaluation of computer-based extraction methods for an automatic melanoma diagnostic system, *Melanoma Research*, vol. 16, no. 2, pp. 183–190, 2006.

7. H. Iyatomi, H. Oka, M. E. Celebi, M. Hashimoto, M. Hagiwara, M. Tanaka, and K. Ogawa, An improved Internet-based melanoma screening system with dermatologist-like tumor area extraction algorithm, *Computerized Medical Imaging and Graphics*, vol. 32, no. 7, pp. 566–579, 2008.

8. R. Melli, C. Grana, and R. Cucchiara, Comparison of color clustering algorithms for segmentation of dermatological images, in *Proceedings of the SPIE Medical Imaging Conference*, pp. 61443S-1–61443S-9, 2006, San Diego, CA.

9. R. Garnavi, M. Aldeen, M. E. Celebi, G. Varigos, and S. Finch, Border detection in dermoscopy images using hybrid thresholding on optimized color channels, *Computerized Medical Imaging and Graphics*, vol. 35, no. 2, pp. 105–115, 2011.

10. P. Wighton, T. K. Lee, H. Lui, D. McLean, and M. S. Atkins, Generalizing common tasks in automated skin lesion diagnosis, *IEEE Transactions on Information Technology in Biomedicine*, vol. 15, no. 4, pp. 622–629, 2011.

11. Q. Abbas, M. E. Celebi, and I. Garcia, Skin tumor area extraction using an improved dynamic programming approach, *Skin Research and Technology*, vol. 18, no. 2, pp. 133–142, 2012.

12. G. A. Hance, S. E. Umbaugh, R. H. Moss, and W. V. Stoecker, Unsupervised color image segmentation: With application to skin tumor borders, *IEEE Engineering in Medicine and Biology Magazine*, vol. 15, no. 1, pp. 104–111, 1996.

13. M. Fleming, C. Steger, J. Zhang, J. Gao, A. Cognetta, I. Pollak, and C. Dyer, Techniques for a structural analysis of dermatoscopic imagery, *Computerized Medical Imaging and Graphics*, vol. 22, no. 5, pp. 375–389, 1998.

14. J. Gao, J. Zhang, M. Fleming, I. Pollak, and A. Cognetta, Segmentation of dermatoscopic images by stabilized inverse diffusion equations, in *Proceedings of the IEEE International Conference on Image Processing (ICIP)*, pp. 823–827, 1998, Chicago, IL.

15. H. Zhou, M. Chen, L. Zou, R. Gass, L. Ferris, L. Drogowski, and J. Rehg, Spatially constrained segmentation of dermoscopy images, in *Proceedings of the IEEE International Symposium on Biomedical Imaging (ISBI): From Nano to Macro*, pp. 800–803, 2008, Paris, France.

16. D. Delgado, C. Butakoff, B. K. Ersboll, and W. V. Stoecker, Independent histogram pursuit for segmentation of skin lesions, *IEEE Transactions on Biomedical Engineering*, vol. 55, no. 1, pp. 157–161, 2008.

17. M. E. Celebi, G. Schaefer, H. Iyatomi, and W. V. Stoecker, Approximate lesion localization in dermoscopy images, *Skin Research and Technology*, vol. 15, no. 3, pp. 314–322, 2009.

18. A. Silletti, E. Peserico, A. Mantovan, E. Zattra, A. Peserico, and A. Belloni Fortina, Variability in human and automatic segmentation of melanocytic lesions, in *Proceedings of the International Conference of the IEEE Engineering in Medicine and Biology Society (EMBC)*, pp. 5789–5792, 2009, Minneapolis, MN.

19. M. E. Celebi, Q. Wen, S. Hwang, H. Iyatomi, and G. Schaefer, Lesion border detection in dermoscopy images using ensembles of thresholding methods, *Skin Research and Technology*, vol. 19, no. 1, pp. e252–e258, 2013.

20. A. Belloni Fortina, E. Peserico, A. Silletti, and E. Zattra, Where's the naevus? Inter-operator variability in the localization of melanocytic lesion border, *Skin Research and Technology*, vol. 18, no. 3, pp. 311–315, 2011. Available at http://ieeexplore.ieee.org/xpl/articleDetails.jsp?arnumber=6612682 (epub year: 2013; issue year: 2014).

21. M. Silveira, J. Nascimento, J. Marques, J. Marcal, T. Mendonca, S. Yamauchi, J. Maeda, and J. Rozeira, Comparison of segmentation methods for melanoma diagnosis in dermoscopy images, *IEEE Journal of Selected Topics in Signal Processing*, vol. 3, no. 1, pp. 35–45, 2009.

22. J. Guillod, P. Schmid, D. Guggisberg, J. Cerottini, R. Braun, J. Krischer, J. Saurat, and K. Murat, Validation of segmentation techniques for digital dermoscopy, *Skin Research and Technology*, vol. 8, no. 4, pp. 240–249, 2002.

23. M. E. Celebi, H. A. Kingravi, H. Iyatomi, Y. A. Aslandogan, W. V. Stoecker, R. H. Moss, J. M. Malters, J. M. Grichnik, A. A. Marghoob, H. S. Rabinovitz, and S. W. Menzies, Border detection in dermoscopy images using statistical region merging, *Skin Research and Technology*, vol. 14, no. 3, pp. 347–353, 2008.

24. G. Schaefer, M. Rajab, M. E. Celebi, and H. Iyatomi, Skin lesion segmentation using cooperative neural network edge detection and colour normalisation, in *Proceedings of the International Conference on Information Technology and Applications in Biomedicine (ITAB)*, vol. IV, pp. 1–4, 2009, Larnaca, Cyprus.

25. G. Schaefer, M. Rajab, M. E. Celebi, and H. Iyatomi, Colour and contrast enhancement for improved skin lesion segmentation, *Computerized Medical Imaging and Graphics*, vol. 35, no. 2, pp. 99–104, 2011.

26. K. A. Norton, H. Iyatomi, M. E. Celebi, S. Ishizaki, M. Sawada, R. Suzaki, K. Kobayashi, M. Tanaka, and K. Ogawa, Three-phase general border detection method for dermoscopy images using non-uniform illumination correction, *Skin Research and Technology*, vol. 18, no. 3, pp. 290–300, 2012.

27. R. Unnikrishnan, C. Pantofaru, and M. Hebert, Toward objective evaluation of image segmentation algorithms, *IEEE Transactions on Pattern Analysis and Machine Intelligence*, vol. 29, no. 6, pp. 929–944, 2007.

28. M. E. Celebi, G. Schaefer, H. Iyatomi, W. V. Stoecker, J. M. Malters, and J. M. Grichnik, An improved objective evaluation measure for border detection in dermoscopy images, *Skin Research and Technology*, vol. 15, no. 4, pp. 444–450, 2009.

29. E. Peserico and A. Silletti, Is (N)PRI suitable for evaluating automated segmentation of skin lesions?, *Pattern Recognition Letters*, vol. 31, no. 16, pp. 2464–2467, 2010.

30. M. E. Celebi, Y. A. Aslandogan, W. V. Stoecker, H. Iyatomi, H. Oka, and X. Chen, Unsupervised border detection in dermoscopy images, *Skin Research and Technology*, vol. 13, no. 4, pp. 454–462, 2007.

31. B. Erkol, R. H. Moss, R. J. Stanley, W. V. Stoecker, and E. Hvatum, Automatic lesion boundary detection in dermoscopy images using gradient vector flow snakes, *Skin Research and Technology*, vol. 11, no. 1, pp. 17–26, 2005.

32. M. E. Celebi, G. Schaefer, H. Iyatomi, and W. V. Stoecker, Lesion border detection in dermoscopy images, *Computerized Medical Imaging and Graphics*, vol. 33, no. 2, pp. 148–153, 2009.

33. P. Good, *Permutation, Parametric and Bootstrap Tests of Hypotheses*, Springer, Berlin, 2005.

34. J. Scharcanski and M. E. Celebi, eds., *Computer Vision Techniques for the Diagnosis of Skin Cancer*, Springer, Berlin, 2013.

35. M. E. Celebi, W. V. Stoecker, and R. H. Moss, eds., *Computerized Medical Imaging and Graphics*, vol. 35, no. 2, pp. 83–166, 2011.

36. K. Korotkov and R. Garcia, Computerized analysis of pigmented skin lesions: A review, *Artificial Intelligence in Medicine*, vol. 56, no. 2, pp. 69–90, 2012.

37. F. Peruch, F. Bogo, M. Bonazza, M. Bressan, V. Cappelleri, and E. Peserico, Simple, fast, accurate melanocytic lesion segmentation in 1D colour space, in *Proceedings of VISAPP*, pp. 191–200, 2013, Barcelona, Spain.

38. H. Zhou, G. Schaefer, M. E. Celebi, F. Lin, and T. Liu, Gradient vector flow with mean shift for skin lesion segmentation, *Computerized Medical Imaging and Graphics*, vol. 35, no. 2, pp. 121–127, 2011.

39. H. Zhou, X. Li, G. Schaefer, M. E. Celebi, and P. Miller, Mean shift based gradient vector flow for image segmentation, *Computer Vision and Image Understanding*, vol. 117, no. 9, pp. 1004–1016, 2013.

40. H. Wang, X. Chen, R. H. Moss, R. J. Stanley, W. V. Stoecker, M. E. Celebi, T. Szalapski, J. M. Malters, J. M. Grichnik, A. A. Marghoob, H. S. Rabinovitz, and S. W. Menzies, Watershed segmentation of dermoscopy images using a watershed technique, *Skin Research and Technology*, vol. 16, no. 3, pp. 378–384, 2010.

41. N. Otsu, A threshold selection method from gray-level histograms, *IEEE Transactions on Systems, Man and Cybernetics*, vol. 9, no. 1, pp. 62–66, 1979.

42. H. Zhou, G. Schaefer, A. Sadka, and M. E. Celebi, Anisotropic mean shift based fuzzy c-means segmentation of dermoscopy images, *IEEE Journal of Selected Topics in Signal Processing*, vol. 3, no. 1, pp. 26–34, 2009.

43. P. Schmid, Segmentation of digitized dermatoscopic images by two-dimensional clustering, *IEEE Transactions on Medical Imaging*, vol. 18, no. 2, pp. 164–171, 1999.

44. R. Cucchiara, C. Grana, S. Seidenari, and G. Pellacani, Exploiting color and topological features for region segmentation with recursive fuzzy c-means, *Machine Graphics and Vision*, vol. 11, no. 2/3, pp. 169–182, 2002.

45. Q. Abbas, M. E. Celebi, and I. Garcia, Hair removal methods: A comparative study for dermoscopy images, *Biomedical Signal Processing and Control*, vol. 6, no. 4, pp. 395–404, 2011.

46. T. K. Lee, V. Ng, R. Gallagher, A. Coldman, and D. McLean, DullRazor: A software approach to hair removal from images, *Computer in Biology and Medicine*, vol. 27, no. 6, pp. 533–543, 1997.

47. N. Nguyen, T. K. Lee, and M. S. Atkins, Segmentation of light and dark hair in dermoscopic images: A hybrid approach using a universal kernel, in *Proceedings of the SPIE Medical Imaging Conference*, pp. 76234N-1–76234N-8, 2010, San Diego, CA.

48. M. Fiorese, E. Peserico, and A. Silletti, VirtualShave: Automated hair removal from digital dermatoscopic images, in *Proceedings of the International Conference of the IEEE Engineering in Medicine and Biology Society (EMBC)*, pp. 5145–5148, 2011, Boston, MA.

49. Q. Abbas, I. Garcia, M. E. Celebi, and W. Ahmad, A feature-preserving hair removal algorithm for dermoscopy images, *Skin Research and Technology*, vol. 19, no. 1, pp. e27–e36, 2013.

50. FotoFinder Systems, Inc., Fotofinder dermoscope, http://www.fotofinder.de/en.html.

51. M. Binder, M. Puespoeck-Schwarz, A. Steiner, H. Kittler, M. Muellner, K. Wolff, and H. Pehamberger, Epiluminescence microscopy of small pigmented skin lesions: Short formal training improves the diagnostic performance of dermatologists, *Journal of the American Academy of Dermatology*, vol. 36, no. 2, pp. 197–202, 1997.

4 A State-of-the-Art Survey on Lesion Border Detection in Dermoscopy Images

M. Emre Celebi
Louisiana State University
Shreveport, Louisiana

Quan Wen
University of Electronic Science and Technology of China
Chengdu, People's Republic of China

Hitoshi Iyatomi
Hosei University
Tokyo, Japan

Kouhei Shimizu
Hosei University
Tokyo, Japan

Huiyu Zhou
Queen's University Belfast
Belfast, United Kingdom

Gerald Schaefer
Loughborough University
Loughborough, United Kingdom

CONTENTS

4.1 INTRODUCTION

Invasive and in situ malignant melanoma together comprise one of the most rapidly increasing cancers in the world. Invasive melanoma alone has an estimated incidence of 73,870 and an estimated total of 9940 deaths in the United States in 2015 [1]. Early diagnosis is particularly important since melanoma can be cured with a simple excision if detected early.

Dermoscopy, also known as epiluminescence microscopy, is a noninvasive skin imaging technique that uses optical magnification and either liquid immersion and low-angle-of-incidence lighting or cross-polarized lighting, making subsurface structures more easily visible than in conventional clinical images [2]. Dermoscopy allows the identification of dozens of morphological features, such as atypical pigment networks, dots/globules, streaks, blue–white areas, and blotches [3]. This reduces screening errors and provides greater differentiation between difficult lesions, such as pigmented Spitz nevi and small, clinically equivocal lesions [4]. However, it has been demonstrated that dermoscopy may actually lower the diagnostic accuracy in the hands of inexperienced dermatologists [5]. Therefore, in order to minimize the diagnostic errors that result from the difficulty and subjectivity of visual interpretation, the development of computerized image analysis techniques is of paramount importance [6].

Border detection is often the first step in the automated analysis of dermoscopy images [7]. It is crucial for image analysis for two main reasons. First, the border structure provides important information for accurate diagnosis, as many clinical features, such as asymmetry [8], border irregularity [9], and abrupt border cutoff [10], are calculated directly from the border. Second, the extraction of other important clinical features, such as atypical pigment networks [6, 11–25], dots [21, 26–28], globules [6, 28], streaks [16, 19, 29, 30], blue–white areas [19, 31–37], blotches [38–42], regression structures [19, 31, 33, 43, 44], and color variegation [45], critically depends on the accuracy of border detection. Automated border detection is a challenging task for several reasons [46]: (1) low contrast between the lesion and the surrounding skin (Figure 4.1a), (2) irregular (Figure 4.1b) and fuzzy lesion borders (Figure 4.1c), (3) artifacts and intrinsic cutaneous features such as black frames (Figure 4.1d), skin lines, blood vessels (Figure 4.1e), air bubbles (Figure 4.1f), and hairs (Figures 4.1g and 4.1h), (4) perspective distortion (Figure 4.1i) (5) variegated coloring inside the lesion (Figure 4.1j), (6) fragmentation due to various reasons such as regression (Figure 4.1k), (7) presence

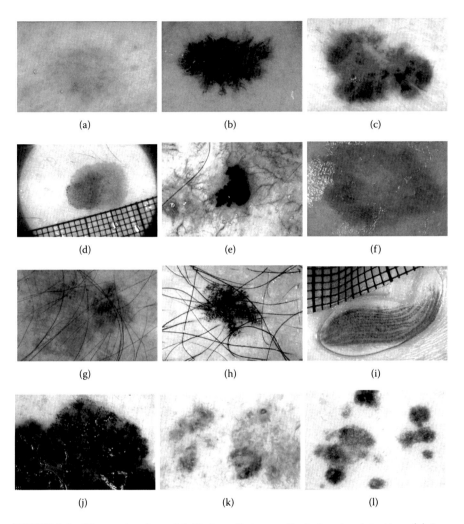

FIGURE 4.1 **(See color insert.)** Factors that complicate border detection. (a) Low contrast [3]. (b) Irregular border [3]. (c) Fuzzy border [2]. (d) Black frame [2]. (e) Blood vessels. (f) Bubbles [2]. (g) Thin hairs [3]. (h) Thick hairs [2]. (i) Distortion [2]. (j) Variegated coloring [2]. (k) Regression [2]. (l) Multiple lesions [2]. (Reprinted with permission from Argenziano, G. et al., *Dermoscopy: A Tutorial*, EDRA Medical Publishing and New Media, Milan, Italy, 2002.)

of multiple lesions (Figure 4.1l), and (8) lesion larger than the field of view (Figure 4.1j).

Since the late 1990s numerous methods have been developed for automated border detection in dermoscopy images [47–50]. Unfortunately, due to the interdisciplinary nature of the field, the existing literature is scattered among numerous medical and engineering journals. In an earlier study, we reviewed

18 methods published between 1998 and 2008 [46]. The amount of research on border detection has been steadily increasing since 2008. As evidence to this is, 5 out of 11 articles in the 2011 *Computerized Medical Imaging and Graphics* special issue "Advances in Skin Cancer Image Analysis" [47] were devoted to border detection. In this chapter, we update our earlier survey with 32 additional methods published between 2009 and 2014. In Sections 4.2 through 4.4, we review the preprocessing, segmentation, and postprocessing phases, respectively. In Section 4.5, we discuss performance evaluation issues. Finally, in Section 4.6, we compare 50 published border detection methods with respect to various criteria and propose guidelines for future studies in automated border detection.

4.2 PREPROCESSING

In this section, we describe the preprocessing steps that facilitate the border detection procedure, namely, color space transformation, contrast enhancement, approximate lesion localization, and artifact removal.

4.2.1 COLOR SPACE TRANSFORMATION

Dermoscopy images are commonly acquired using a digital camera with a dermoscope attachment. Due to the computational simplicity and convenience of scalar (single-channel) processing, the resulting RGB (red–green–blue) color image is often converted to a scalar image using one of the following methods:

- Retaining only the blue channel [51] (lesions are often more prominent in this channel, but typically, this is also the noisiest channel)
- Retaining the channel with the highest entropy [52]
- Applying a fixed luminance transformation, for example, [53, p. 122], such as
  Luminance (Rec. 601) $= 0.2990 \times \text{Red} + 0.5870 \times \text{Green} + 0.1140 \times \text{Blue}$
  or
  Luminance (Rec. 709) $= 0.2126 \times \text{Red} + 0.7152 \times \text{Green} + 0.0722 \times \text{Blue}$
- Applying an adaptive luminance transformation [54, 55]
- Applying the Karhunen–Loéve (KL) transformation [56] and retaining the channel with the highest variance [57]

In applications where vector (multichannel) processing is desired, the RGB image can be used directly or it can be transformed to a different color space for various reasons, including (1) reducing the number of channels, (2) decoupling luminance and chromaticity information, (3) ensuring (approximate) perceptual uniformity, and (4) achieving invariance to various imaging conditions, such as viewing direction, illumination intensity, and highlights [58]. Common target color spaces [59] in this case include CIELAB, CIELUV, KL, and HSI (hue–saturation–intensity) [60]. Note that there are various formulations of the HSI color space in the literature [61], and therefore it is good practice to cite an appropriate reference when using this color space or its variants.

4.2.2 CONTRAST ENHANCEMENT

As mentioned in Section 4.1, one of the factors that complicate the detection of borders in dermoscopy images is insufficient contrast. There are two main approaches to address this issue: hardware-based techniques [62–67] and software-based techniques. The former approach is generally preferable to the latter. However, in many cases, for example, web-based systems [68], acquisition cannot be controlled, and thus software-based postacquisition enhancement is the only option.

Gomez et al. [69] proposed a contrast enhancement method based on independent histogram pursuit. This algorithm linearly transforms the input RGB image to a decorrelated color space in which the lesion and the background skin are maximally separated. Given an input RGB image, Celebi et al.'s method [54] determines the optimal weights to convert it to grayscale by maximizing a histogram bimodality measure. The authors demonstrated that their adaptive optimization scheme increases the contrast between the lesion and background skin, leading to a more accurate separation of the two regions using Otsu's thresholding method [70]. Madooei et al. [55] proposed a physics-based color-to-grayscale conversion method that attenuates shading as well as thin and short hairs. As in Celebi et al.'s study [54], the authors showed that the resulting grayscale image allows for a more accurate segmentation. Iyatomi et al. [71] proposed a color correction method based on the HSV (hue–saturation–value) color space. First, a multiple linear regression model for each of the H, S, and V channels is built using various low-level features extracted from a training image set. Using these regression models, the method then automatically adjusts the hue and saturation of a previously unseen image. Schaefer et al. [72] presented a two-stage scheme that removes color variations and enhances the contrast of the images by combining Grayworld and MaxRGB normalization techniques [73]. Abbas et al. [74, 75] and Norton et al. [76] proposed the use of homomorphic filtering [77] and contrast-limited adaptive histogram equalization [78], respectively. Barata et al. [79] compared the performance of several color constancy algorithms on the task of color normalization. Finally, Lu et al. [80] proposed a no-reference uneven illumination assessment measure based on a variational formulation of Retinex [81].

4.2.3 APPROXIMATE LESION LOCALIZATION

Although dermoscopy images can be quite large, lesions often occupy a relatively small area. An accurate bounding box (the smallest axis-aligned rectangular box that encloses the lesion) might be useful for various reasons [82]: (1) it provides an estimate of the lesion size (certain image segmentation methods, such as region growing and morphological flooding [83, 84], can use this information as part of their termination criteria), (2) it might improve the accuracy of border detection since the procedure is focused on a region that is guaranteed to contain the lesion (active contour-based segmentation methods can be initialized inside/outside this region [74, 85, 86]), (3) it speeds up border detection since the procedure is performed in a region that is often smaller than the entire image [87], and (4) its surrounding might be used in the estimation of the background skin color, which is useful for various operations, including the elimination of spurious regions that are discovered during border detection [88] and the extraction of dermoscopic features such as streaks and blue–white areas. Several authors employed histogram thresholding methods such as Otsu's method [70] and Kittler and Illingworth's method [89] to localize lesions in dermoscopy images [52, 74, 85–87]. Celebi et al. [82], on the other hand, proposed the use of an *ensemble* of thresholding methods. This method was shown to be significantly more robust than pathological cases (e.g., unimodal histograms) when compared to individual thresholding methods. Wang et al. [83, 84] determined the bounding box by fitting a least-squares quadratic polynomial [90] to each of the horizontal and vertical projections [91, pp. 355–356] of the luminance image.

4.2.4   ARTIFACT REMOVAL

Dermoscopy images often contain artifacts such as black frames, ink markings, rulers, air bubbles, and intrinsic cutaneous features that can affect border detection, such as skin lines, blood vessels, and hairs. These elements complicate the border detection procedure, resulting in loss of accuracy as well as increase in computational time. The most straightforward way to remove these artifacts is to smooth the image using a general-purpose filter such as the Gaussian (GF), mean ($\overline{\text{MF}}$), median ($\widetilde{\text{MF}}$), or anisotropic diffusion (ADF) filter. Several issues should be considered while using these filters:

- **Scalar versus vector processing**: These filters are originally formulated for scalar images. For vector images, one can apply a scalar filter to each channel independently and then combine the results, a strategy referred to as *marginal* filtering. Although fast, this scheme introduces color artifacts into the output. An alternative solution is to use filters that treat the pixels as vectors [92].
- **Mask size**: The amount of smoothing is proportional to the mask size. Therefore, excessively large masks result in the blurring of edges, which might reduce the accuracy of border detection. Setting the mask size proportional to the image size appears to be a reasonable strategy [88, 93].
- **Computational time**: For the GF, $\overline{\text{MF}}$, and $\widetilde{\text{MF}}$, algorithms that require constant time regardless of the mask size are available [94–96].

As for the ADF, the computational time depends on the mask size and the number of iterations.

An alternative strategy for artifact removal is to use a specialized method for each artifact type. For the removal of rectangular black frames, Celebi et al. [88] proposed an iterative algorithm based on the lightness component of the HSL (hue–saturation–lightness) color space. Similar approaches can be found in [52, 76, 83, 97]. It should be noted that a systematic method to remove circular black frames (see Figure 4.1d) appears to be missing. In most cases, image smoothing effectively removes the skin lines and blood vessels. A method that can remove bubbles with bright edges was introduced in [6], where the authors utilized a morphological top-hat operator [98] followed by a radial search procedure.

Hair detection/removal received the most attention in the literature. An ideal hair detection/removal method should (1) detect/remove light and thin as well as dark and thick hairs [99], (2) deal with intersecting hairs [99], (3) not cause excessive blurring and color bleeding [100], (4) be evaluated both qualitatively and quantitatively using synthetic as well as real images with and without hair [101, 102], and (5) be computationally efficient.

Lee et al. [99] used morphological closing to detect hairs, which were then removed using bilinear interpolation. Schmid-Saugeon et al. [103] transformed the RGB image to CIELUV color space and then detected hairs using morphological closing on the L channel followed by thresholding. The hair pixels were replaced by their values after morphological closing. Wighton et al. [101], Xie et al. [104], and Fiorese et al. [102] also used morphological operators for detection, but used partial differential equation (PDE)–based inpainting [105, 106] for removal. Fleming et al. [6] and Zhou et al. [100] detected hairs using curvilinear structure detection [107] with various constraints. The latter authors removed the detected hairs using exemplar-based inpainting [108]. Nguyen et al. [109] employed matched filtering [110] followed by Gaussian smoothing, entropic thresholding [111], morphological thinning, and curve fitting for detection and bilinear interpolation [99] for removal. Mollersen et al. [64] thresholded the red channel using Otsu's method [70] and applied a sequence of morphological operators along various directions to detect hairs. Abbas et al. [75] used a two-dimensional derivative of the Gaussian filter [112] for detection and exemplar-based inpainting [108] for removal. Kiani and Sharafat [113] used the radon transform [114] followed by edge detection using the Prewitt operator [115] for detection and interpolation by averaging for removal. Wighton et al. [23] employed linear discriminant analysis [116] and maximum a posteriori estimation [117] for detecting hairs. Barata et al. [24] used a bank of directional filters for detection and PDE-based inpainting [106] for removal. Thon et al. [28] detected hairs using Bayesian multiscale analysis with an intrinsic second-order Gaussian Markov random field (MRF) [118] prior. Afonso and Silveira [119] applied the morphological top-hat operator on the channel with the greatest entropy and then thresholded the result using

Otsu's method. The hairs were then detected using percolation [120] subject to shape constraints. Abbas et al. [121] used modified matched filtering [122] followed by morphological closing for detection and fast marching-based inpainting [123] for removal. Toossi et al. [124] converted the RGB image to a grayscale one using the KL transform and then smoothed the latter image using the Wiener filter [125]. The edges in the smoothed image were detected using Canny's algorithm [126] with the high threshold determined using Rosenfeld and de la Torre's thresholding method [127]. The hairs were then detected using morphological dilation and removed using fast marching-based inpainting [123]. Abbas et al. [128] presented a comparative study of four recent hair detection/removal methods. Mirzaalian et al. [129] presented a method to detect light and dark hairs with varying thickness using dual-channel matched filters [130] and multilabel MRF optimization [131].

4.3 SEGMENTATION

Segmentation refers to the partitioning of an image into disjoint regions that are homogeneous with respect to a chosen property such as luminance, color, and texture [91, p. 178]. Segmentation methods can be roughly classified into the following categories:

- Histogram thresholding [52, 64, 74, 76, 85, 86, 97, 132–140]: These methods involve the determination of one or more histogram threshold values that separate the objects from the background [141–145].
- Clustering [69, 93, 134, 135, 137, 146–159]: These methods involve the partitioning of a color (feature) space into homogeneous regions using unsupervised clustering algorithms [160–162].
- Edge based [75, 97]: These methods involve the detection of edges between the regions using edge operators [163–168].
- Region based [52, 57, 87, 88]: These methods involve the grouping of pixels into homogeneous regions using region merging, region splitting, or a combination of the two [169–171].
- Morphological [83, 84, 172]: These methods involve the detection of object contours from predetermined seeds using the watershed transform [173–179].
- Model based [57]: These methods involve the modeling of images as random fields [180–182] whose parameters are determined using various optimization procedures.
- Active contours (snakes and their variants) [52, 74, 85, 86, 147, 152, 183]: These methods involve the detection of object contours using curve evolution techniques [184–186].
- Fuzzy logic [52]: These methods involve the classification of pixels using fuzzy rules [187].
- Supervised learning [23, 72, 84, 188–191]: These methods involve the application of models obtained by training classifiers such as decision trees, artificial neural networks, and support vector machines.

Several issues should be considered when choosing a segmentation method:

- Scalar versus vector processing: Most segmentation methods are designed for scalar images [192–195]. Although numerous vector image segmentation methods have been developed during the past two decades [196–198], their use is hindered by various factors, including excessive computational requirements and difficulty of choosing an appropriate color space [199].
- Automatic versus semiautomatic: Some segmentation methods are completely automated, whereas others require human interaction [200]. For example, active contour methods often require the manual delineation of the initial contour, whereas seeded region growing methods [201, 202] require the specification of the initial region seeds. Since there are only a few semiautomatic methods proposed in the literature [52, 203], in this chapter, we focus on automatic methods.
- Number of parameters: Most segmentation methods have several parameters whose values need to be determined by the user. In general, the more the number of parameters, the harder the model selection (i.e., the determination of the optimal parameters). Among the methods listed above, histogram thresholding methods are often the simplest ones, as they require very few parameters. In contrast, segmentation methods based on active contours and supervised learning, in particular neural networks, often involve a large number of tunable parameters. Many clustering algorithms, such as k-means and fuzzy c-means, require the number of clusters to be specified by the user [204, 205]. In addition, these algorithms are often highly sensitive to initialization [206–209]. Density-based clustering algorithms [210, 211] such as mean shift [212] and DBSCAN (density based spatial clustering of applications with noise) [213] do not have these limitations. These algorithms, however, involve additional parameters, some of which are difficult to determine.

4.4   POSTPROCESSING

The result of the segmentation procedure is typically either a label image or a binary edge map. In order to obtain the lesion border, the segmentation output should be postprocessed. The precise sequence of postprocessing operations depends on the particular choice of the segmentation method. However, certain operations seem to be generally useful. These include the following:

- **Region merging**: The segmentation procedure should ideally produce two regions: the lesion and the background skin. However, since these regions are rarely homogeneous, segmentation methods often partition them into multiple subregions. In order to obtain a single lesion object, subregions that are part of the lesion should first be identified and then merged. This can be accomplished in several ways:

- If the black frame of the image has already been removed, the background skin color can be estimated from the corners of the image and the subregions with similar color to the background skin can be eliminated, leaving only those subregions that are part of the lesion [87, 88, 157, 214].
- Various color and texture features can be extracted from each region and a classifier can be trained to determine which features effectively discriminate between the regions that are part of the lesion and those that are part of the background skin [6].
- The optimal border can be determined by maximizing the normalized texture gradient [215] and minimizing the total similarity [216] between pairs of subregions inside the border and between pairs of subregions outside the border.

- **Island removal**: Islands (small isolated regions) in the label image can be eliminated using a binary area opening filter [98, p. 113].
- **Border smoothing**: Most segmentation methods produce regions with ragged borders. More natural borders can be obtained by using a variety of operations, including majority filtering [88], morphological filtering [69, 93, 134, 217, 218], and curve fitting [75, 83–85, 97]. Note that it might be better to calculate the border-related features, such as asymmetry, border irregularity, and abrupt border cutoff prior to smoothing.
- **Border expansion**: In several studies, it was observed that the computer-detected borders were mostly contained within the dermatologist-determined borders. This is because the automated segmentation methods tend to find the sharpest pigment change, whereas the dermatologists choose the outmost detectable pigment. The discrepancy between the two borders can be reduced by expanding the computer-detected border using morphological filtering [76, 88], Euclidean distance transform [88], or iterative region growing [68, 136, 139].

4.5   EVALUATION

Evaluation of the results seems to be one of the least explored aspects of the border detection task. As in the case of the more general image segmentation problem, there are two major evaluation methods: subjective and objective. The former involves the visual assessment of the border detection results by one or more dermatologists. Since there is no objective measure of quality involved, this technique does not permit parameter tuning or comparisons among automated border detection methods. On the other hand, objective

TABLE 4.1

Definitions of True/False Positive/Negative

		Detected Pixel	
		Lesion	**Background**
Actual	Lesion	True pos. (TP)	False neg. (FN)
Pixel	Background	False pos. (FP)	True neg. (TN)

evaluation involves the quantification of the border detection errors using dermatologist-determined borders. In the rest of this discussion, we refer to the computer-detected borders as *automatic borders* and those determined by dermatologists as *manual borders*.

Most of the quantitative evaluation measures are based on the concepts of true/false positive/negative given in Table 4.1 (here actual and detected pixels refer to a pixel in the ground-truth image and the corresponding pixel in the border detection output, respectively). These include the following [219]:

- XOR measure (XOR) [220] $= \dfrac{FP + FN}{TP + FN}$

- Sensitivity (SE) $= \dfrac{TP}{TP + FN}$ and specificity (SP) $= \dfrac{TN}{FP + TN}$

- False positive rate (FPR) $= \dfrac{FP}{FP + TN}$

- False negative rate (FNR) $= \dfrac{FN}{TP + FN}$

- Precision (PR) $= \dfrac{TP}{TP + FP}$

- F measure (F) $= 2 \times \dfrac{\text{Precision} \times \text{Recall}}{\text{Precision} + \text{Recall}}$

- Accuracy (AC) $= \dfrac{TP + TN}{TP + FN + FP + TN}$

- Error probability (EP) $= 1 - AC$

- Jaccard index (J) [221] $= \dfrac{TP}{TP + FN + FP}$

- Hammoude distance (HM)* [222] $= \dfrac{FN + FP}{TP + FN + FP}$

---

* In his dissertation, Hammoude actually divides by the perimeter of the ground-truth border [222, p. 102]. Dividing by the area of the ground-truth border appears to have been mistakenly attributed to him by Chalana and Kim [223].

In addition, the following relations hold:

- Recall $\equiv$ True positive rate (TPR) $\equiv$ True detection rate (TDR) $\equiv$ Sensitivity
- Sensitivity $= 1 -$ False negative rate
- {Specificity $\equiv$ True negative rate (TNR)} $= 1 -$ False positive rate
- Precision $\equiv$ Positive predictive value (PPV)
- Hammoude distance $= 1 -$ Jaccard index

In a comprehensive study, Guillod et al. [224] demonstrated that a single dermatologist, even one who is experienced in dermoscopy, cannot be used as an absolute reference for evaluating the accuracy of border detection. In addition, they emphasized that manual borders are not precise, with interdermatologist borders and even borders determined by the same dermatologist at different times showing significant disagreement, so that a probabilistic model of the border is preferred to an absolute gold-standard model. Accordingly, they used 15 sets of borders drawn by five dermatologists over a minimum period of 1 month. A probability image for each lesion was constructed by associating a misclassification probability $p(i, j) = 1 - n(i, j)/N$ with each pixel (N, number of observations; $n(i, j)$, number of times pixel (i, j) was selected as part of the lesion). For each automatic border B, the detection error was calculated as the mean probability of misclassification over the pixels inside the border, that is, $\sum_{(i,j) \in B} p(i, j)/(\text{TP} + \text{FP})$.

Iyatomi et al. [68, 76, 139] modified Guillod et al.'s approach by combining multiple manual borders that correspond to each lesion into one using the majority vote rule. The automatic borders were then compared against these combined ground-truth images. Garnavi et al. [136] used the intersection of the border areas, whereas Garnavi and Aldeen [225] used their union. Celebi et al. [88] compared each automatic border against multiple manual borders independently. Unfortunately, these methods do not accurately capture the variations in manual borders. For example, according to Guillod et al.'s measure, an automated border that is entirely within the manual borders gets a very low error. Iyatomi et al. and Garnavi et al.'s methods discount the variation in the manual borders by reducing them to a single border. On the other hand, Celebi et al.'s approach does not produce a scalar error value, which makes comparisons more difficult.

Celebi et al. [226] proposed the use of an objective measure, the Normalized Probabilistic Rand Index (NPRI) [227], which takes into account the variations in the manual borders. They demonstrated that differences among four of the evaluated border detection methods were in fact smaller than those predicted by the commonly used XOR measure. For a critique of the NPRI, the reader is referred to Peserico and Silletti [228].

Garnavi et al. [229] proposed the weighted performance index (WPI), which is an average of six commonly used weighted measures: sensitivity, specificity, accuracy, precision, similarity, and XOR. Each of these measures involves a subset of $\{\mathrm{TP}, \mathrm{FN}, \mathrm{FP}, \mathrm{TN}\}$ with the following subjective weights: $w_{TP} = 1.5$, $w_{FN} = w_{TN} = 1$, and for the calculation of precision, $w_{FP} = 1$, otherwise $w_{FP} = 0.5$. In a follow-up study, Garnavi and Aldeen [225] utilized a constrained nonlinear multivariable optimization scheme to determine these weights. Their findings were similar to those of Celebi et al. [226] in that with the optimized weights, differences among five automated border detection methods were smaller than those predicted using the fixed weights.

Fortina et al. [230] investigated the level of agreement among 12 dermatologists with differing levels of experience. On a set of 77 images, they determined that, on average, the area of disagreement was about 15% of the lesion area. In addition, more experienced dermatologists exhibited greater agreement among themselves than with less experienced dermatologists and a slight tendency toward tighter borders. They concluded that the agreement among experienced dermatologists could provide an upper bound for the accuracy achievable by the automated border detection methods.

None of the above measures quantify the effect of border detection error upon the accuracy of the classifier. Loss of classification accuracy due to automatic border error can be measured as the difference between the classification accuracy using the manual borders and that using the automatic borders.

4.6   COMPARISONS AND DISCUSSION

Table 4.2 compares recent border detection methods based on their color space (and, if applicable, the number of color channels), preprocessing steps, and segmentation method. Note that only those methods that are adequately described in the literature are included and the postprocessing steps are omitted since they are often not reported in detail. The following observations are in order:

- 15/50 methods do not require any preprocessing. It is possible that in some studies the authors have omitted the details of this crucial phase.
- 25/50 methods operate on multiple color channels. It is, however, unclear whether or not the use of color information improves the accuracy of border detection [133].
- 25/50 methods use a smoothing filter. Some segmentation methods, such as those based on thresholding, are inherently robust against noise, while others, for example, active contour-based methods, are highly sensitive to noise. Note that smoothing can also be performed as part of the hair removal step [99].
- Clustering (19/50) and thresholding (18/50) are the most popular segmentation methods, possibly due to the availability of simple and robust algorithms.

Table 4.3 compares the border detection methods based on their evaluation methodology: the number of human experts who determined the manual

TABLE 4.2

Characteristics of Border Detection Methods

Ref.	Year	Color Space (# Channels)	Preprocessing	Segmentation
[132]	2014	KL{RGB} (1)	$\overline{\text{MF}}$, IC, HR	Thresholding
[133]	2013	B/RGB (1)	nr	Thresholding
[147]	2013	Luminance	nr	Active contours + clustering
[134]	2013	B/RGB (1)	OF	Clustering + thresholding
[135]	2013	LAB (3)	HR, CR, GF	Clustering + thresholding
[188]	2013	RGB (3)	nr	Supervised learning
[146]	2013	RGB (3)	HR	Clustering + supervised Learning
[76]	2013	B or G/RGB (1)	$\overline{\text{MF}}$, IC, CE, BFR	Thresholding
[86]	2012	J/JCh (1)	CE, IC, HR	Thresholding + active contours
[97]	2012	LAB (3)	CE, IC, HR, BFR	Thresholding + edge detection
[148]	2012	RGB (3)	nr	Clustering
[149]	2012	RGB (3)	GF	Clustering + supervised Learning
[150]	2012	HSI (3)	ADF, CE	Clustering
[74]	2011	Luminance	$\widetilde{\text{MF}}$, CE, IC, HR	Thresholding + active contours
[75]	2011	Luminance	CE, IC, HR	Edge detection
[136]	2011	Misc.	GF, CE	Thresholding
[137]	2011	L/HSL (1)	ALL	Thresholding + clustering
[72]	2011	Luminance	CE	Supervised learning
[151]	2011	RGB (3)	nr	Clustering
[84]	2011	B/RGB (1)	IC, BFR, HR, ALL	Morphological + supervised learning
[66]	2011	LAB (3)	IC, GF	Supervised learning
[23]	2011	LAB (3)	GF	Supervised learning
[152]	2011	Luminance	nr	Active contours + clustering
[189]	2011	LUV (3)	$\widetilde{\text{MF}}$, IC	Supervised learning
[153]	2010	RGB (3)	nr	Clustering
[183]	2010	L/HSL (1)	OF, ALL	Active contours
[64]	2010	KL{RGB} (1)	IC, HR	Thresholding
[83]	2010	B/RGB (1)	IC, BFR, HR, ALL	Morphological
[190]	2010	RGB (3)	nr	Supervised learning
[52]	2009	ENT{RGB} (1)	OF, $\widetilde{\text{MF}}$, BFR	Thresholding
[52]	2009	Luminance	OF, $\widetilde{\text{MF}}$, BFR	Thresholding + active contours
[52]	2009	LAB (3)	OF, $\widetilde{\text{MF}}$, BFR	Fuzzy logic + region-based
[154]	2009	RGB (3)	nr	Clustering
[138]	2009	Luminance	nr	Thresholding
[155]	2009	RGB (3)	nr	Clustering
[88]	2008	RGB (3)	$\widetilde{\text{MF}}$, BFR	Region-based
[69]	2008	IHP{RGB} (1)	CE, HR	Clustering
[156]	2008	LAB (3)	nr	Clustering
[87]	2007	RGB (3)	$\widetilde{\text{MF}}$, ALL	Region-based
[139]	2006	B/RGB (1)	GF	Thresholding
[157]	2006	RGB (3)	nr	Clustering

(Continued)

TABLE 4.2 (*Continued*)
Characteristics of Border Detection Methods

Ref.	Year	Color Space (# Channels)	Preprocessing	Segmentation
[85]	2005	Luminance	GF, ALL	Thresholding + active contours
[158]	2003	LUV (3)	$\widetilde{\text{MF}}$	Clustering
[159]	2002	KL{LAB} (2)	GF	Clustering
[140]	2001	KL{RGB} (1)	$\widetilde{\text{MF}}$	Thresholding
[191]	2000	I/HSI (1)	$\widetilde{\text{MF}}$	Supervised learning
[93]	1999	KL{LUV} (2)	$\widetilde{\text{MF}}$	Clustering
[172]	1999	LAB (3)	ADF, HR	Morphological
[57]	1998	RGB (3)	nr	Region-based
[57]	1998	KL{RGB}(1)	nr	Model-based

Note: nr, not reported; KL{C}, KL transform of the color space C; GF, Gaussian filter; $\overline{\text{MF}}$, mean filter; $\widetilde{\text{MF}}$, median filter; ADF, anisotropic diffusion filter; OF, other filter; CE, contrast enhancement; IC, illumination correction; BFR, black frame removal; HR, hair removal; ALL, approximate lesion localization.

borders, the number of images used in the evaluations (and, if available, the diagnostic distribution of these images), the number of automated methods used in the comparisons (only comparisons against *published* border detection methods are considered), and the measure used to quantify the accuracy of border detection. It can be seen that

- Only 15/50 studies used borders determined by multiple dermatologists.
- Only 26/50 studies reported the diagnostic distribution of their test images. This information is valuable given that not every diagnostic category is equally challenging from a border detection perspective. For example, it is often more difficult to detect the borders of melanomas and dysplastic nevi due to their irregular and fuzzy border structure.
- 16/50 studies did not compare their results to those of other studies. This is partly due to the unavailability of public border detection software, as well as the scarcity of public dermoscopy image databases.
- Recent studies used objective measures to determine the quality of their results, whereas earlier studies relied on visual assessment. XOR is still the most popular quantitative evaluation measure despite the fact that it is biased against small lesions and it is not trivial to extend this measure to capture the variations in manual borders [224, 230, 231].

TABLE 4.3

Evaluation of Border Detection Methods (b, Benign; m, Malignant; HS, Hausdorff Distance [234])

Ref.	# Experts	# Images (Distribution)	# Comp.	Evaluation Measure
[132]	4	60	2	XOR
[133]	1	90 (67 b/23 m)	9	XOR
[147]	3	100 (70 b/30 m)	1	SE, SP, XOR
[134]	1	100 (70 b/30 m)	2	TPR, FPR, EP
[135]	1	100 (70 b/30 m)	3	TPR, FPR, EP
[188]	1	25	3	Misc.
[146]	1	125 (57 b/68 m), 181 (128 b/53 m)	1	XOR, J, HS
[76]	4–5	426 (351 b/75 m)	5	PR, RE, F
[86]	1	270 (80 b/190 m)	0	XOR
[97]	1	100 (70 b/30 m)	3	SE, SP, EP
[148]	1	50	0	SE, SP
[149]	1	116	6	SE, SP, AUC
[150]	3	57	2	Tanimoto [235]
[74]	1	320 (210 b/110 m)	2	HM, SE, FPR, HS, XOR
[75]	1	240 (170 b/70 m)	3	SE, SP, EP
[136]	4	85	3	ACC, PR, SE, SP, AUC
[137]	3	100 (70 b/30 m)	0	PR, RE, XOR
[72]	1	100 (70 b/30 m)	0	XOR
[151]	1	100 (70 b/30 m)	1	PR, RE, XOR
[84]	3	100 (70 b/30 m)	4	XOR
[66]	1	116	6	SE, SP
[23]	1	118	5	SE, SP
[152]	3	100 (70 b/30 m)	0	SE, SP
[189]	3	122 (100 b/22 m)	2	SE, SP, HS
[153]	1	100 (70 b/30 m)	0	PR, RE, XOR
[183]	1	50	0	PR, RE, XOR
[64]	3	91 (80 b/11 m)	0	Visual
[83]	3	100 (70 b/30 m)	3	XOR
[190]	1	178	3	XOR
[52]	1	100 (70 b/30 m)	4	HM, SE, FPR, HS
[154]	1	120	1	PR, RE, F, XOR
[138]	0	nr	0	Visual
[155]	1	100 (70 b/30 m)	3	SE, SP
[88]	3	90 (67 b/23 m)	4	XOR
[69]	1	100 (70 b/30 m)	3	XOR
[156]	1	67	0	XOR
[87]	2	100 (70 b/30 m)	3	XOR
[139]	5	319 (244 b/75 m)	1	PR, RE
[157]	nr	117	3	SE, SP
[85]	2	100 (70 b/30 m)	1	XOR
[158]	0	nr	0	nr
[159]	0	600	0	Visual
[140]	0	nr	0	nr

(Continued)

TABLE 4.3 (*Continued*)

Evaluation of Border Detection Methods (b, Benign; m, Malignant; HS, Hausdorff Distance [234])

Ref.	# Experts	# Images (Distribution)	# Comp.	Evaluation Measure
[191]	1	30	0	Visual
[93]	1	400	0	Visual
[172]	1	300	0	Visual
[57]	1	57	5	XOR

Unsolved problems in border detection include the following:

- Incorporation of textural information into the border detection process [87, 156, 232]
- Detection of borders in nonmelanocytic lesions such as seborrheic keratoses and basal/squamous cell carcinomas [76]
- Fusion of multiple border detection methods [133]
- Adaptive expansion of the automatic borders [68, 76, 88, 136, 139]
- Development of clinically oriented evaluation measures that take into account the variations in multiple manual borders

We believe that in a systematic border detection study

1. The image acquisition procedure should be described in sufficient detail.
2. The test image set should be selected randomly from a large and diverse image database.
3. The test image set should be large enough to ensure statistically valid conclusions.
4. The test image set should not be used to train/tune the border detection method.
5. The diagnostic distribution of the test image set should be specified.
6. Algorithms with reasonable computational requirements should be used.
7. The results should be evaluated using borders determined by multiple dermatologists.
8. The results should be compared to those of other published studies.
9. The border detection method should be described in sufficient detail.
10. The implementation of the border detection method should be made publicly available.

Note that all of the aforementioned criteria except (4), (6), (9), and (10) can be satisfied by using a public dermoscopy image set. Therefore, the creation of such a benchmark database should be prioritized in order to improve the quality of future border detection studies. A promising step in this direction is the publicly available PH^2 database [233], which contains 200 annotated dermoscopy images.

ACKNOWLEDGMENTS

This publication was made possible by grants from the U.S. National Science Foundation (0959583, 1117457) and National Natural Science Foundation of China (61050110449, 61073120).

REFERENCES

1. R. L. Siegel, K. D. Miller, and A. Jemal, Cancer Statistics, 2015, *CA: A Cancer Journal for Clinicians*, vol. 65, no. 1, pp. 5–29, 2015.
2. G. Argenziano, H. Soyer, and V. De Giorgi, *Dermoscopy: A Tutorial*, EDRA Medical Publishing and New Media, Milan, Italy, 2002.
3. S. Menzies, K. Crotty, C. Ingvar, and W. McCarthy, *Dermoscopy: An Atlas*, 3rd ed., McGraw-Hill, 2009.
4. K. Steiner, M. Binder, M. Schemper, K. Wolff, and H. Pehamberger, Statistical Evaluation of Epiluminescence Microscopy Criteria for Melanocytic Pigmented Skin Lesions, *Journal of the American Academy of Dermatology*, vol. 29, no. 4, pp. 581–588, 1993.
5. M. Binder, M. Schwarz, A. Winkler, A. Steiner, A. Kaider, K. Wolff, and H. Pehamberger, Epiluminescence Microscopy: A Useful Tool for the Diagnosis of Pigmented Skin Lesions for Formally Trained Dermatologists, *Archives of Dermatology*, vol. 131, no. 3, pp. 286–291, 1995.
6. M. G. Fleming, C. Steger, J. Zhang, J. Gao, A. B. Cognetta, I. Pollak, and C. R. Dyer, Techniques for Structural Analysis of Dermatoscopic Imagery, *Computerized Medical Imaging and Graphics*, vol. 22, no. 5, pp. 375–389, 1998.
7. M. E. Celebi, H. A. Kingravi, B. Uddin, H. Iyatomi, A. Aslandogan, W. V. Stoecker, and R. H. Moss, A Methodological Approach to the Classification of Dermoscopy Images, *Computerized Medical Imaging and Graphics*, vol. 31, no. 6, pp. 362–373, 2007.
8. P. Schmid-Saugeon, Symmetry Axis Computation for Almost-Symmetrical and Asymmetrical Objects: Application to Pigmented Skin Lesions, *Medical Image Analysis*, vol. 4, no. 3, pp. 269–282, 2000.
9. T. K. Lee, D. I. McLean, and M. S. Atkins, Irregularity Index: A New Border Irregularity Measure for Cutaneous Melanocytic Lesions, *Medical Image Analysis*, vol. 7, no. 1, pp. 47–64, 2003.
10. G. R. Day, How Blurry Is That Border? An Investigation into Algorithmic Reproduction of Skin Lesion Border Cut-Off, *Computerized Medical Imaging and Graphics*, vol. 24, no. 1, pp. 69–72, 2000.
11. S. Fischer, P. Schmid, and J. Guillod, Analysis of Skin Lesions with Pigmented Networks, in *Proceedings of the International Conference on Image Processing*, vol. 1, pp. 323–326, 1996.
12. M. G. Fleming, C. Steger, A. B. Cognetta, and J. Zhang, Analysis of the Network Pattern in Dermatoscopic Images, *Skin Research and Technology*, vol. 5, no. 1, pp. 42–48, 1999.

13. B. Caputo, V. Panichelli, and G. E. Gigante, Toward a Quantitative Analysis of Skin Lesion Images, *Studies in Health Technology and Informatics*, vol. 90, pp. 509–513, 2002.
14. M. Anantha, R. H. Moss, and W. V. Stoecker, Detection of Pigment Network in Dermatoscopy Images Using Texture Analysis, *Computerized Medical Imaging and Graphics*, vol. 28, no. 5, pp. 225–234, 2004.
15. C. Grana, R. Cucchiara, G. Pellacani, and S. Seidenari, Line Detection and Texture Characterization of Network Patterns, in *Proceedings of the 18th International Conference on Pattern Recognition*, vol. 2, pp. 275–278, 2006.
16. G. Betta, G. Di Leo, G. Fabbrocini, A. Paolillo, and M. Scalvenzi, Automated Application of the "7-Point Checklist" Diagnosis Method for Skin Lesions: Estimation of Chromatic and Shape Parameters, in *Proceedings of the IEEE Instrumentation and Measurement Technology Conference*, vol. 3, pp. 1818–1822, 2005.
17. G. Betta, G. Di Leo, G. Fabbrocini, A. Paolillo, and P. Sommella, Dermoscopic Image-Analysis System: Estimation of Atypical Pigment Network and Atypical Vascular Pattern, in *Proceedings of the IEEE International Workshop on Medical Measurement and Applications*, pp. 63–67, 2006.
18. G. Di Leo, C. Liguori, A. Paolillo, and P. Sommella, An Improved Procedure for the Automatic Detection of Dermoscopic Structures in Digital ELM Images of Skin Lesions, in *IEEE International Conference on Virtual Environments, Human-Computer Interfaces, and Measurement Systems*, pp. 190–194, 2008.
19. G. Di Leo, A. Paolillo, P. Sommella, and G. Fabbrocini, Automatic Diagnosis of Melanoma: A Software System Based on the 7-Point Check-List, in *Proceedings of the 43rd Hawaii International Conference on System Sciences*, pp. 1–10, 2010.
20. B. Shrestha, J. Bishop, K. Kam, X. Chen, R. H. Moss, W. V. Stoecker, S. Umbaugh et al., Detection of Atypical Texture Features in Early Malignant Melanoma, *Skin Research and Technology*, vol. 16, no. 1, pp. 60–65, 2010.
21. S. O. Skrovseth, T. R. Schopf, K. Thon, M. Zortea, M. Geilhufe, K. Mollersen, H. M. Kirchesch, and F. Godtliebsen, A Computer-Aided Diagnosis System for Malignant Melanomas, in *Proceedings of the 3rd International Symposium on Applied Sciences in Biomedical and Communication Technologies*, pp. 1–5, 2010.
22. M. Sadeghi, M. Razmara, T. K. Lee, and M. S. Atkins, A Novel Method for Detection of Pigment Network in Dermoscopic Images, *Computerized Medical Imaging and Graphics*, vol. 35, no. 2, pp. 137–143, 2011.
23. P. Wighton, T. K. Lee, H. Lui, D. I. McLean, and M. S. Atkins, Generalizing Common Tasks in Automated Skin Lesion Diagnosis, *IEEE Transactions on Information Technology in Biomedicine*, vol. 15, no. 4, pp. 622–629, 2011.
24. C. Barata, J. S. Marques, and J. Rozeira, A System for the Detection of Pigment Network in Dermoscopy Images Using Directional Filters, *IEEE Transactions on Biomedical Engineering*, vol. 59, no. 10, pp. 2744–2754, 2012.
25. J. L. G. Arroyo and B. G. Zapirain, Detection of Pigment Network in Dermoscopy Images Using Supervised Machine Learning and Structural Analysis, *Computers in Biology and Medicine*, vol. 44, pp. 144–157, 2014.
26. S. Sigurdsson, L. K. Hansen, and K. Drzewiecki, Identifying Black Dots in Dermatoscopic Images Using Template Matching, Tech. Rep. 2003-21, Technical University of Denmark, 2003.

27. S. Yoshino, T. Tanaka, M. Tanaka, and H. Oka, Application of Morphology for Detection of Dots in Tumor, in *Proceedings of the SICE 2004 Annual Conference*, vol. 1, pp. 591–594, 2004.

28. K. Thon, H. Rue, S. O. Skrovseth, and F. Godtliebsen, Bayesian Multiscale Analysis of Images Modeled as Gaussian Markov Random Fields, *Computational Statistics and Data Analysis*, vol. 56, no. 1, pp. 49–61, 2012.

29. H. Mirzaalian, T. K. Lee, and G. Hamarneh, Learning Features for Streak Detection in Dermoscopic Color Images using Localized Radial Flux of Principal Intensity Curvature, in *Proceedings of the IEEE Workshop on Mathematical Methods for Biomedical Image Analysis*, pp. 97–101, 2012.

30. M. Sadeghi, T. K. Lee, D. I. McLean, H. Lui, and M. S. Atkins, Detection and Analysis of Irregular Streaks in Dermoscopic Images of Skin Lesions, *IEEE Transactions on Medical Imaging*, vol. 32, no. 5, pp. 849–861, 2013.

31. G. Di Leo, G. Fabbrocini, C. Liguori, A. Pietrosanto, and M. Sclavenzi, ELM Image Processing for Melanocytic Skin Lesion Diagnosis Based on 7-Point Checklist: A Preliminary Discussion, in *Proceedings of the 13th International Symposium on Measurements for Research and Industry Applications*, vol. 2, pp. 474–479, 2004.

32. M. E. Celebi, H. Iyatomi, W. V. Stoecker, R. H. Moss, H. S. Rabinovitz, G. Argenziano, and H. P. Soyer, Automatic Detection of Blue-White Veil and Related Structures in Dermoscopy Images, *Computerized Medical Imaging and Graphics*, vol. 32, no. 8, pp. 670–677, 2008.

33. G. Di Leo, G. Fabbrocini, A. Paolillo, O. Rescigno, and P. Sommella, Towards an Automatic Diagnosis System for Skin Lesions: Estimation of Blue-Whitish Veil and Regression Structures, in *Proceedings of the 6th International Multi-Conference on Systems, Signals and Devices*, pp. 1–6, 2009.

34. J. L. G. Arroyo, B. G. Zapirain, and A. M. Zorrilla, Blue-White Veil and Dark-Red Patch of Pigment Pattern Recognition in Dermoscopic Images Using Machine-Learning Techniques, in *Proceedings of the 2011 IEEE International Symposium on Signal Processing and Information Technology*, pp. 196–201, 2011.

35. A. Madooei and M. S. Drew, A Colour Palette for Automatic Detection of Blue-White Veil, in *Proceedings of the 21st Color and Imaging Conference*, pp. 200–205, 2013.

36. A. Madooei, M. S. Drew, M. Sadeghi, and M. S. Atkins, Automatic Detection of Blue-White Veil by Discrete Colour Matching in Dermoscopy Images, in *Proceedings of the 16th International Conference on Medical Image Computing and Computer-Assisted Intervention*, vol. 3, pp. 453–460, 2013.

37. M. Lingala, R. J. Stanley, R. K. Rader, J. Hagerty, H. S. Rabinovitz, M. Oliviero, I. Choudhry, and W. V. Stoecker, Fuzzy Logic Color Detection: Blue Areas in Melanoma Dermoscopy Images, *Computerized Medical Imaging and Graphics*, vol. 38, no. 5, pp. 403–410, 2014.

38. M. Anantha, W. V. Stoecker, and R. H. Moss, Detection of Solid Pigment in Dermatoscopy Images Using Texture Analysis, *Skin Research and Technology*, vol. 6, no. 4, pp. 193–198, 2000.

39. G. Pellacani, C. Grana, R. Cucchiara, and S. Seidenari, Automated Extraction and Description of Dark Areas in Surface Microscopy Melanocytic Lesion Images, *Dermatology*, vol. 208, no. 1, pp. 21–26, 2004.

40. W. V. Stoecker, G. Gupta, R. J. Stanley, R. H. Moss, and B. Shrestha, Detection of Asymmetric Blotches (Asymmetric Structureless Areas) in Dermoscopy Images of Malignant Melanoma Using Relative Color, *Skin Research and Technology*, vol. 11, no. 3, pp. 179–184, 2005.

41. A. Khan, K. Gupta, R. J. Stanley, W. V. Stoecker, R. H. Moss, G. Argenziano, H. P. Soyer, H. S. Rabinovitz, and A. B. Cognetta, Fuzzy Logic Techniques for Blotch Feature Evaluation in Dermoscopy Images, *Computerized Medical Imaging and Graphics*, vol. 33, no. 1, pp. 50–57, 2009.

42. V. K. Madasu and B. C. Lovell, Blotch Detection in Pigmented Skin Lesions Using Fuzzy Co-Clustering and Texture Segmentation, in *Proceedings of the International Conference on Digital Image Computing: Techniques and Applications*, pp. 25–31, 2009.

43. W. V. Stoecker, M. Wronkiewiecz, R. Chowdhury, R. J. Stanley, J. Xu, A. Bangert, B. Shrestha et al., Detection of Granularity in Dermoscopy Images of Malignant Melanoma Using Color and Texture Features, *Computerized Medical Imaging and Graphics*, vol. 35, no. 2, pp. 144–147, 2011.

44. A. Dalal, R. H. Moss, R. J. Stanley, W. V. Stoecker, K. Gupta, D. A. Calcara, J. Xu et al., Concentric Decile Segmentation of White and Hypopigmented Areas in Dermoscopy Images of Skin Lesions Allows Discrimination of Malignant Melanoma, *Computerized Medical Imaging and Graphics*, vol. 35, no. 2, pp. 148–154, 2011.

45. C. Barata, M. A. T. Figueiredo, M. E. Celebi, and J. S. Marques, Color Identification in Dermoscopy Images Using Gaussian Mixture Models, in *Proceedings of the IEEE International Conference on Acoustics, Speech, and Signal Processing*, pp. 3611–3615, 2014.

46. M. E. Celebi, H. Iyatomi, G. Schaefer, and W. V. Stoecker, Lesion Border Detection in Dermoscopy Images, *Computerized Medical Imaging and Graphics*, vol. 33, no. 2, pp. 148–153, 2009.

47. M. E. Celebi, W. V. Stoecker, and R. H. Moss, Advances in Skin Cancer Image Analysis, *Computerized Medical Imaging and Graphics*, vol. 35, no. 2, pp. 83–84, 2011.

48. M. E. Celebi and G. Schaefer, eds., *Color Medical Image Analysis*, Springer, Berlin, 2012.

49. K. Korotkov and R. Garcia, Computerized Analysis of Pigmented Skin Lesions: A Review, *Artificial Intelligence in Medicine*, vol. 56, no. 2, pp. 69–90, 2012.

50. J. Scharcanski and M. E. Celebi, eds., *Computer Vision Techniques for the Diagnosis of Skin Cancer*, Springer, Berlin, 2013.

51. D. Gutkowicz-Krusin, M. Elbaum, P. Szwaykowski, and A. W. Kopf, Can Early Malignant Melanoma Be Differentiated from Atypical Melanocytic Nevus by In Vivo Techniques? Part II. Automatic Machine Vision Classification, *Skin Research and Technology*, vol. 3, no. 1, pp. 15–22, 1997.

52. M. Silveira, J. C. Nascimento, J. S. Marques, A. R. S. Marcal, T. Mendonca, S. Yamauchi, J. Maeda, and J. Rozeira, Comparison of Segmentation Methods for Melanoma Diagnosis in Dermoscopy Images, *IEEE Journal of Selected Topics in Signal Processing*, vol. 3, no. 1, pp. 35–45, 2009.

53. C. Poynton, *Digital Video and HD: Algorithms and Interfaces*, 2nd ed., Morgan Kaufmann, 2012.

54. M. E. Celebi, H. Iyatomi, and G. Schaefer, Contrast Enhancement in Dermoscopy Images by Maximizing a Histogram Bimodality Measure, in

Proceedings of the 16th IEEE International Conference on Image Processing, pp. 2601–2604, 2009.

55. A. Madooei, M. S. Drew, M. Sadeghi, and M. S. Atkins, Automated Pre-Processing Method for Dermoscopic Images and Its Application to Pigmented Skin Lesion Segmentation, in *Proceedings of the 20th Color and Imaging Conference: Color Science and Engineering Systems, Technologies, and Applications*, pp. 158–163, 2012.

56. W. K. Pratt, Spatial Transform Coding of Color Images, *IEEE Transactions on Communication Technology*, vol. 19, no. 6, pp. 980–992, 1971.

57. J. Gao, J. Zhang, M. G. Fleming, I. Pollak, and A. B. Cognetta, Segmentation of Dermatoscopic Images by Stabilized Inverse Diffusion Equations, in *Proceedings of the 1998 International Conference on Image Processing*, vol. 3, pp. 823–827, 1998.

58. T. Gevers and A. W. M. Smeulders, Color-Based Object Recognition, *Pattern Recognition*, vol. 32, no. 3, pp. 453–464, 1999.

59. L. Busin, N. Vandenbroucke, and L. Macaire, Color Spaces and Image Segmentation, in *Advances in Imaging and Electron Physics* (P. W. Hawkes, ed.), vol. 151, pp. 65–168, Academic Press, 2008.

60. M. E. Celebi, H. A. Kingravi, and F. Celiker, Fast Color Space Transformations Using Minimax Approximations, *IET Image Processing*, vol. 4, no. 2, pp. 70–79, 2010.

61. T. Y. Shih, The Reversibility of Six Geometric Color Spaces, *Photogrammetric Engineering and Remote Sensing*, vol. 61, no. 10, pp. 1223–1232, 1995.

62. Y. V. Haeghen, J. M. A. D. Naeyaert, I. Lemahieu, and W. Philips, An Imaging System with Calibrated Color Image Acquisition for Use in Dermatology, *IEEE Transactions on Medical Imaging*, vol. 19, no. 7, pp. 722–730, 2000.

63. C. Grana, G. Pellacani, and S. Seidenari, Practical Color Calibration for Dermoscopy, *Skin Research and Technology*, vol. 11, no. 4, pp. 242–247, 2005.

64. K. Mollersen, H. M. Kirchesch, T. G. Schopf, and F. Godtliebsen, Unsupervised Segmentation for Digital Dermoscopic Images, *Skin Research and Technology*, vol. 16, no. 4, pp. 401–407, 2010.

65. J. Quintana, R. Garcia, and L. Neumann, A Novel Method for Color Correction in Epiluminescence Microscopy, *Computerized Medical Imaging and Graphics*, vol. 35, no. 7/8, pp. 646–652, 2011.

66. P. Wighton, T. K. Lee, H. Lui, D. McLean, and M. S. Atkins, Chromatic Aberration Correction: An Enhancement to the Calibration of Low-Cost Digital Dermoscopes, *Skin Research and Technology*, vol. 17, no. 3, pp. 339–347, 2011.

67. A. Delalleau, J. M. Lagarde, and J. George, An *A Priori* Shading Correction Technique for Contact Imaging Devices, *IEEE Transactions on Image Processing*, vol. 20, no. 10, pp. 2876–2885, 2011.

68. H. Iyatomi, H. Oka, M. E. Celebi, M. Hashimoto, M. Hagiwara, M. Tanaka, and K. Ogawa, An Improved Internet-Based Melanoma Screening System with Dermatologist-Like Tumor Area Extraction Algorithm, *Computerized Medical Imaging and Graphics*, vol. 32, no. 7, pp. 566–579, 2008.

69. D. D. Gomez, C. Butakoff, B. K. Ersboll, and W. V. Stoecker, Independent Histogram Pursuit for Segmentation of Skin Lesions, *IEEE Transactions on Biomedical Engineering*, vol. 55, no. 1, pp. 157–161, 2008.

70. N. Otsu, A Threshold Selection Method from Gray Level Histograms, *IEEE Transactions on Systems, Man and Cybernetics*, vol. 9, no. 1, pp. 62–66, 1979.

71. H. Iyatomi, M. E. Celebi, G. Schaefer, and M. Tanaka, Automated Color Calibration Method for Dermoscopy Images, *Computerized Medical Imaging and Graphics*, vol. 35, no. 2, pp. 89–98, 2011.

72. G. Schaefer, M. I. Rajab, M. E. Celebi, and H. Iyatomi, Colour and Contrast Enhancement for Improved Skin Lesion Segmentation, *Computerized Medical Imaging and Graphics*, vol. 35, no. 2, pp. 99–104, 2011.

73. A. Rizzi, C. Gatta, and D. Marini, A New Algorithm for Unsupervised Global and Local Color Correction, *Pattern Recognition Letters*, vol. 24, no. 11, pp. 1663–1677, 2003.

74. Q. Abbas, I. Fondon, and M. Rashid, Unsupervised Skin Lesions Border Detection via Two-Dimensional Image Analysis, *Computer Methods and Programs in Biomedicine*, vol. 104, no. 3, 2011.

75. Q. Abbas, M. E. Celebi, I. F. Garcia, and M. Rashid, Lesion Border Detection in Dermoscopy Images Using Dynamic Programming, *Skin Research and Technology*, vol. 17, no. 1, pp. 91–100, 2011.

76. K. A. Norton, H. Iyatomi, M. E. Celebi, S. Ishizaki, M. Sawada, R. Suzaki, K. Kobayashi, M. Tanaka, and K. Ogawa, Three-Phase General Border Detection Method for Dermoscopy Images Using Non-Uniform Illumination Correction, *Skin Research and Technology*, vol. 18, no. 3, pp. 290–300, 2012.

77. T. G. Stockham, Image Processing in the Context of a Visual Model, *Proceedings of the IEEE*, vol. 60, no. 7, pp. 828–842, 1972.

78. S. M. Pizer, E. P. Amburn, J. D. Austin, R. Cromartie, A. Geselowitz, T. Greer, B. Romeny, J. B. Zimmerman, and K. Zuiderveld, Adaptive Histogram Equalization and Its Variations, *Computer Vision, Graphics, and Image Processing*, vol. 39, no. 3, pp. 355–368, 1987.

79. C. Barata, M. E. Celebi, and J. S. Marques, Improving Dermoscopy Image Classification Using Color Constancy, *IEEE Journal of Biomedical and Health Informatics*, vol. 19, no. 3, pp. 1146–1152, 2015.

80. Y. Lu, F. Xie, Y. Wu, Z. Jiang, and R. Meng, No Reference Uneven Illumination Assessment for Dermoscopy Images, *IEEE Signal Processing Letters*, vol. 22, no. 5, pp. 534–538, 2015.

81. R. Kimmel, M. Elad, D. Shaked, R. Keshet, and I. Sobel, A Variational Framework for Retinex, *International Journal of Computer Vision*, vol. 52, no. 1, pp. 7–23, 2003.

82. M. E. Celebi, H. Iyatomi, G. Schaefer, and W. V. Stoecker, Approximate Lesion Localization in Dermoscopy Images, *Skin Research and Technology*, vol. 15, no. 3, pp. 314–322, 2009.

83. H. Wang, X. Chen, R. H. Moss, R. J. Stanley, W. V. Stoecker, M. E. Celebi, T. M. Szalapski et al., Segmentation of Dermoscopy Images Using a Watershed Technique, *Skin Research and Technology*, vol. 16, no. 3, pp. 378–384, 2010.

84. H. Wang, R. H. Moss, X. Chen, R. J. Stanley, W. V. Stoecker, M. E. Celebi, J. M. Malters et al., Modified Watershed Technique and Post-Processing for Segmentation of Skin Lesions in Dermoscopy Images, *Computerized Medical Imaging and Graphics*, vol. 35, no. 2, pp. 116–120, 2011.

85. B. Erkol, R. H. Moss, R. J. Stanley, W. V. Stoecker, and E. Hvatum, Automatic Lesion Boundary Detection in Dermoscopy Images Using Gradient Vector Flow Snakes, *Skin Research and Technology*, vol. 11, no. 1, pp. 17–26, 2005.

86. Q. Abbas, M. E. Celebi, and I. F. Garcia, A Novel Perceptually-Oriented Approach for Skin Tumor Segmentation, *International Journal of Innovative Computing, Information and Control*, vol. 8, no. 3, pp. 1837–1848, 2012.

87. M. E. Celebi, Y. A. Aslandogan, W. V. Stoecker, H. Iyatomi, H. Oka, and X. Chen, Unsupervised Border Detection in Dermoscopy Images, *Skin Research and Technology*, vol. 13, no. 4, pp. 454–462, 2007.

88. M. E. Celebi, H. A. Kingravi, H. Iyatomi, A. Aslandogan, W. V. Stoecker, R. H. Moss, J. M. Malters et al., Border Detection in Dermoscopy Images Using Statistical Region Merging, *Skin Research and Technology*, vol. 14, no. 3, pp. 347–353, 2008.

89. J. Kittler and J. Illingworth, Minimum Error Thresholding, *Pattern Recognition*, vol. 19, no. 1, pp. 41–47, 1986.

90. G. E. Forsythe, Generation and Use of Orthogonal Polynomials for Data-Fitting with a Digital Computer, *Journal of the Society for Industrial and Applied Mathematics*, vol. 5, no. 2, pp. 74–88, 1957.

91. M. Sonka, V. Hlavac, and R. Boyle, *Image Processing, Analysis, and Machine Vision*, 4th ed., Cengage Learning, 2014.

92. M. E. Celebi, H. A. Kingravi, and Y. A. Aslandogan, Nonlinear Vector Filtering for Impulsive Noise Removal from Color Images, *Journal of Electronic Imaging*, vol. 16, no. 3, p. 033008, 2007.

93. P. Schmid, Segmentation of Digitized Dermatoscopic Images by Two-Dimensional Color Clustering, *IEEE Transactions on Medical Imaging*, vol. 18, no. 2, pp. 164–171, 1999.

94. J. M. Geusebroek, A. W. M. Smeulders, and J. van de Weijer, Fast Anisotropic Gauss Filtering, *IEEE Transactions on Image Processing*, vol. 12, no. 8, pp. 938–943, 2003.

95. S. Nakariyakul, Fast Spatial Averaging: An Efficient Algorithm for 2D Mean Filtering, *Journal of Supercomputing*, vol. 65, no. 1, pp. 262–273, 2013.

96. S. Perreault and P. Hebert, Median Filtering in Constant Time, *IEEE Transactions on Image Processing*, vol. 16, no. 9, pp. 2389–2394, 2007.

97. Q. Abbas, M. E. Celebi, and I. F. Garcia, Skin Tumor Area Extraction Using an Improved Dynamic Programming Approach, *Skin Research and Technology*, vol. 18, no. 2, pp. 133–142, 2012.

98. P. Soille, *Morphological Image Analysis: Principles and Applications*, 2nd ed., Springer, Berlin, 2004.

99. T. K. Lee, V. Ng, R. Gallagher, A. Coldman, and D. McLean, DullRazor: A Software Approach to Hair Removal from Images, *Computers in Biology and Medicine*, vol. 27, no. 6, pp. 533–543, 1997.

100. H. Zhou, M. Chen, R. Gass, J. M. Rehg, L. Ferris, J. Ho, and L. Drogowski, Feature-Preserving Artifact Removal from Dermoscopy Images, in *Proceedings of the SPIE Medical Imaging 2008 Conference*, pp. 69141B-1–69141B-9, 2008.

101. P. Wighton, T. K. Lee, and M. S. Atkins, Dermascopic Hair Disocclusion Using Inpainting, in *Proceedings of the SPIE Medical Imaging 2008 Conference*, pp. 691427-1–691427-8, 2008.

102. M. Fiorese, E. Peserico, and A. Silletti, VirtualShave: Automated Hair Removal from Digital Dermatoscopic Images, in *Proceedings of the 33rd Annual International Conference of the IEEE Engineering in Medicine and Biology Society*, pp. 5145–5148, 2011.

103. S. Schmid-Saugeon, J. Guillod, and J. P. Thiran, Towards a Computer-Aided Diagnosis System for Pigmented Skin Lesions, *Computerized Medical Imaging and Graphics*, vol. 27, no. 1, pp. 65–78, 2003.

104. F. Y. Xie, S. Y. Qin, Z. G. Jiang, and R. S. Meng, PDE-Based Unsupervised Repair of Hair-Occluded Information in Dermoscopy Images of Melanoma, *Computerized Medical Imaging and Graphics*, vol. 33, no. 4, pp. 275–282, 2009.

105. P. Perona and J. Malik, Scale-Space and Edge Detection Using Anisotropic Diffusion, *IEEE Transactions on Pattern Analysis and Machine Intelligence*, vol. 12, no. 7, pp. 629–639, 1990.

106. M. Bertalmio, G. Sapiro, V. Caselles, and C. Ballester, Image Inpainting, in *Proceedings of the 27th Annual Conference on Computer Graphics and Interactive Techniques*, pp. 417–424, 2000.

107. C. Steger, An Unbiased Detector of Curvilinear Structures, *IEEE Transactions on Pattern Analysis and Machine Intelligence*, vol. 20, no. 2, pp. 113–125, 1998.

108. A. Criminisi, P. Perez, and K. Toyama, Region Filling and Object Removal by Exemplar-Based Image Inpainting, *IEEE Transactions on Image Processing*, vol. 13, no. 9, pp. 1200–1212, 2004.

109. N. H. Nguyen, T. K. Lee, and M. S. Atkins, Segmentation of Light and Dark Hair in Dermoscopic Images: A Hybrid Approach Using a Universal Kernel, in *Proceedings of the SPIE Medical Imaging 2010 Conference*, pp. 76234N-1–76234N-8, 2010.

110. S. Chaudhuri, S. Chatterjee, N. Katz, M. Nelson, and M. Goldbaum, Detection of Blood Vessels in Retinal Images Using Two-Dimensional Matched Filters, *IEEE Transactions on Medical Imaging*, vol. 8, no. 3, pp. 263–269, 1989.

111. N. R. Pal and S. K. Pal, Entropic Thresholding, *Signal Processing*, vol. 16, no. 2, pp. 97–108, 1989.

112. Q. Li, L. Zhang, J. You, D. Zhang, and P. Bhattacharya, Dark Line Detection with Line Width Extraction, in *Proceedings of the 15th IEEE International Conference on Image Processing*, pp. 621–624, 2008.

113. K. Kiani and A. R. Sharafat, E-Shaver: An Improved DullRazor for Digitally Removing Dark and Light-Colored Hairs in Dermoscopic Images, *Computers in Biology and Medicine*, vol. 41, no. 3, pp. 139–145, 2011.

114. K. Jafari-Khouzani and H. Soltanian-Zadeh, Radon Transform Orientation Estimation for Rotation Invariant Texture Analysis, *IEEE Transactions on Pattern Analysis and Machine Intelligence*, vol. 27, no. 6, pp. 1004–1008, 2005.

115. J. M. S. Prewitt, Object Enhancement and Extraction, in *Picture Processing and Psychopictorics* (B. S. Lipkin and A. Rosenfeld, eds.), pp. 75–149, Academic Press, 1970.

116. K. Fukunaga, *Introduction to Statistical Pattern Recognition*, 2nd ed., Academic Press, 1990.

117. S. K. Kopparapu and U. B. Desai, *Bayesian Approach to Image Interpretation*, Kluwer Academic Publishers, 2001.

118. H. Rue and L. Held, *Gaussian Markov Random Fields: Theory and Applications*, Chapman & Hall/CRC, Boca Raton, FL, 2005.

119. A. Afonso and M. Silveira, Hair Detection in Dermoscopic Images Using Percolation, in *Proceedings of the 34th Annual International Conference of the IEEE Engineering in Medicine and Biology Society*, pp. 4378–4381, 2012.

120. T. Yamaguchi, S. Nakamura, and S. Hashimoto, An Efficient Crack Detection Method Using Percolation-Based Image Processing, in *Proceedings of the 3rd*

IEEE Conference on Industrial Electronics and Applications, pp. 1875–1880, 2008.

121. Q. Abbas, I. F. Garcia, M. E. Celebi, and W. Ahmad, A Feature-Preserving Hair Removal Algorithm for Dermoscopy Images, *Skin Research and Technology*, vol. 19, no. 1, pp. e27–e36, 2013.

122. B. Zhang, L. Zhang, L. Zhang, and F. Karray, Retinal Vessel Extraction by Matched Filter with First-Order Derivative of Gaussian, *Computers in Biology and Medicine*, vol. 40, no. 4, pp. 438–445, 2010.

123. F. Bornemann and T. Marz, Fast Image Inpainting Based on Coherence Transport, *Journal of Mathematical Imaging and Vision*, vol. 28, no. 3, pp. 259–278, 2007.

124. M. T. B. Toossi, H. R. Pourreza, H. Zare, M. H. Sigari, P. Layegh, and A. Azimi, An Effective Hair Removal Algorithm for Dermoscopy Images, *Skin Research and Technology*, vol. 19, no. 3, pp. 230–235, 2013.

125. W. K. Pratt, Generalized Wiener Filtering Computation Techniques, *IEEE Transactions on Computers*, vol. C-21, no. 7, pp. 636–641, 1972.

126. F. Canny, A Computational Approach to Edge Detection, *IEEE Transactions on Pattern Analysis and Machine Intelligence*, vol. 8, no. 6, pp. 679–698, 1986.

127. A. Rosenfeld and P. de la Torre, Histogram Concavity Analysis as an Aid in Threshold Selection, *IEEE Transactions on Systems, Man and Cybernetics*, vol. 13, no. 2, pp. 231–235, 1983.

128. Q. Abbas, M. E. Celebi, and I. F. Garcia, Hair Removal Methods: A Comparative Study for Dermoscopy Images, *Biomedical Signal Processing and Control*, vol. 6, no. 4, pp. 395–404, 2011.

129. H. Mirzaalian, T. K. Lee, and G. Hamarneh, Hair Enhancement in Dermoscopic Images Using Dual-Channel Quaternion Tubularness Filters and MRF-Based Multi-Label Optimization, *IEEE Transactions on Image Processing*, vol. 23, no. 12, pp. 5486–5496, 2014.

130. A. F. Frangi, W. J. Niessen, K. L. Vincken, and M. A. Viergever, Multiscale Vessel Enhancement Filtering, in *Proceedings of the First International Conference on Medical Image Computing and Computer-Assisted Intervention*, pp. 130–137, 1998.

131. Y. Boykov, O. Veksler, and R. Zabih, Fast Approximate Energy Minimization via Graph Cuts, *IEEE Transactions on Pattern Analysis and Machine Intelligence*, vol. 23, no. 11, pp. 1222–1239, 2001.

132. F. Peruch, F. Bogo, M. Bonazza, V. M. Cappelleri, and E. Peserico, Simpler, Faster, More Accurate Melanocytic Lesion Segmentation through MEDS, *IEEE Transactions on Biomedical Engineering*, vol. 61, no. 2, pp. 557–565, 2014.

133. M. E. Celebi, Q. Wen, S. Hwang, H. Iyatomi, and G. Schaefer, Lesion Border Detection in Dermoscopy Images Using Ensembles of Thresholding Methods, *Skin Research and Technology*, vol. 19, no. 1, pp. e252–e258, 2013.

134. Q. Abbas, I. F. Garcia, M. E. Celebi, W. Ahmad, and Q. Mushtaq, Unified Approach for Lesion Border Detection Based on Mixture Modeling and Local Entropy Thresholding, *Skin Research and Technology*, vol. 19, no. 3, pp. 314–319, 2013.

135. Q. Abbas, I. F. Garcia, M. E. Celebi, W. Ahmad, and Q. Mushtaq, A Perceptually Oriented Method for Contrast Enhancement and Segmentation of Dermoscopy Images, *Skin Research and Technology*, vol. 19, no. 1, pp. e490–e497, 2013.

136. R. Garnavi, M. Aldeen, M. E. Celebi, G. Varigos, and S. Finch, Border Detection in Dermoscopy Images Using Hybrid Thresholding on Optimized Color Channels, *Computerized Medical Imaging and Graphics*, vol. 35, no. 2, pp. 105–115, 2011.

137. M. Mete, S. Kockara, and K. Aydin, Fast Density-Based Lesion Detection in Dermoscopy Images, *Computerized Medical Imaging and Graphics*, vol. 35, no. 2, pp. 128–136, 2011.

138. M. E. Yuksel and M. Borlu, Accurate Segmentation of Dermoscopic Images by Image Thresholding Based on Type-2 Fuzzy Logic, *IEEE Transactions on Fuzzy Systems*, vol. 17, no. 4, pp. 976–982, 2009.

139. H. Iyatomi, H. Oka, M. Saito, A. Miyake, M. Kimoto, J. Yamagami, S. Kobayashi et al., Quantitative Assessment of Tumor Extraction from Dermoscopy Images and Evaluation of Computer-Based Extraction Methods for Automatic Melanoma Diagnostic System, *Melanoma Research*, vol. 16, no. 2, pp. 183–190, 2006.

140. M. Hintz-Madsen, L. K. Hansen, J. Larsen, and K. Drzewiecki, A Probabilistic Neural Network Framework for the Detection of Malignant Melanoma, in *Artificial Neural Networks in Cancer Diagnosis, Prognosis and Patient Management* (R. N. G. Naguib and G. V. Sherbet, eds.), pp. 141–183, CRC Press, Boca Raton, FL, 2001.

141. J. S. Weszka, A Survey of Threshold Selection Techniques, *Computer Graphics and Image Processing*, vol. 7, no. 2, pp. 259–265, 1978.

142. P. K. Sahoo, S. Soltani, and A. K. C. Wong, A Survey of Thresholding Techniques, *Computer Vision, Graphics, and Image Processing*, vol. 41, no. 2, pp. 233–260, 1988.

143. C. A. Glasbey, An Analysis of Histogram-Based Thresholding Algorithms, *CVGIP: Graphical Models and Image Processing*, vol. 55, no. 6, pp. 532–537, 1993.

144. M. Sezgin and B. Sankur, Survey over Image Thresholding Techniques and Quantitative Performance Evaluation, *Journal of Electronic Imaging*, vol. 13, no. 1, pp. 146–165, 2004.

145. C. I. Chang, Y. Du, J. Wang, S. M. Guo, and P. D. Thouin, Survey and Comparative Analysis of Entropy and Relative Entropy Thresholding Techniques, *IEE Proceedings—Vision, Image and Signal Processing*, vol. 153, no. 6, pp. 837–850, 2006.

146. F. Xie and A. C. Bovik, Automatic Segmentation of Dermoscopy Images Using Self-Generating Neural Networks Seeded by Genetic Algorithm, *Pattern Recognition*, vol. 46, no. 3, pp. 1012–1019, 2013.

147. H. Zhou, X. Li, G. Schaefer, M. E. Celebi, and P. Miller, Mean Shift Based Gradient Vector Flow for Image Segmentation, *Computer Vision and Image Understanding*, vol. 117, no. 9, pp. 1004–1016, 2013.

148. H. Castillejos, V. Ponomaryov, L. Nino de Rivera, and V. Golikov, Wavelet Transform Fuzzy Algorithms for Dermoscopic Image Segmentation, *Computational and Mathematical Methods in Medicine*, vol. 2012, 2012.

149. S. Khakabi, P. Wighton, T. K. Lee, and M. S. Atkins, Multi-Level Feature Extraction for Skin Lesion Segmentation in Dermoscopic Images, in *Proceedings of the SPIE Medical Imaging 2012 Conference*, pp. 83150E-1–83150E-7, 2012.

150. Z. Liu, J. Sun, M. Smith, L. Smith, and R. Warr, Unsupervised Sub-Segmentation for Pigmented Skin Lesions, *Skin Research and Technology*, vol. 18, no. 1, pp. 77–87, 2012.

151. S. Suer, S. Kockara, and M. Mete, An Improved Border Detection in Dermoscopy Images for Density Based Clustering, *BMC Bioinformatics*, vol. 12, suppl. 10, 2011.

152. H. Zhou, G. Schaefer, M. E. Celebi, F. Lin, and T. Liu, Gradient Vector Flow with Mean Shift for Skin Lesion Segmentation, *Computerized Medical Imaging and Graphics*, vol. 35, no. 2, pp. 121–127, 2011.

153. S. Kockara, M. Mete, V. Yip, B. Lee, and K. Aydin, A Soft Kinetic Data Structure for Lesion Border Detection, *Bioinformatics*, vol. 26, no. 12, pp. i21–i28, 2010.

154. P. Wighton, M. Sadeghi, T. K. Lee, and M. S. Atkins, A Fully Automatic Random Walker Segmentation for Skin Lesions in a Supervised Setting, in *Proceedings of the 12th International Conference on Medical Image Computing and Computer Assisted Intervention*, pp. 1108–1115, 2009.

155. H. Zhou, G. Schaefer, A. Sadka, and M. E. Celebi, Anisotropic Mean Shift Based Fuzzy C-Means Segmentation of Dermoscopy Images, *IEEE Journal of Selected Topics in Signal Processing*, vol. 3, no. 1, pp. 26–34, 2009.

156. H. Zhou, M. Chen, L. Zou, R. Gass, L. Ferris, L. Drogowski, and J. M. Rehg, Spatially Constrained Segmentation of Dermoscopy Images, in *Proceedings of the 5th IEEE International Symposium on Biomedical Imaging: From Nano to Macro*, pp. 800–803, 2008.

157. R. Melli, C. Grana, and R. Cucchiara, Comparison of Color Clustering Algorithms for Segmentation of Dermatological Images, in *Proceedings of the SPIE Medical Imaging 2006 Conference*, pp. 1211–1219, 2006.

158. H. Galda, H. Murao, H. Tamaki, and S. Kitamura, Skin Image Segmentation Using a Self-Organizing Map and Genetic Algorithms, *IEEJ Transactions on Electronics, Information and Systems*, vol. 123, no. 11, pp. 2056–2062, 2003.

159. R. Cucchiara, C. Grana, S. Seidenari, and G. Pellacani, Exploiting Color and Topological Features for Region Segmentation with Recursive Fuzzy C-Means, *Machine Graphics and Vision*, vol. 11, no. 2/3, pp. 169–182, 2002.

160. A. K. Jain and P. J. Flynn, Image Segmentation Using Clustering, in *Advances in Image Understanding: A Festschrift for Azriel Rosenfeld* (K. W. Bowyer and N. Ahuja, eds.), pp. 65–83, IEEE Computer Society Press, 1996.

161. A. K. Jain, M. N. Murty, and P. J. Flynn, Data Clustering: A Review, *ACM Computing Surveys*, vol. 31, no. 3, pp. 264–323, 1999.

162. M. A. Sutton, Image Segmentation by Fuzzy Clustering: Methods and Issues, in *Handbook of Medical Image Processing and Analysis*, 2nd ed. (I. N. Bankman, ed.), pp. 91–111, Academic Press, 2008.

163. L. S. Davis, A Survey of Edge Detection Techniques, *Computer Graphics and Image Processing*, vol. 4, no. 3, pp. 248–270, 1975.

164. M. Petrou, The Differentiating Filter Approach to Edge Detection, in *Advances in Electronics and Electron Physics* (P. W. Hawkes, ed.), vol. 88, pp. 297–345, Academic Press, 1994.

165. D. Ziou and S. Tabbone, Edge Detection Techniques—An Overview, *Pattern Recognition and Image Analysis*, vol. 8, no. 4, pp. 537–559, 1998.

166. M. Basu, Gaussian-Based Edge-Detection Methods—A Survey, *IEEE Transactions on Systems, Man, and Cybernetics, Part C: Applications and Reviews*, vol. 32, no. 3, pp. 252–260, 2002.

167. P. A. Mlsna and J. J. Rodriguez, Gradient and Laplacian Edge Detection, in *The Essential Guide to Image Processing* (A. Bovik, ed.), pp. 495–524, Academic Press, 2009.

168. S. T. Acton, Diffusion Partial Differential Equations for Edge Detection, in *The Essential Guide to Image Processing* (A. Bovik, ed.), pp. 525–552, Academic Press, 2009.

169. S. W. Zucker, Region Growing: Childhood and Adolescence, *Computer Graphics and Image Processing*, vol. 5, no. 3, pp. 382–399, 1976.

170. X. Cufi, X. Munoz, J. Freixenet, and J. Marti, A Review of Image Segmentation Techniques Integrating Region and Boundary Information, in *Advances in Imaging and Electron Physics* (P. W. Hawkes, ed.), vol. 120, pp. 1–39, Academic Press, 2002.

171. X. Munoz, J. Freixenet, X. Cufi, and J. Marti, Strategies for Image Segmentation Combining Region and Boundary Information, *Pattern Recognition Letters*, vol. 24, no. 1–3, pp. 375–392, 2003.

172. P. Schmid, Lesion Detection in Dermatoscopic Images Using Anisotropic Diffusion and Morphological Flooding, in *Proceedings of the 1999 IEEE International Conference on Image Processing*, vol. 3, pp. 449–453, 1999.

173. F. Meyer and S. Beucher, Morphological Segmentation, *Journal of Visual Communication and Image Representation*, vol. 1, no. 1, pp. 21–46, 1990.

174. F. Meyer, C. Vachier, A. Oliveras, and P. Salembier, Morphological Tools for Segmentation: Connected Filters and Watersheds, *Annales Des Telecommunications*, vol. 52, no. 7–8, pp. 367–379, 1997.

175. J. B. T. M. Roerdink and A. Meijster, The Watershed Transform: Definitions, Algorithms and Parallelization Strategies, *Fundamenta Informaticae*, vol. 41, no. 1–2, pp. 187–228, 2000.

176. I. R. Terol-Villalobos, Morphological Image Enhancement and Segmentation, in *Advances in Imaging and Electron Physics* (P. W. Hawkes, ed.), vol. 118, pp. 207–273, Academic Press, 2001.

177. F. Meyer, An Overview of Morphological Segmentation, *International Journal of Pattern Recognition and Artificial Intelligence*, vol. 15, no. 7, pp. 1089–1118, 2001.

178. F. Meyer, Morphological Segmentation Revisited, in *Space, Structure and Randomness: Contributions in Honor of Georges Matheron in the Field of Geostatistics, Random Sets and Mathematical Morphology* (M. Bilodeau, F. Meyer, and M. Schmitt, eds.), vol. 183 of *Lecture Notes in Statistics*, pp. 315–347, Springer, Berlin, 2005.

179. J. Serra, Advances in Mathematical Morphology: Segmentation, in *Advances in Imaging and Electron Physics* (P. W. Hawkes, ed.), vol. 150, pp. 185–219, Academic Press, 2008.

180. R. C. Dubes and A. K. Jain, Random Field Models in Image Analysis, *Journal of Applied Statistics*, vol. 16, no. 2, pp. 131–164, 1989.

181. G. Winkler, *Image Analysis, Random Fields and Markov Chain Monte Carlo Methods: A Mathematical Introduction*, 2nd ed., Springer, Berlin, 2003.

182. S. Z. Li, *Markov Random Field Modeling in Image Analysis*, 3rd ed., Springer, Berlin, 2009.

183. M. Mete and N. M. Sirakov, Lesion Detection in Dermoscopy Images with Novel Density-Based and Active Contour Approaches, *BMC Bioinformatics*, vol. 11, suppl. 6, p. S23, 2010.

184. C. Xu, D. L. Pham, and J. L. Prince, Image Segmentation Using Deformable Models, in *Handbook of Medical Imaging: Medical Image Processing and Analysis*, vol. 2 (M. Sonka and J. M. Fitzpatrick, eds.), pp. 129–174, SPIE Press, 2000.

185. S. Osher and N. Paragios, eds., *Geometric Level Set Methods in Imaging, Vision, and Graphics*, Springer, Berlin, 2003.

186. V. Caselles, R. Kimmel, and G. Sapiro, Geometric Active Contours for Image Segmentation, in *Handbook of Image and Video Processing*, 2nd ed. (A. Bovik, ed.), pp. 613–627, Academic Press, 2005.

187. O. Basir, H. Zhu, and F. Karray, Fuzzy Based Image Segmentation, in *Fuzzy Filters for Image Processing* (M. Nachtegael, D. Van der Weken, E. E. Kerre, and D. Van De Ville, eds.), Springer, Berlin, 2003.

188. A. R. Sadri, M. Zekri, S. Sadri, N. Gheissari, M. Mokhtari, and F. Kolahdouzan, Segmentation of Dermoscopy Images Using Wavelet Networks, *IEEE Transactions on Biomedical Engineering*, vol. 60, no. 4, pp. 1134–1141, 2013.

189. M. Zortea, S. O. Skrovseth, T. R. Schopf, H. M. Kirchesch, and F. Godtliebsen, Automatic Segmentation of Dermoscopic Images by Iterative Classification, *International Journal of Biomedical Imaging*, vol. 2011, 2011.

190. H. Zhou, J. M. Rehg, and M. Chen, Exemplar-Based Segmentation of Pigmented Skin Lesions from Dermoscopy Images, in *Proceedings of the 2010 IEEE International Symposium on Biomedical Imaging: From Nano to Macro*, pp. 225–228, 2010.

191. T. Donadey, C. Serruys, A. Giron, G. Aitken, J. P. Vignali, R. Triller, and B. Fertil, Boundary Detection of Black Skin Tumors Using an Adaptive Radial-Based Approach, in *Proceedings of the SPIE Medical Imaging 2000 Conference*, pp. 800–816, 2000.

192. K. S. Fu and J. K. Mui, A Survey on Image Segmentation, *Pattern Recognition*, vol. 13, no. 1, pp. 3–16, 1981.

193. S. Di Zenzo, Advances in Image Segmentation, *Image and Vision Computing*, vol. 1, no. 4, pp. 196–210, 1983.

194. R. M. Haralick and L. G. Shapiro, Image Segmentation Techniques, *Computer Vision, Graphics, and Image Processing*, vol. 29, no. 1, pp. 100–132, 1985.

195. N. R. Pal and S. K. Pal, A Review on Image Segmentation Techniques, *Pattern Recognition*, vol. 26, no. 9, pp. 1277–1294, 1993.

196. L. Lucchese and S. K. Mitra, Color Image Segmentation: A State-of-the-Art Survey, *Proceedings of the Indian National Science Academy*, vol. 67A, no. 2, pp. 207–221, 2001.

197. H. D. Cheng, X. H. Jiang, Y. Sun, and J. Wang, Color Image Segmentation: Advances and Prospects, *Pattern Recognition*, vol. 34, no. 12, pp. 2259–2281, 2001.

198. S. R. Vantaram and E. Saber, Survey of Contemporary Trends in Color Image Segmentation, *Journal of Electronic Imaging*, vol. 21, no. 4, pp. 040901-1–040901-28, 2012.

199. N. Vandenbroucke, L. Macaire, and J. G. Postaire, Color Image Segmentation by Pixel Classification in an Adapted Hybrid Color Space: Application to Soccer Image Analysis, *Computer Vision and Image Understanding*, vol. 90, no. 2, pp. 190–216, 2003.

200. K. McGuinness and N. E. O'Connor, A Comparative Evaluation of Interactive Segmentation Algorithms, *Pattern Recognition*, vol. 43, no. 2, pp. 434–444, 2010.
201. R. Adams and L. Bischof, Seeded Region Growing, *IEEE Transactions on Pattern Analysis and Machine Intelligence*, vol. 16, no. 6, pp. 641–647, 1994.
202. A. Mehnert and P. Jackway, An Improved Seeded Region Growing Algorithm, *Pattern Recognition Letters*, vol. 18, no. 10, pp. 1065–1071, 1997.
203. Y. V. Haeghen, J. M. Naeyaert, and I. Lemahieu, Development of a Dermatological Workstation: Preliminary Results on Lesion Segmentation in CIE $L^*A^*B^*$ Color Space, in *Proceedings of the International Conference on Color in Graphics and Image Processing*, pp. 328–333, 2000.
204. L. Vendramin, R. J. G. B. Campello, and E. R. Hruschka, Relative Clustering Validity Criteria: A Comparative Overview, *Statistical Analysis and Data Mining*, vol. 3, no. 4, pp. 209–235, 2010.
205. O. Arbelaitz, I. Gurrutxaga, J. Muguerza, J. M. Perez, and I. Perona, An Extensive Comparative Study of Cluster Validity Indices, *Pattern Recognition*, vol. 46, no. 1, pp. 243–256, 2013.
206. M. E. Celebi, Improving the Performance of K-Means for Color Quantization, *Image and Vision Computing*, vol. 29, no. 4, pp. 260–271, 2011.
207. M. E. Celebi and H. Kingravi, Deterministic Initialization of the K-Means Algorithm Using Hierarchical Clustering, *International Journal of Pattern Recognition and Artificial Intelligence*, vol. 26, no. 7, p. 1250018, 2012.
208. M. E. Celebi, H. Kingravi, and P. A. Vela, A Comparative Study of Efficient Initialization Methods for the K-Means Clustering Algorithm, *Expert Systems with Applications*, vol. 40, no. 1, pp. 200–210, 2013.
209. M. E. Celebi and H. A. Kingravi, Linear, Deterministic, and Order-Invariant Initialization Methods for the K-Means Clustering Algorithm, in *Partitional Clustering Algorithms* (M. E. Celebi, ed.), pp. 79–98, Springer, Berlin, 2014.
210. H. P. Kriegel, P. Kroger, J. Sander, and A. Zimek, Density-Based Clustering, *Wiley Interdisciplinary Reviews: Data Mining and Knowledge Discovery*, vol. 1, no. 3, pp. 231–240, 2011.
211. M. Ester, Density-Based Clustering, in *Data Clustering: Algorithms and Applications* (C. C. Aggarwal and C. K. Reddy, eds.), pp. 111–126, Chapman & Hall/CRC, Boca Raton, FL, 2013.
212. D. Comaniciu and P. Meer, Mean Shift: A Robust Approach toward Feature Space Analysis, *IEEE Transactions on Pattern Analysis and Machine Intelligence*, vol. 24, no. 5, pp. 603–619, 2002.
213. J. Sander, M. Ester, H. P. Kriegel, and X. Xu, Density-Based Clustering in Spatial Databases: The Algorithm GDBSCAN and Its Applications, *Data Mining and Knowledge Discovery*, vol. 2, no. 2, pp. 169–194, 1998.
214. P. M. Ferreira, T. Mendonca, and P. Rocha, A Wide Spread of Algorithms for Automatic Segmentation of Dermoscopic Images, in *Proceedings of the 6th Iberian Conference on Pattern Recognition and Image Analysis*, pp. 592–599, 2013.
215. D. R. Martin, C. C. Fowlkes, and J. Malik, Learning to Detect Natural Image Boundaries Using Local Brightness, Color, and Texture Cues, *IEEE Transactions on Pattern Analysis and Machine Intelligence*, vol. 26, no. 5, pp. 530–549, 2004.

216. Y. Rubner, C. Tomasi, and L. J. Guibas, The Earth Mover's Distance as a Metric for Image Retrieval, *International Journal of Computer Vision*, vol. 40, no. 2, pp. 99–121, 2000.

217. P. M. Ferreira, T. Mendonca, P. Rocha, and J. Rozeira, A New Interface for Manual Segmentation of Dermoscopic Images, in *Proceedings of the 3rd ECCOMAS Thematic Conference on Computational Vision and Medical Image Processing*, pp. 399–404, 2011.

218. P. M. Ferreira, T. Mendonca, J. Rozeira, and P. Rocha, An Annotation Tool for Dermoscopic Image Segmentation, in *Proceedings of the 1st International Workshop on Visual Interfaces for Ground Truth Collection in Computer Vision Applications*, 2012, Article 5.

219. T. Fawcett, An Introduction to ROC Analysis, *Pattern Recognition Letters*, vol. 27, no. 8, pp. 861–874, 2006.

220. G. A. Hance, S. E. Umbaugh, R. H. Moss, and W. V. Stoecker, Unsupervised Color Image Segmentation with Application to Skin Tumor Borders, *IEEE Engineering in Medicine and Biology Magazine*, vol. 15, no. 1, pp. 104–111, 1996.

221. P. Jaccard, Distribution de la Flore Alpine dans le Bassin des Dranses et dans Quelques Régions Voisines, *Bulletin de la Société Vaudoise des Sciences Naturelles*, vol. 37, no. 140, pp. 241–272, 1901.

222. A. Hammoude, Computer-Assisted Endocardial Border Identification from a Sequence of Two-Dimensional Echocardiographic Images, PhD thesis, University of Washington, 1988.

223. V. Chalana and Y. Kim, A Methodology for Evaluation of Boundary Detection Algorithms on Medical Images, *IEEE Transactions on Medical Imaging*, vol. 16, no. 5, pp. 642–652, 1997.

224. J. Guillod, P. Schmid-Saugeon, D. Guggisberg, J. P. Cerottini, R. Braun, J. Krischer, J. H. Saurat, and M. Kunt, Validation of Segmentation Techniques for Digital Dermoscopy, *Skin Research and Technology*, vol. 8, no. 4, pp. 240–249, 2002.

225. R. Garnavi and M. Aldeen, Optimized Weighted Performance Index for Objective Evaluation of Border-Detection Methods in Dermoscopy Images, *IEEE Transactions on Information Technology in Biomedicine*, vol. 15, no. 6, pp. 908–917, 2011.

226. M. E. Celebi, G. Schaefer, H. Iyatomi, W. V. Stoecker, J. M. Malters, and J. M. Grichnik, An Improved Objective Evaluation Measure for Border Detection in Dermoscopy Images, *Skin Research and Technology*, vol. 15, no. 4, pp. 444–450, 2009.

227. R. Unnikrishnan, C. Pantofaru, and M. Hebert, Toward Objective Evaluation of Image Segmentation Algorithms, *IEEE Transactions on Pattern Analysis and Machine Intelligence*, vol. 29, no. 6, pp. 929–944, 2007.

228. E. Peserico and A. Silletti, Is (N)PRI Suitable for Evaluating Automated Segmentation of Cutaneous Lesions? *Pattern Recognition Letters*, vol. 31, no. 16, pp. 2464–2467, 2010.

229. R. Garnavi, M. Aldeen, and M. E. Celebi, Weighted Performance Index for Objective Evaluation of Border Detection Methods in Dermoscopy Images, *Skin Research and Technology*, vol. 17, no. 1, pp. 35–44, 2011.

230. A. B. Fortina, E. Peserico, A. Silletti, and E. Zattra, Where's the Naevus? Inter-Operator Variability in the Localization of Melanocytic Lesion Border, *Skin Research and Technology*, vol. 18, no. 3, pp. 311–315, 2012.

231. A. Silletti, E. Peserico, A. Mantovan, E. Zattra, A. Peserico, and A. B. Fortina, Variability in Human and Automatic Segmentation of Melanocytic Lesions, in *Proceedings of the 31st Annual International Conference of the IEEE Engineering in Medicine and Biology Society*, pp. 5789–5792, 2009.
232. S. Hwang and M. E. Celebi, Texture Segmentation of Dermoscopy Images Using Gabor Filters and G-Means Clustering, in *Proceedings of the 2010 International Conference on Image Processing, Computer Vision, and Pattern Recognition*, pp. 882–886, 2010.
233. T. Mendonca, P. M. Ferreira, J. S. Marques, A. R. S. Marcal, and J. Rozeira, PH^2: A Dermoscopic Image Database for Research and Benchmarking, in *Proceedings of the 35th Annual International Conference of the IEEE Engineering in Medicine and Biology Society*, pp. 5437–5440, 2013.
234. D. P. Huttenlocher, G. A. Klanderman, and W. J. Rucklidge, Comparing Images Using the Hausdorff Distance, *IEEE Transactions on Pattern Analysis and Machine Intelligence*, vol. 15, no. 9, pp. 850–863, 1993.
235. D. J. Rogers and T. T. Tanimoto, A Computer Program for Classifying Plants, *Science*, vol. 132, no. 3434, pp. 1115–1118, 1960.

5 Comparison of Image Processing Techniques for Reticular Pattern Recognition in Melanoma Detection

Jose Luis García Arroyo
University of Deusto
Bilbao, Spain

Begoña García Zapirain
University of Deusto
Bilbao, Spain

CONTENTS

5.1   INTRODUCTION

5.1.1   RETICULAR PATTERN IN DERMOSCOPY IMAGES

Melanoma is a type of skin cancer that accounts for approximately 1.6% of the total number of cancer cases worldwide [1]. In the fight against this type of cancer, early detection is a key factor: if detected early, before the tumor has penetrated the skin (noninvasive melanoma or melanoma in situ), the survival rate is 98%, falling to 15% in advanced cases (invasive melanoma), when the tumor has spread (metastasized) [2].

In order to carry out the diagnosis, the most frequently used method is the Two-step procedure, in which, as its name suggests, the diagnosis is carried out in two steps. In the first step, the dermatologist must discern whether it is a melanocytic lesion or not, on the basis of a series of criteria. If not, the lesion is not a melanoma. In the affirmative case, the dermatologist goes on to the second step, in which a diagnostic method is used to calculate the degree of malignancy, determining whether a biopsy should be performed [3]. The most commonly used methods are Pattern Analysis [4] or the so-called medical algorithms, such as the ABCD Rule [5], the Menzies Method [6], and the 7-point Checklist [7]. All of them aim to quantitatively detect and characterize a series of indicators observed by doctors and to proceed to diagnosis based on preestablished ranges of values. Some of the most relevant indicators are the dermoscopic patterns or structures, such as pigment network, streaks, globules, dots, blue–white veil, blotches, or regression structures. It should be noted, however, that their objectification is particularly difficult and, in many cases, extremely biased due to dermatologists' subjective opinions.

One of the key dermoscopic structures is the pigment network, also called the reticular pattern, whose presence is an indicator of melanin deep inside the layers of the skin. It is of great importance since it is one of the key criteria for identifying melanocytic lesions in the first step of the so-called Two-step procedure. Moreover, it is an indicator present in all the medical methods for diagnosis of melanoma. The name is derived from the shape of this structure, which resembles a net and is darker in color than the "holes" it forms, which make up part of the lesion's background. There are two types of pigment networks: the most typical one, with a light to dark-brown net with small, uniformly spaced holes and thin lines distributed more or less evenly, and the atypical one, which is a black, brown, or gray net with irregular holes and thick lines and is frequently an indicator of melanoma [3]. Four examples of pigment network are shown in Figure 5.1.

This chapter shows a comparison of the state-of-the-art reticular pattern recognition methods.

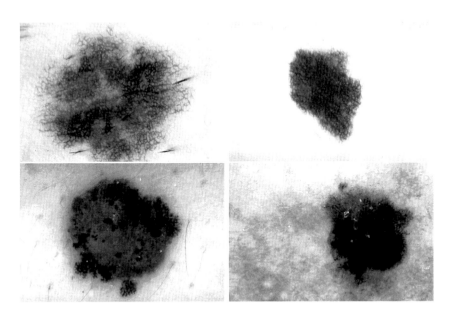

FIGURE 5.1   Four examples of pigment network: the two uppermost examples are typical, while the ones below are atypical. (Reprinted with permission from Argenziano, G. et al., *Dermoscopy: A Tutorial*, EDRA Medical Publishing and New Media, Milan, Italy, 2002.)

5.1.2   CONTEXTUALIZATION OF THE AUTOMATIC DETECTION OF PIGMENT NETWORK

Various computer-aided diagnosis (CAD) systems have been presented recently for the automated detection of melanoma from dermoscopic images. This is a subject of current research [8–10].

As can be seen in Figure 5.2, the life cycle of a CAD of this type consists of the following stages: (1) image acquisition; (2) image preprocessing, the main task of which is the detection and removal of artifacts, especially hairs; (3) skin lesion segmentation; (4) detection and characterization of indicators; and (5) diagnosis.

In the design of stages 4 and 5 there are two different approaches. A first approach, used, for example, in the classic work [11] or in more recent ones [12, 13], uses supervised machine learning, consisting firstly of the extraction of different types of features from the dermoscopic image and subsequently carrying out the diagnosis by means of the classifier generated. A second approach, used, for example, in [14–16] and in most of the commercial systems described in [17], consists of reproducing as faithfully as possible a medical algorithm, calculating the values of the indicators and obtaining the degree of malignancy, using the corresponding formula. This approach is the most common one, since physicians make the final decision and prefer to rely on a well-known algorithm. In all of them, some of the most relevant indicators are the dermoscopic patterns or structures. Some relevant works on their detection and characterization are examined in pigment network (described in later sections of this chapter), streaks [18–20], globules and dots [21–23], blue–white veil [24–27]), vascular [28], blotches [29–31], hypopigmentation [32], regression structures [25, 33], and parallel pattern [34].

Automated detection of the pigment network pattern would be considered as algorithm within a CAD in the second approach. As was mentioned above, there are two types of reticular patterns, typical and atypical. Therefore, the key objectives in this field of research are detection of both types.

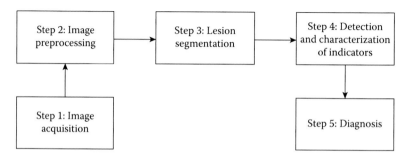

FIGURE 5.2 Stages of the life cycle of an automated system for the detection of melanoma.

Automated detection of the pigment network, both typical and atypical, is a complex problem, for several reasons. There is sometimes a low contrast between the net and the background. Moreover, the size of the net holes may differ considerably in different images. Even in the same image there are often important irregularities in shape and size and, finally, distinguishing between typical and atypical is often very difficult.

5.2   STATE-OF-THE-ART METHODS

A complete review of the different methods was carried out, and the most important to date were chosen for this comparative study. The selected methods focus on reticular pattern detection, either exclusively or within a family of algorithms or a CAD, contributing an innovative algorithm and from which detailed information on the system design can be obtained. Therefore, software systems used to detect pigment networks that do not give information about their design have not been included, even those reporting good results.

The works that are the end result of a series of related studies are dealt with as one. In some cases, they are broader versions of preliminary studies; in other cases, they are based on other studies. The works are presented in chronological order. In the case of several related studies, the date given is that of the latest relevant work.

Only in two cases, Sadeghi et al. and Serrano et Acha/Abbas et al./Sáez et al., are presented separately more than one different work of the same research group. In the first case, they are presented because of their importance and the fact that they study different problems: the first work, pigment network detection, and the second, atypical pigment network detection, basing the design of the second work on the first one. In the second case, they are presented because of their importance and because the different works use different approaches with different techniques, although they share parts between them.

5.2.1   FISCHER ET AL. (1996)

In [35], Fischer et al. present a method for obtaining the pigment network from a dermoscopy image. They first converted the image to grayscale, using the Karhunen–Loeve transform [36]. After segmenting the image (this chapter does not examine the techniques used for this purpose), they went on to use local histogram equalization to improve contrast. Thirdly, they used gray-level morphological operations, which enabled them to eliminate noise and obtain the pigment network from a threshold value obtained.

They did not give data about the images used to test the method or the results obtained. However, for later works classifying images as either reticular or nonreticular, the authors propose obtaining features extracted from the binary image corresponding to the pigment network obtained using structural analysis.

5.2.2 FLEMING ET AL. (1999)

In [37], Fleming et al. detect the pigment network, combining two techniques. Firstly, the image is converted to grayscale, selecting the first plane of the CIEXYZ transform. Secondly, they use the Steger (one of the authors) curvilinear line detection algorithm [38] on the image to extract the net, which also provides a measure of the line widths, according to preestablished parameters. Thirdly, they use Lobregt–Viergever's snake algorithm [39] to segment the holes and measure them. Figure 5.3 shows a diagram of how the pigment network is obtained in this study.

Sixty-nine images (16 common nevi, 22 dysplastic nevi, and 31 melanoma) were used to test the algorithm. Interesting statistical results were found with analysis of variance (ANOVA), related to the correlations between these images and net line widths and hole areas. The different indicators related to these values were studied, and the most important were the mean line width (common nevi, 6.72; dysplastic nevi, 7.03; melanoma, 8.58) and the mean hole area (common nevi, 251; dysplastic nevi, 308; melanoma, 345), obtaining the correct classification between nevus and melanoma in 80% of the cases, based on a generated linear discrimination function. Nevertheless, no outcome concerning the behavior of the system in reticular pattern detection, that is, the differentiation between pigment network and no-pigment network, was reported.

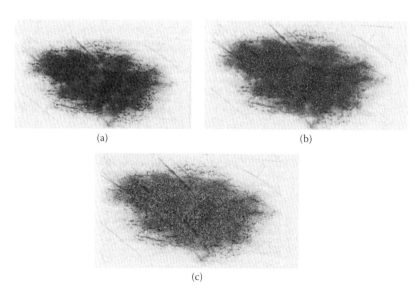

(a)   (b)

(c)

FIGURE 5.3 In the method proposed by Fleming et al., network detection algorithms were applied to a compound dysplastic nevus. (a) Grayscale version of the original image; (b) centers of detected network lines; (c) boundaries of network lines. (Reprinted with permission from Fleming, M. G. et al., *Skin Research and Technology*, vol. 5, no. 1, pp. 42–48, 1999.)

5.2.2.1 Other Related Studies

This work explains the reticular pattern detection method proposed by the authors. Following this work, the same authors published another study in [40] that dealt with other dermatoscopic structures and in which the section on pigment network detection cites the work described.

5.2.3 CAPUTO ET AL. (2002)

In [41], Caputo et al. present a method to obtain the pigment network and the quantitative analysis of its structure. The method consists of four stages: (1) prefiltering, (2) extraction of the network structure, (3) computing of the number and areas of meshes, and (4) computing of the statistical indicators. A Wiener filter [42] is used in the first stage to remove the noise, followed by image enhancing using a histogram stretching operation [42] to make the network structure easily detectable. The network structure is extracted in the second stage, using adaptive thresholding techniques [42]. A validation of the mesh correction is performed in the third stage, comparing the mask obtained with the original image. Based on the histograms of the images and masks obtained, the statistical indicators are calculated in the fourth stage. An example of the stages is shown in Figure 5.4.

The process was tested on 14 images, selected from a total of 100 by expert dermatologists. Of the 14 images, 7 were labeled as regular (regular pigment network structure) and 7 as irregular (irregular pigment network structure), based on the values obtained for the threshold classification statistics. Using this threshold, six of the seven images were correctly classified, thus obtaining 85.71% accuracy.

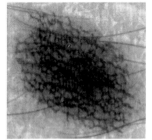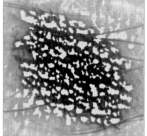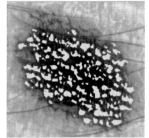

FIGURE 5.4 In Caputo et al.'s method, an example of network structure extracted from an original image. The original image (left) is first filtered and binarized (center). The false positive meshes are then eliminated by hand (right). (Reprinted with permission from Caputo, B. et al., *Studies in Health Technology and Informatics*, vol. 90, pp. 509–513, 2002.)

5.2.4   ANANTHA ET AL. (2004)

In [43], Anantha et al. use the Dullrazor software [44] for detecting, removing, and repairing hair, followed by two different texture analysis methods for pigment network detection. The first one uses Laws' energy masks [45]. In this method, texture measurements are based on co-occurrence, correlation, and statistical moment methods and the relationships between them. Masks of $n \times n$ pixels are the result, which are used to convolve the images and compute the energy of the results [45]. The second one uses the neighborhood gray-level dependence matrix (NGLDM) [46]. This is a rotation-invariant texture determination method that defines an $m \times m$ matrix size that includes the relationship between a pixel and all its neighbors, based on five texture attributes: small number emphasis, large number emphasis, number nonuniformity, second moment, and entropy [46]. Both methods are run on the dermatoscopic image that has previously been converted to grayscale using the common formula $(I_G(x, y) = 0.2989\,I_{RGB}(x, y, 0) + 0.587\,I_{RGB}(x, y, 1) + 0.114\,I_{RGB}(x, y, 2))$, obtaining the optimal n and m sizes for each one and the texture blocks when determining the pigment network.

The system was tested on a total of 155 images, which are divided into blocks of 64×64 pixels, classified by expert dermatologists as no-pigment network, partial pigment network, and full-pigment network. Better results were obtained with the first method, Laws' energy masks, yielding the best classification using a weight of 40% for the 9×9 and 60% for the 11×11 masks, as shown in Figure 5.5. Approximately 80% accuracy was obtained when classifying the blocks, based on optimal threshold values. The main problem was differentiating between a partial, on the one hand, and a no-pigment network or full-pigment network on the other. Determining a texel width of 10 pixels

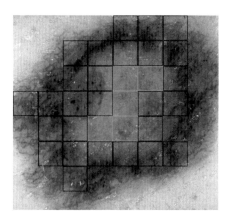

FIGURE 5.5   In Anantha et al.'s method, result of pigment network finder using the weighted combination of 9×9 and 11×11 of Laws' energy masks. (Reprinted with permission from Anantha, M. et al., *Computerized Medical Imaging and Graphics*, vol. 28, pp. 225–234, 2004.)

(0.22 mm, in the resolution of the images used) as the optimal texture unit in reticular pattern recognition is another important result. This is the first study reviewed that systematically examines a large number of images to study reticular pattern detection.

Perhaps the main weakness is due to use of the Dullrazor software, firstly because the method depends on this preprocessing software and secondly due to the errors made by this software, which leads to failure of the reticular detection algorithm. In fact, this is the cause of some of the errors reported by the authors.

5.2.4.1 Other Related Studies

This work continues the study [47], by the same research team.

5.2.5 GRANA ET AL. (2007)

In [48], Grana et al. use three steps to detect pigment networks. Their approach is quite similar to that in the work by Fleming et al. [37].

Firstly, they use the Steger curvilinear line detection algorithm [38], on an image previously converted to grayscale, to detect the net points. Secondly, they link these points into a line, taking into account the direction of the line at its endpoints and the number of line points connected to these. They choose the best points, based on the optimal thresholds in the delineation of the structure, using Fisher linear discriminant analysis. Then they link them using bilinear interpolation and gray-level morphological operations. Thirdly, they validate the meshes obtained, using as criteria whether they can be closed with the lines and have the right area and circularity values. Figure 5.6 shows two graphs of the results obtained.

The number of the valid meshes and their area with respect to the whole area of the lesion are the inputs of a linear discriminant function that classifies the lesions into reticular and nonreticular. A group of 100 images was used: 50 with a pigment network and 50 without, obtaining 82% sensitivity, 94% specificity, and 88% accuracy.

5.2.5.1 Other Related Studies

This work continues with the preliminary study [49], by the same research team.

5.2.6 TANAKA ET AL. (2008)

In [50], Tanaka et al. present an algorithm to detect the following pattern types: homogeneous, globular, and reticular.

Firstly, they segmented the lesion (this paper does not examine the techniques used for this purpose) and went on to analyze the texture and classify it. Different feature types are used to determine if it is homogenous or reticular and globular: 7 intensity histogram features, 7 differential statistical features,

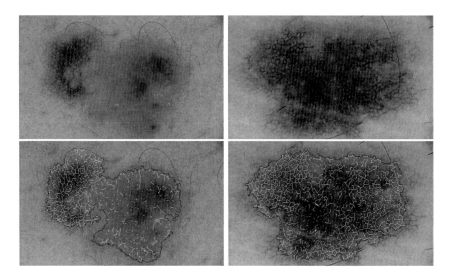

FIGURE 5.6 In Grana et al.'s method, two examples of pigment network detection, at the top the original images and at the bottom the pigment networks detected. (Reprinted with permission from Grana, R. et al., Line detection and texture characterization of network patterns, in *18th International Conference on Pattern Recognition (ICPR '06)*, Hong Kong, China, vol. 2, pp. 275–278, 2006.)

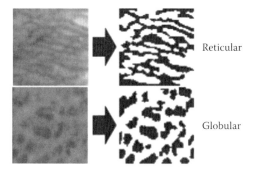

Reticular

Globular

FIGURE 5.7 In Tanaka et al.'s method, two examples of reticular pattern (above) and globular pattern (below), showing the original image and the generated mask for each one. Sixty-four features are extracted from these images to differentiate between the two patterns. (Reprinted with permission from Tanaka, T. et al., *IEEJ Transactions on Electrical and Electronic Engineering*, vol. 3, no. 1, pp. 143–150, 2008.)

14 Fourier power spectrum features, 5 run-length matrix features, and 13 co-occurrence matrix features, up to a total of 46 features. Sixty-four features extracted from the following processes are proposed to differentiate between reticular and globular: run-length matrix using intensity and a connected component of black and white after binarization, as shown in Figure 5.7.

A total of 213 images were divided into subimages, with the different patterns. A statistical analysis of the 110 features was run on the subimages with the following methods: F-test, t-test, stepwise method, and finally, discriminant method for pattern classification. 94% accuracy was achieved, correctly classifying the three categories out of a total of 852 subimages.

5.2.6.1   Other Related Studies

The content of this paper is basically the same as [51], and was written by the same research team.

5.2.7   DI LEO ET AL. (2008)

In [52], Di Leo et al. detect the atypical pigment network by combining two techniques, as shown in Figure 5.8: a structural one, in which morphological methods are used, and a spectral one, based on a Fourier analysis, in which fast Fourier transform (FFT), high-pass filters, inverse FFT, and finally thresholding techniques are used. The result was the pigment network mask, which was in turn combined with the mask resulting from segmentation of the skin lesion, based on Otsu's method [53]. The management of distortive artifacts (hairs, etc.) is not reported. Examples of pigment network detection are shown in Figure 5.9.

Nine chromatic and four spatial features related to the structures obtained were later defined for classification of the pigment network using supervised machine learning. In order to discriminate between the absent, typical, and atypical categories, the C4.5 decision tree classifier [54] was run on a total of 173 images (43, 53, and 77 of each type). Numerical results of the classification

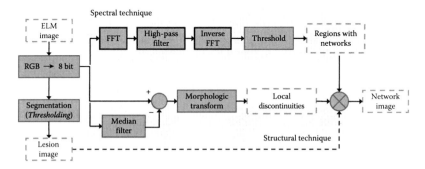

FIGURE 5.8 High-level view of Di Leo et al.'s method. (Reprinted with permission from Di Leo, G. et al., An improved procedure for the automatic detection of dermoscopic structures in digital ELM images of skin lesions, in *2008 IEEE Conference on Virtual Environments, Human-Computer Interfaces and Measurement Systems*, Istanbul, Turkey, pp. 190–194, 2008.)

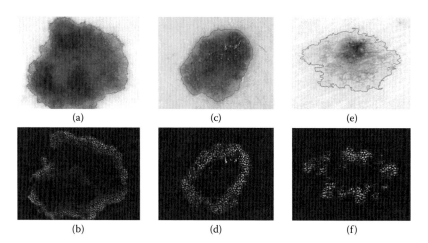

(a)   (c)   (e)

(b)   (d)   (f)

FIGURE 5.9 Examples of atypical pigment network in Di Leo et al.'s method. Lesion contour (a, c, e) and corresponding detected pigment network (b, d, f). (Reprinted with permission from Di Leo, G. et al., An improved procedure for the automatic detection of dermoscopic structures in digital ELM images of skin lesions, in *2008 IEEE Conference on Virtual Environments, Human-Computer Interfaces and Measurement Systems*, Istanbul, Turkey, pp. 190–194, 2008.)

by decision tree were not shown. Differentiation between nonatypical (absent and typical) and atypical (atypical) was examined, obtaining more than 85% sensitivity and specificity (no exact values are set). This is a relevant work, which has been integrated to form a complete CAD.

5.2.7.1   Other Related Studies

This research team developed a CAD to detect melanoma based on the medical algorithm 7-point checklist [7], which was mentioned in the introduction. One of the most important indicators in this work is the atypical pigment network. The team has published many papers on the CAD. However, the key publication on pigment network is [52], as it contains in-depth information about this team's final version of the method they propose for reticular pattern detection. The others are considered to be preliminary publications [28], or publications about the CAD, which in some cases were preceded by versions on reticular pattern detection [55, 56] and other final versions [15, 57, 58]. Reference [15] of the work cited is considered to be the most relevant to date about the CAD.

5.2.8   SERRANO AND ACHA (2009)

In [59], Serrano and Acha propose an algorithm based on Markov random fields (MRFs) [60] extended for color images that classifies images representing

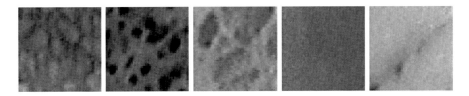

FIGURE 5.10 (See color insert.) In Serrano and Acha's method, five dermoscopic 40×40 image samples of each type of pattern to classify: reticular, globular, cobblestone, homogeneous, and parallel. (Reprinted with permission from Serrano, C. and Acha, B., *Pattern Recognition*, vol. 42, no. 6, pp. 1052–1057, 2009.)

different dermoscopic patterns: reticular, globular, cobblestone, homogeneous, and parallel.

In this method, the image is converted to different color spaces (RGB, YIQ, HSV, and L*a*b*) and each plane is modeled as an MRF, following a finite symmetric conditional model (FSCM). Once this has been completed, supervised machine learning is run on a database with 100 pieces of images with a size of 40×40, 20 of each pattern. See the diagram in Figure 5.10. No detailed information, sources, or how these image tiles were selected is given.

The statistical analysis is performed supposing that the MRF features in the three color planes follow a multivariate normal distribution, testing the models with two different assumptions: method 1, with the interplane independence assumption and method 2, without the interplane independence assumption. The k-nearest-neighbor method is also tested.

The best results are obtained with the L*a*b* color space and method 2, without the interplane independence assumption, reaching an average accuracy of 86% for the classification problem between the five patterns. For reticular pattern detection, 90% accuracy was achieved.

5.2.8.1 Other Related Studies

This work is a continuation of the preliminary study [61], by the same research team.

5.2.9 SKROVSETH ET AL. (2010)

In [62], Skrovseth et al. present a CAD to detect melanoma. One of the modules of this software detects the pigment network, classifying the image's different pixels and identifying those that belong to a pigment network and those that do not. It defines 20 texture measures (no information is given on what they are) and uses a linear classifier to select the three most significant, obtaining the optimal thresholds for each classification.

This work does not give information about the database used or the results obtained.

5.2.10   SHRESTHA ET AL. (2010)

In [63], Shrestha et al. use 5 of the statistical texture measures from the gray-level co-occurrence matrix (GLCM) presented by Haralick et al. [64]: energy, inertia, correlation, inverse difference, and entropy, computing the average and range of each of these variables, defining a total of 10 texture measures. The purpose of the study is to detect atypical pigment networks (APNs).

A total of 106 images were used, showing benign and malignant lesions (the number of each is not specified). An expert dermatologist marked the part of the lesion with the most irregular texture in all of them. These are called APN areas, as can be observed in Figure 5.11. In the case of melanoma, these areas contained one or more of the following features: thickened and dark pigment networks, branch streaks, radial streaming, or pseudopods. For the benign lesions, the areas chosen as APN areas were the most irregular areas. Using the 10 features described above, the APN areas were discriminated from those that were not. As part of the study, efforts were made to obtain the best distance (d-value) between the pixels for the GLCM matrices when calculating the texture.

The supervised machine learning process is run using six classifiers: BayesNet, ADTree, DecisionStump, J48, NBTree, and Random Forest, all of which are implemented on the data mining software tool WEKA [65]. The best feature is obtained for discrimination, which is the correlation average, yielding a result of 95.4% accuracy. For images of 768×512 pixels, 20 is found to be the optimal distance in the discrimination with an estimated resolution of 4–5 texels per mm, which is equivalent to a texel size of 0.2 mm, and is very important in the model generation, with no significant differences shown between the different classifiers. As in the previously mentioned study by

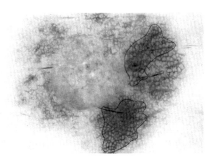
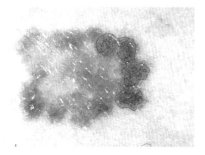

FIGURE 5.11   Shrestha et al.'s method, examples of areas marked by experts. Benign dysplastic nevus is shown on the left, with the atypical network area marked. On the right, melanoma in situ, with the atypical network area marked. (Reprinted with permission from Shrestha, B. et al., *Skin Research and Technology*, vol. 16, pp. 60–65, 2010.)

Anantha et al. [43], the conclusion is that the d-value, which determines the texel size, is critical in discrimination, with similar optimal values also being obtained in the two studies (0.22 mm in the study by Anantha et al. and 0.2 mm in the study by Shrestha et al.).

5.2.11   SADEGHI ET AL. (2011): WORK 1

In [66], Sadeghi et al. detect the pigment network in several steps. Firstly, they use a high-pass filter to sharpen the image to highlight the net of the pigment network, converted to grayscale, choosing the green channel of the RGB. Then they use a Laplacian of Gaussian (LoG) filter in order to properly capture the clear–dark–clear changes, obtaining a mask with the pixels that may be part of the structure. Once this has been done, a graph-based structure is created, linking the eight-connected components. The cyclical subgraphs are searched using the iterative loop counting algorithm (ILCA) [67], removing other round structures such as globules, dots, and oil bubbles, based on their size and color. Upon completion, another high-level graph is created from each correctly extracted subgraph, with a node corresponding to a hole in the pigment network. The nodes are connected by edges according to the distances between them. Finally, the image is classified according to the density ratio of the graph: $Density = |E|/(|V| \log[LesionSize])$, where $|E|$ is the number of edges in the graph, $|V|$ is the number of nodes of the graph, and $|LesionSize|$ is the size of the area of the image within the lesion boundary. Images containing a density ratio higher than a threshold (set to 1.5) are classified as present and the rest as absent. An overview of this process is shown in Figure 5.12. Two examples of pigment network detection are shown in Figure 5.13. Five hundred images were tested with 94.3% accuracy.

5.2.12   SADEGHI ET AL. (2010): WORK 2

In [68], Sadeghi et al. improve the algorithm and extend the previous study, presenting a new method for classification between absent, typical, and atypical. An overview of the system can be seen in Figure 5.14. As can be observed, the first stage is preprocessing, performing an image enhancement, which is followed by segmentation. The next stage is pigment network detection, the results of which are used to detect holes and nets. Thirdly, the structural, geometric, chromatic, and texture features are extracted. They make it possible to generate the classification model (stage 4).

In the preprocessing stage, a contrast-limited adaptive histogram equalization is applied to the image, which is then sharpened by removing a blurred version of it. Segmentation is performed using the method proposed by Wighton et al. [69].

Sadeghi et al.'s method [66] is used in the pigment network detection stage. As described above, this technique obtains a mask with the holes of the pigment network. The LoG filter is then applied to the green channel of the

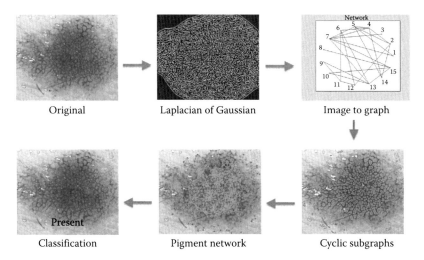

FIGURE 5.12 **(See color insert.)** Overview of the algorithm proposed by Sadeghi et al.: work 1. (Reprinted with permission from Sadeghi, M. et al., *Computerized Medical Imaging and Graphics*, vol. 35, pp. 137–143, 2011.)

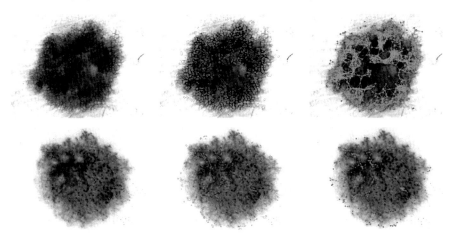

FIGURE 5.13 **(See color insert.)** Two examples with the algorithm proposed by Sadeghi et al.: work 1. Firstly, the original images; in the second place, the cyclic subgraphs; and thirdly, the diagnosis (present in the first lesion and absent in the second one). (Reprinted with permission from Sadeghi, M. et al., *Computerized Medical Imaging and Graphics*, vol. 35, pp. 137–143, 2011.)

image; 0.15 is set as the threshold value of this filter (although it can be tuned according to resolution and magnification), and the average thickness of the network and the average size of the holes can be observed. The LoG window size is also set to half of the average hole size in the image. The average window size over all the images in the dataset is 11 pixels. A threshold is

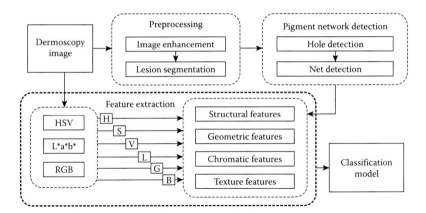

FIGURE 5.14   High-level view of the classification method proposed by Sadeghi et al.: work 2. (Reprinted with permission from Sadeghi, M. et al., *Lecture Notes in Computer Science*, vol. 6326, pp. 467–474, 2010.)

set for the filter response, resulting in a net mask that indicates which pixels belong to the net of the pigment network. The mask is also skeletonized.

In the feature extraction stage, a total of 69 features of four types are defined in the image in order to discriminate between absent, typical, and atypical. Firstly, the structural features for characterization is the typical pigment network (TPN) and atypical pigment network (APN): net thickness and variation in thickness as well as the size and variation in size of the network holes. Secondly, the geometric features were examined to characterize the uniformity of the network to discriminate TPN and APN. More specifically, the density ratio of the holes used in the study [66] and the hole irregularity added to it because the density ratio did not allow for correct discrimination between typical and atypical. Thirdly, the chromatic features are obtained. They are based on color characteristics, from the RGB, HSV, and L*a*b* spaces. Finally, textural features are obtained in the fourth stage. More specifically, these were five of the statistical texture measures of the GLCM presented by Haralick et al. in their classic work [64]: entropy, energy, contrast, correlation, and homogeneity.

Once the values of the features have been extracted, the classification model is generated with the LogitBoost algorithm. Of a total of 436 images (161 absent, 154 typical, and 121 atypical) 82.3% accuracy is obtained for the classification problem between absent, typical, and atypical, and in the experiments concerning both the absent and present categories, 93.3% accuracy is obtained. Two examples of pigment network detection are shown in Figure 5.15.

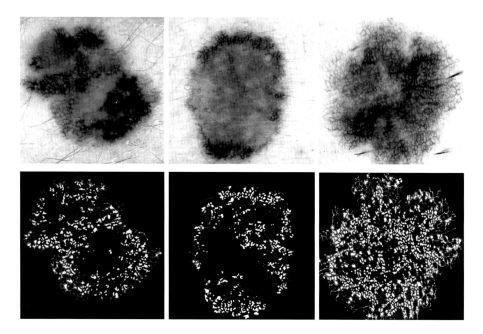

FIGURE 5.15 (See color insert.) In the method proposed by Sadeghi et al.: work 2, three images: the top row shows the original ones of APN, APN, and TPN; the bottom row shows their corresponding pigment networks. (Reprinted with permission from Sadeghi, M. et al., *Lecture Notes in Computer Science*, vol. 6326, pp. 467–474, 2010.)

5.2.12.1   Other Related Studies

This research team has published numerous works to date on this subject, both preliminary versions and later descriptions. Of all the works published to the present time, the most important are [66], in which the team develops a new pigment network detection method, and [68], in which the study is extended to cover atypical pigment network detection. Study [70] is considered to be a preliminary version of the first, and [71] (which also examines irregular streak detection) is the preliminary version of the second [72], a book chapter, which explains the team's work on pigment network detection.

5.2.13   GOLA ET AL. (2011)

In [23], Gola et al. presents a software system for detection of melanoma based on the ABCD rule [5], mentioned in the introduction of this paper, with the reticular pattern as an indicator.

In this approach the pigment network detection is conducted in three steps. Firstly, they convert the image to gray, using the formula $I_G(x, y) = 1/3\, I_{RGB}(x, y, 0) + 1/3\, I_{RGB}(x, y, 1) + 1/3\, I_{RGB}(x, y, 2)$. Secondly, they combine spectral techniques and the Canny edge detection algorithm [73], obtaining several masks as the result. Thirdly, they perform several morphological operations on these masks, obtaining the pigment network mask as a result. From this mask, they obtain the holes in the net, the number of which is used as a feature in discrimination between a reticular pattern present or absent in the lesion. An example showing the different steps of the algorithm is shown in Figure 5.16.

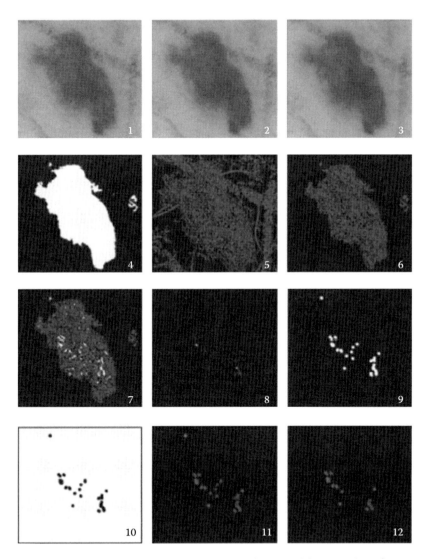

FIGURE 5.16 Example of the different steps in Gola et al.'s algorithm. (Reprinted with permission from Isasi, A. G. et al., *Computers in Biology and Medicine*, vol. 41, pp. 742–755, 2011.)

A 150-image dataset is used to tune and test the algorithm, 20 images having reticular pattern. A linear discriminant function is used to obtain the optimal threshold for the values of the number of holes in the nets detected. The method achieved 90% accuracy in detecting images with pigment network.

5.2.13.1 Other Related Studies

This work further develops a preliminary study [74] in which, like the study presented, other dermatoscopic structures are examined.

5.2.14 WIGHTON ET AL. (2011)

In [69], Wighton et al. present an algorithm for the detection of hair and pigment network based on supervised machine learning, using color features (CIEL*a*b* features) and spectral features (Gaussian and Laplacian of Gaussian filters at various scales features extracted), followed by linear discriminant analysis (LDA) for the reduction of dimensionality and the maximum a posteriori probability (MAP) Bayesian method, based on multivariate Gaussian distributions for generation of the model. A diagram of the training phase can be seen in Figure 5.17, and the classification process can be seen in Figure 5.18.

The aim is to differentiate between absent and present in pigment network detection. A total of 20 images with pigment network across the entire lesion and another 20 with no-pigment network were selected for this purpose. The masks of the skin lesions were obtained to identify the different pixels in the 40 images as background (pixels outside the lesion), absent (nonreticular pixels of the skin lesion), and present (reticular pixels of the skin lesion). An example of this analysis can be seen in Figure 5.19.

The test was run on a total of 734 images, without reported results in the pigment network detection.

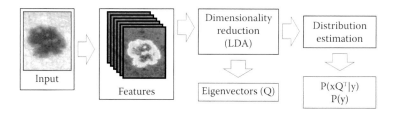

FIGURE 5.17 The training phase of Wighton et al.'s method. Features are computed from a training set whose dimensionality is then reduced via LDA. The posterior probabilities of the labels are modeled as multivariate Gaussian distributions and saved along with the eigenvectors obtained from LDA. (Wighton, P. et al., *IEEE Transactions on Information Technology in Biomedicine*, vol. 15, pp. 622–629. © 2011 IEEE.)

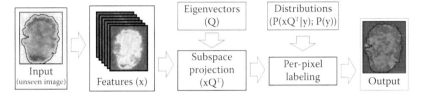

FIGURE 5.18   Classification phase of Wighton et al.'s method. For a previously unseen image, features are computed as in the previous stage and the dimensionality of the feature space is reduced using the eigenvectors obtained in the training phase. MAP estimation is then used along with the posterior probabilities from the training phase to label the image. (Wighton, P. et al., *IEEE Transactions on Information Technology in Biomedicine*, vol. 15, pp. 622–629. © 2011 IEEE.)

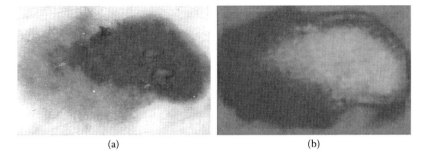

(a)   (b)

FIGURE 5.19   Example of the classification obtained with Wighton et al.'s method. (a) Original dermoscopic images. (b) The likelihoods of pixels to be background, absent, and present. (Wighton, P. et al., *IEEE Transactions on Information Technology in Biomedicine*, vol. 15, pp. 622–629. © 2011 IEEE.)

5.2.15   BARATA ET AL. (2012)

In the study [75], Barata et al. present a pigment network detection method. As can be seen in Figure 5.20, which presents the high-level view of the system, the process consists of three stages. Firstly, the image is preprocessed. Secondly, the pigment network detection is performed. The third stage is classification, determining if the lesion has a pigment network or not.

In the preprocessing stage, the researchers convert the images to a grayscale, using the results of a previous study [76], which makes an automatic selection of the color component based on its entropy, choosing the one which has the highest entropy. They then perform reflection and hair detection and removal (this paper will not study the techniques used in this task).

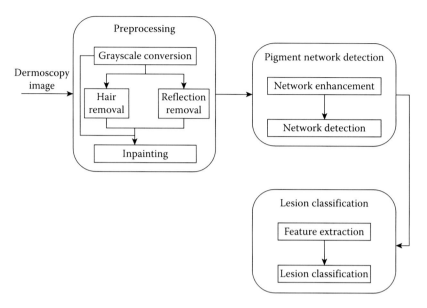

FIGURE 5.20 High-level view of Barata et al.'s method. (Barata, C. et al., *IEEE Transactions on Biomedical Engineering*, vol. 59, pp. 2744–2754. © 2012 IEEE.)

The first step in the pigment network detection stage is image enhancement, in which the lines associated with pigment network are sharpened in relation to their background. A bank of N directional filters is used for this purpose. Optimal values are set empirically for these filters, and the pixels that form the pigment network are selected, based on a set threshold value T_R. Morphological operations based on the 8-connectivity criterion are used next to determine the mask resulting from the union of all the submasks that have an area larger than a minimum area A_{min}, which is an empirically set threshold. An example of this procedure can be seen in Figure 5.21. In the tests, the pigment network obtained is compared to the ground truths that have been previously segmented manually by expert dermatologists, as shown in Figure 5.22.

Once the pigment network has been detected, the mask generated is used to begin the image classification stage. Five different morphological features are calculated from it. They are used to train the AdaBoost classifier in a supervised machine learning process with a database containing 200 images, 88 of which have a pigment network and 112 that do not. The ground truths segmented by the experts and the image labeling are used to tune the model.

The method is tested, trying different N, T_R, and A_{min} parameter values and by running a receiver operating characteristic (ROC) analysis. Lastly, having established values of 9, 0.0185, and 900 for these parameters, respectively, the optimal sensitivity value of 91.1% and a specificity of 82.1% are obtained

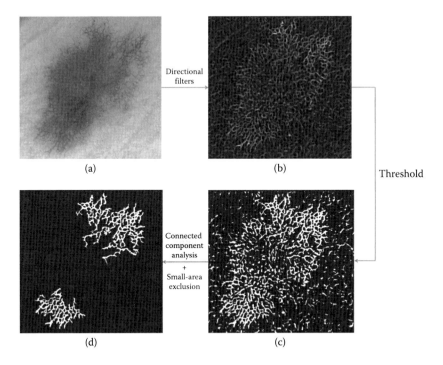

FIGURE 5.21 Example of pigment network detection with Barata et al.'s method: (a) original image in gray; (b) applying directional filters; (c) binarization using threshold values; (d) 8-connected component analysis and removing small areas. (Barata, C. et al., *IEEE Transactions on Biomedical Engineering*, vol. 59, pp. 2744–2754. © 2012 IEEE.)

with the 200-image database, and also obtaining good results in the detection of reticular pixels, with respect to the ground truths segmented by the experts: a sensitivity of 57.6% and a specificity of 85.4%.

5.2.15.1 Other Related Studies

This study can be considered the culmination of the previous works [77–79].

5.2.16 ABBAS ET AL. (2012): WORK 1

In [80], Abbas et al. present an algorithm that classifies images of six dermoscopic patterns: reticular, globular, cobblestone, homogeneous, parallel ridge, and starbust. Firstly, they transform to CIEL*a*b* color space and then perform the preprocessing, detecting, and removing of disturbing artifacts, followed by segmentation of the skin lesion. From this area color features are extracted, related to the percentage of occurrence of the six typical skin lesion colors and the degree of symmetry thereof, as well as texture features,

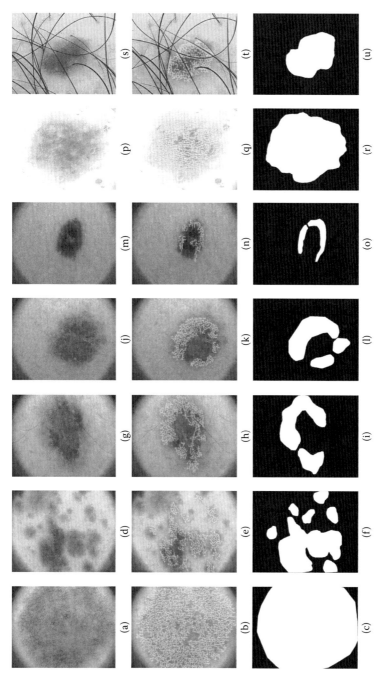

FIGURE 5.22 Barata et al.'s method, seven examples of pigment network detection: original image (top), output of the detection system—with pigment network (middle), medical ground truth (bottom). (Barata, C. et al., *IEEE Transactions on Biomedical Engineering*, vol. 59, pp. 2744–2754. © 2012 IEEE.)

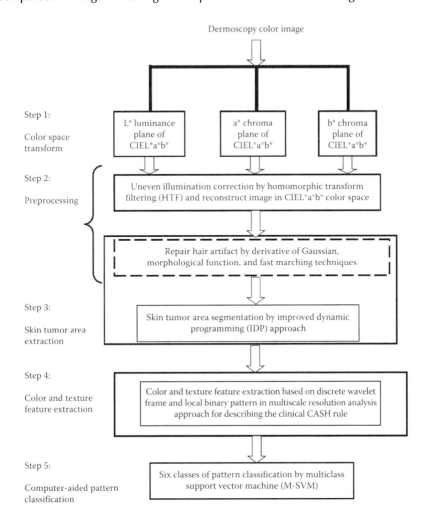

FIGURE 5.23 Flow diagram of the method proposed by Abbas et al.: work 1. (Reprinted with permission from Abbas, Q. et al., *Skin Research and Technology*, vol. 18, no. 3, pp. 278–289, 2012.)

extracted using discrete wavelet frame (DWF) [81] and local binary pattern (LBP) [82]. Both color and texture features are extracted with a sliding window of 16×16 pixels. As a final result, there is a vector with two color and six texture features. In Figure 5.23 the design of the method can be observed.

The dataset has 180 images, 30 of each pattern. The training and testing are performed using a multiclass support vector machine (M-SVM) [83], obtaining reticular pattern detection with results of 90% sensitivity, 93% specificity, and 0.94 area under the curve (AUC).

5.2.17 ABBAS ET AL. (2012): WORK 2

In [84], Abbas et al. from the same research group of the previous work [80] and also from Serrano and Acha's group [59], present a method that performs the classification between seven dermoscopic patterns: reticular, globular, cobblestone, homogeneous, parallel ridge, starbust, and multicomponent.

The high-level view can be seen in Figure 5.24. As shown, the method is performed over image tiles of 450×450, carrying out in the first place a transformation to the CIECAM02 color space, and then extracting color and texture features. The color features are the same as in the previous work [80]. For the extraction of texture features, the method uses a steerable pyramid transformation (SPT) decomposition algorithm [85, 86], performing a multiscale texture feature extraction, as can be seen in Figure 5.25. From these features a selection process is done using principal component analysis (PCA), obtaining the most significant ones.

Using a multilabel learning with the extracted data, a pattern classification model is generated. For this task an extension of the AdaBoost.MH [87] algorithm to multiclass output, called AdaBoost.MC, is used, implementing maximum a posterior (MAP) and ranking strategies.

Over an image database of 350 image tiles, 50 of each pattern, the results in the reticular pattern detection are 87.11% sensitivity, 97.96% specificity, and 0.981 AUC. The generated model is also tested against two other ones, generated by multilabel SVM (ML-SVM) and multilabel k-nearest neighbor (ML-kNN), respectively, obtaining the best accuracy with the model generated by AdaBoost.MC.

5.2.18 ABBAS ET AL. (2013)

In [16], Abbas et al. from the same research group of the previous works [80, 84] present a melanoma recognition system based on the ABCD rule [5], the reticular pattern being one of its indicators. With respect to reticular pattern, in the first place there is a transformation to CIEL*a*b* space, and after performing the preprocessing (detecting and removing disturbing artifacts), followed by segmentation of the skin lesion, the pigment network detection is done. For this purpose, color and texture features are extracted. The color features are the same as in the previous works [80, 84]. The texture features are obtained using the radon-like transform [88] and LBP [82], different from those extracted in the work [80], though inspired by the same idea. The features corresponding to this indicator are saved with the other ones corresponding to the other indicators of ABCD, in a vector of features.

On the vector of features a selection process using sequential floating forward selection (SFFS) is performed and the model is generated with the SVM classifier. Over a database of 120 images (60 melanomas, 10 blue nevi, 15 Clark nevi, 10 combined nevi, 15 congenital nevi, and 10 dermal nevi) the method

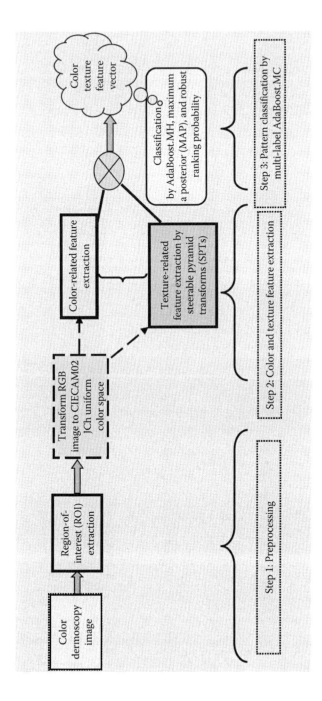

FIGURE 5.24 Flowchart of the pattern classification model for dermoscopy images proposed by Abbas et al.: work 2. (Reprinted with permission from Abbas, Q. et al., *Pattern Recognition*, vol. 46, no. 1, pp. 86–97, 2012.)

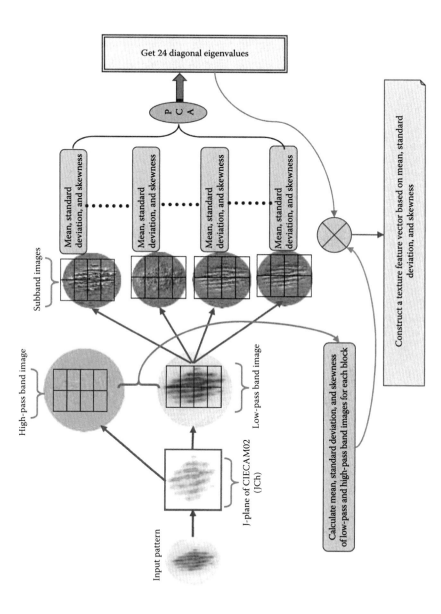

FIGURE 5.25 Design of the multiscale texture feature extraction in the method proposed by Abbas et al.: work 2. (Reprinted with permission from Abbas, Q. et al., *Pattern Recognition*, vol. 46, no. 1, pp. 86–97, 2012.)

obtains 88.2% sensitivity, 91.30% specificity, and 0.880 AUC in melanoma detection. Regarding the detection of pigment network, no result is reported.

5.2.19   SÁEZ ET AL. (2014)

In [89], Sáez et al. from the same research group of the previous works [59, 84] carry out the classification of dermoscopic images between three global patterns: reticular, globular, and homogeneous.

Two different training sets of images are used, as can be seen in Figure 5.26: the first one with the complete lesions and the second one with image patches extracted from the original images, corresponding to the different patterns. The test set is composed of complete lesions. In order to analyze each whole lesion, the lesion is divided into overlapping patches of optimal size, found experimentally, set to 81×81 pixels (proposed in [90]).

In the method, the image is first converted to L*a*b* color space. Then, after making the segmentation, the skin lesion is modeled as Markov random fields (MRFs) [60] following, as suggested by Xia et al. [91], a finite symmetric conditional model (FSCM) [92]. In order to obtain texture features, three different models are used, in both training sets for image patches and images of whole lesions: Gaussian model, Gaussian mixture model, and a bag-of-features (BoF) model. For each case, the classification is done with an image retrieval approach, using different distance metrics, followed by the k-nearest-neighbor algorithm (kNN) for the final classification.

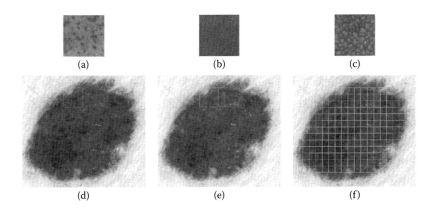

FIGURE 5.26 (**See color insert.**) Examples of the two image sets used. (a–c) First set: Individual patches. 81×81 dermoscopic individual patches belonging to (a) globular pattern, (b) homogeneous pattern, and (c) reticular pattern. (d–f) Second image set: Complete lesions. (d) 81×81 sample extracted from the whole lesion. (e) Displacement equal to 27 rows or 27 columns is applied to obtain the following sample. (f) Overlapping samples to analyze the whole lesion. (Sáez, A. et al., *IEEE Transactions on Medical Imaging*, vol. 33, pp. 1137–1147. © 2014 IEEE.)

A 90-image dataset is used to test the algorithm, 30 images per pattern. The best results were obtained using the Gaussian mixture model and the distance metric proposed in [93], obtaining 75.33% accuracy in reticular recognition and 78.44% accuracy in the three-pattern classification problem.

5.2.20 GARCÍA ET AL. (2014)

In [94], García et al. present an algorithm for detection of the reticular pattern from dermoscopic images, consisting of two blocks, as can be seen in Figure 5.27. In the first one, a supervised machine learning process is carried out generating a set of rules that, when applied to the image, make it possible to obtain a mask with the pixels that are candidates to be part of the pigment network. In the second one, this mask is processed by conducting a structural analysis process to detect the reticular pattern. The purpose is to obtain the diagnosis, that is, determine whether it has a pigment network, and to generate the mask corresponding to that structure, if any.

The design of block 1 can be observed in Figure 5.28. As shown, the process consists of four stages. In the first place, the training data are set. Secondly, the features are extracted in order to feed the machine learning process. Obviously, the features chosen are those considered to be the most suitable for the characterization of the pixels that are part of a pigment network. There are two types of features: color features, based on RGB and rgb (RGB normalized) color spaces; HSV, CIEXYZ, CIEL*a*b*, and CIEL*u*v*, based on the median values in a neighborhood of 5×5; and texture features (spectral and statistical), taken from the image converted to gray with the formula $I_G(x,y) = 0.2989\,I_{RGB}(x,y,0) + 0.587\,I_{RGB}(x,y,1) + 0.114\,I_{RGB}(x,y,2)$. The spectral texture features are taken by applying a bank of Gaussian filters $\sigma = 1, 2, 4, \ldots, \sigma_{max}$, with $\sigma_{max} = 8$, and the Sobel,

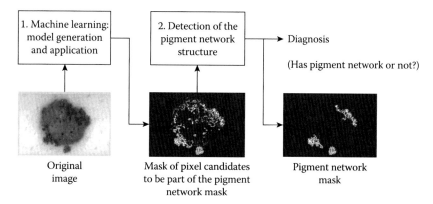

1. Machine learning: model generation and application	2. Detection of the pigment network structure	Diagnosis

(Has pigment network or not?)

Original image	Mask of pixel candidates to be part of the pigment network mask	Pigment network mask

FIGURE 5.27 High-level view of the method proposed by García et al. (Reprinted with permission from García Arroyo, J. L. and García Zapirain, B., *Computers in Biology and Medicine*, vol. 44, pp. 144–157, 2014.)

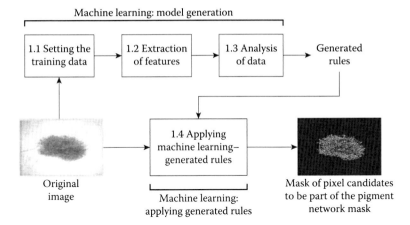

FIGURE 5.28 High-level view of the block 1: Machine learning: model generation and application of the method proposed by García et al. (Reprinted with permission from García Arroyo, J. L. and García Zapirain, B., *Computers in Biology and Medicine*, vol. 44, pp. 144–157, 2014.)

Hessian, Gaussian, and difference of Gaussian (DoG) features are collected later. The statistical features are taken from the calculation of the GLCM by Haralick et al. in [64], for matrix sizes $n = 1, 3, \ldots, n_{max}$, with $n_{max} = 7$, and for variance and entropy. Once this is completed, the third step is analysis of the data, using the C4.5 [54] method. The result is the construction of a classification model and implementation of the generated rules, as a decision tree. Finally, in the fourth place, the generated rules are applied to the image in an iterative process over all the pixels in the image, obtaining the mask corresponding to the pixels that are candidates to be part of the pigment network.

The design of block 2 can be observed in Figure 5.29. As shown, the process of detecting the pigment network structure consists of four stages:

- Stage 1: the 8-connected components higher than a threshold area $numPixelsSubRegion_{min}$ value of 100 are obtained.
- Stage 2: each one of them is iterated, determining whether they have a reticular structure (firstly by looking for holes larger than a threshold $numPixelsHole_{min}$ value of 20 and secondly by checking the conditions so that the percentage of the area of these holes is higher than the threshold $percentHolesSubmask_{min}$ value of 0.04 and the number of holes is higher than the threshold $numHolesSubmask_{min}$ value of 3) and also calculating the number of holes.
- Stage 3: the diagnosis is carried out, determining whether it has a reticular structure and if the number and total number of holes are higher than the threshold $numHolesTotal_{min}$ value of 5.
- Stage 4: if positive, the mask of the pigment network is generated.

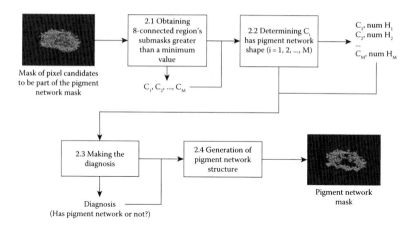

FIGURE 5.29 High-level view of block 2: Detection of the pigment network structure in the method proposed by García et al. (Reprinted with permission from García Arroyo, J. L. and García Zapirain, B., *Computers in Biology and Medicine*, vol. 44, pp. 144–157, 2014.)

The reliability of the method was tested by analyzing the results obtained with the image database consisting of 220 images, comprising 120 without a reticular structure and 100 with such a structure. All the images were catalogued by expert dermatologists. The method showed 83.64% accuracy, 86% sensitivity, and 81.67% specificity. Examples of pigment network detection are shown in Figure 5.30.

5.3 SUMMARY OF THE USED TECHNIQUES

This section summarizes the different techniques used in the state-of-the-art methods described in Section 5.2.

The techniques used have been classified into two categories:

1. Image processing
2. Statistical techniques and data mining

Table 5.1 shows the techniques used in each study by groups, presenting the category, description of the task performed, and the name of the technique.

As can be seen, most of the works included the following techniques. Firstly, images are converted to grayscale (using different color spaces), with texture analysis carried out on the image in gray, together with other types of analysis, and usually combined with morphological operations. Secondly, over the result, as the mask with the region that is candidate to be a pigment network, different types of features (including in most cases morphological/geometric/structural) are extracted for the characterization of whether it has a reticular pattern, and if it is reticular, whether it is typical or atypical. Finally, this is fed into a supervised machine learning process by either performing

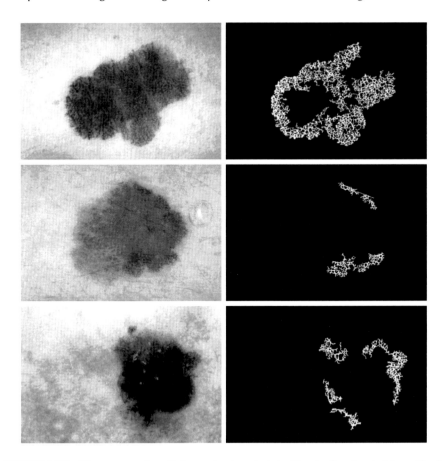

FIGURE 5.30   Three examples of pigment network detection in García et al.'s method. (Reprinted with permission from García Arroyo, J. L. and García Zapirain, B., *Computers in Biology and Medicine*, vol. 44, pp. 144–157, 2014.)

an empirical selection of threshold values or using a statistical function or a classifier.

In general terms, this is the technique–pattern that most of the studies follow. Notwithstanding, as can be observed, other different techniques are often used and different objectives are pursued.

In order to obtain the pigment network, there are different types of techniques: color [16, 52, 66, 69, 80, 84, 94], line detection [16, 23, 35, 37, 48], thresholding [35, 41, 50, 52], spectral features [23, 50, 52, 66, 68, 69, 75, 94], GLCM [63, 68, 94], LBP [16, 80], snakes [37], Laws' energy masks [43], NGLDM [43], MRF [59, 89], DWF [80], and SPT [84].

Almost all of the works use morphological techniques when working with the pigment network detected. As mentioned, the main objective of most of the studies is determining whether it has a reticular pattern or discerning

TABLE 5.1

Techniques Used in the Most Relevant Works

Proposed Work	Type	Task	Techniques
Fischer et al. 1996 [35]	IP	Transformation to grayscale	Karhunen–Loeve transformation [36]
	IP	Contrast enhancement for the network detection	Local histogram equalization
	IP	Noise removal	Gray-level morphological operations
	IP	Obtaining the pigment network	Obtaining threshold
Fleming et al. 1999 [37]	IP	Transformation to grayscale	First plane of the CIEXYZ transform
	IP	Extraction of the net	Steger curvilinear line detection algorithm [38]
	IP	Segmentation of the holes	Snake Lobregt–Viergever model [39]
	SD	Statistical analysis	ANOVA, linear discrimination function
Caputo et al. 2002 [41]	IP	Prefiltering, removing the noise	Wiener filter [42]
	IP	Prefiltering, image enhancing	Histogram stretching operation [42]
	IP	Extraction of the network structure	Adaptative thresholding [42]
	IP	Characterization of the network	Calculation of statistical indicators
	SD	Statistical analysis	Selection of thresholds and application
Anantha et al. 2004 [43]	IP	Texture analysis for obtaining pigment network	Laws' energy masks [45]
	IP	Texture analysis for obtaining pigment network	Neighborhood gray-level dependence matrix (NGLDM) [46]
	IP	Characterization of the network	Structural features
	SD	Statistical analysis	Selection of thresholds and application
Grana et al. 2007 [48]	IP	Detection of the net points	Steger curvilinear line detection algorithm [38]
	SD	Selection of the best points belonging to the net	Fisher linear discriminant analysis
	IP	Linking the points of the net	Bilinear interpolation and gray-level morphological operations
	IP	Validation of meshes	Area and circularity values
	SD	Statistical analysis	Linear discriminant function

(Continued)

TABLE 5.1 (*Continued*)
Techniques Used in the Most Relevant Works

Proposed Work	Type	Task	Techniques
Tanaka et al. 2008 [50]	IP	Discrimination between homogeneous, and reticular and globular	Intensity histogram, differential statistical, Fourier power spectrum, run-length matrix and co-occurrence matrix features
	IP	Discrimination between reticular and globular	Run-length matrix using intensity and connected component of black and white after binarization features
	SD	Statistical analysis	F-test, t-test, stepwise method, and discriminant method
Di Leo et al. 2008 [52]	IP	Obtaining the atypical pigment network	Morphological methods
	IP	Obtaining the atypical pigment network	Spectral methods based on Fourier analysis: FFT, high-pass filters, inverse FFT, and thresholding techniques
	IP	Pigment network characterization	Chromatic and spatial features
	SD	Model generation	C4.5 decision tree classifier [54]
Serrano and Acha 2009 [59]	IP	Transformation to grayscale	Transformation to L*a*b* color space
	IP	Pattern characterization	Markov random field (MRF) [60]
	SD	Statistical analysis (selected)	Multivariate normal distribution, without the interplane independence assumption
	SD	Statistical analysis (not selected)	Multivariate normal distribution, with the interplane independence assumption, and the K-nearest neighbor
Skrovseth et al. 2010 [62]	IP	Pigment network pixel characterization	Texture measures
	SD	Statistical analysis	Linear classifier
Shrestha et al. 2010 [63]	IP	Obtaining the pigment network	Texture measures from GLCM [64]
	IP	Characterization of the network	Structural features
	SD	Model generation	Six classifiers implemented in WEKA [65]: BayesNet, ADTree, DecisionStump, J48, NBTree, and Random Forest

(Continued)

TABLE 5.1 (*Continued*)
Techniques Used in the Most Relevant Works

Proposed Work	Type	Task	Techniques
Sadeghi et al. 2011 [66]	IP	Pigment network enhancement	Sharpening high-pass filter
	IP	Pigment network detection: capture the clear–dark–clear changes	Laplacian of Gaussian (LoG) filter
	IP	Pigment network detection: graph-based structure	8-connected components' morphological operations
	IP	Pigment network detection: select the correct submasks	Cyclical subgraphs searched using the iterative loop counting algorithm (ILCA) algorithm [67]
	IP	Characterization of the net	Graph-based density feature
	SD	Decision between absent and present	Based on threshold value of density
Sadeghi et al. 2010 [68]	IP	Pigment network enhancement	Contrast-limited adaptive histogram equalization
	IP	Pigment network enhancement	Sharpening high-pass filter
	IP	Pigment network detection: capture the clear–dark–clear changes	Laplacian of Gaussian (LoG) filter
	IP	Pigment network detection: graph-based structure	8-connected components' morphological operations
	IP	Pigment network detection: select the correct submasks	Cyclical subgraphs searched using the ILCA algorithm [67]
	IP	Characterization of the net	Structural features: variations in thickness of net and size of network holes
	IP	Characterization of the net	Geometric features: graph-based density and hole irregularity features
	IP	Characterization of the net	Chromatic features: corresponding to RGB, HSV, and L*a*b* color spaces
	IP	Characterization of the net	Texture features: based on GLCM [64]
	SD	Model generation	LogitBoost algorithm
Gola et al. 2011 [23]	IP	Pigment network shape detection	Spectral techniques
	IP	Pigment network line detection	Canny edge detection algorithm [73]
	IP	Obtaining the pigment network	Morphological methods
	IP	Characterization of the network	Structural features
	SD	Statistical analysis	Linear discriminant function

(Continued)

TABLE 5.1 (*Continued*)
Techniques Used in the Most Relevant Works

Proposed Work	Type	Task	Techniques
Wighton et al. 2011 [69]	IP	Pigment network pixel color characterization	Color features (CIEL*a*b* features)
	IP	Pigment network pixel texture characterization	Spectral features (Gaussian and Laplacian of Gaussian filter features)
	IP	Characterization of the network	Structural features
	SD	Reduction of dimensionality	Linear discriminant analysis (LDA)
	SD	Model generation	Multivariate Gaussian distributions, maximum a posteriori probability (MAP) Bayesian method
Barata et al. 2012 [75]	IP	Transformation to grayscale	Selection of the color component with highest entropy
	IP	Pigment network detection	Bank of directional filters
	IP	Pigment network detection	Morphological methods
	IP	Pigment network characterization	Structural features
	SD	Model generation	AdaBoost, ROC analysis
Abbas et al. 2012 [80]	IP	Transformation to color space	Transformation to CIEL*a*b* color space
	IP	Pigment network characterization	Color features: percentage of occurrence and degree of symmetry, respect to the 6 typical colors in skin lesions
	IP	Pigment network characterization	Texture features based on discrete wavelet frame (DWF) decomposition [81]
	IP	Pigment network characterization	Texture features based on local binary pattern (LBP) [82]
	SD	Model generation	Multiclass support vector machine (M-SVM) [83]
Abbas et al. 2012 [84]	IP	Transformation to color space	Transformation to CIEL*a*b* color space
	IP	Pigment network characterization	Color features: percentage of occurrence and degree of symmetry, respect to the 6 typical colors in skin lesions
	IP	Pigment network characterization	Multiscale texture features based on steerable pyramid transformation (SPT) decomposition algorithm [85, 86]

(Continued)

TABLE 5.1 (*Continued*)
Techniques Used in the Most Relevant Works

Proposed Work	Type	Task	Techniques
	SD	Selection of features	Principal component analysis (PCA)
	SD	Model generation	AdaBoost.MC: extension of the AdaBoost.MH algorithm Reference [87] to multiclass output, implementing maximum a posterior (MAP) and ranking strategies
Abbas et al. 2013 [16]	IP	Transformation to color space	Transformation to CIEL*a*b* color space
	IP	Pigment network characterization	Color features: percentage of occurrence and degree of symmetry, respect to the 6 typical colors in skin lesions
	IP	Pigment network characterization	Texture features based on radon-like transform [88] and local binary pattern (LBP) [82]
	SD	Selection of features	Sequential floating forward selection (SFFS)
	SD	Model generation	SVM classifier
Sáez et al. 2014 [89]	IP	Transformation to grayscale	Transformation to L*a*b* color space
	IP	Pattern characterization	Markov random field (MRF) [60]
	IP	Pattern characterization	Texture features based on Gaussian model
	IP	Pattern characterization	Texture features based on Gaussian mixture model
	IP	Pattern characterization	Texture features based on BoF model
	SD	Model generation	kNN algorithm
García et al. 2014 [94]	IP	Characterization of pigment network pixels	Color features: based on RGB, rgb (RGB normalized), HSV, CIEXYZ, CIEL*a*b*, and CIEL*u*v* color spaces
	IP	Characterization of pigment network pixels	Spectral texture features: bank of Gaussian filters, Sobel, Hessian, Gaussian, and difference of Gaussian (DoG) features
	IP	Characterization of pigment network pixels	Statistical texture features: from GLCM [64]
	SD	Model generation for the extraction of the pigment network pixels	C4.5 decision tree classifier [54]

(Continued)

TABLE 5.1 (*Continued*)
Techniques Used in the Most Relevant Works

Proposed Work	Type	Task	Techniques
	SD	Detection of the network structure	Morphological operations
	IP	Characterization of the network	Structural features
	SD	Model generation	C4.5 decision tree classifier [54]

Note: IP, image processing; SD, statistical or data mining.

between typical and atypical in the case of reticular patterns. For this purpose, most of them include morphological/structural/geometric characterizations of the pigment network [23, 41, 43, 48, 52, 63, 66, 68, 69, 75, 94] and, in some cases, mapping of the network structure to a graph-based structure [66, 68]. Sometimes chromatic features are used [16, 52, 66, 69, 80, 84, 89, 94].

The statistical and data mining models generated in some cases simply give threshold values used in decision making [41, 66], while statistical functions are used in others [23, 37, 48, 50, 59, 62, 69]. Lastly, other studies use classifiers [16, 52, 59, 63, 68, 75, 80, 84, 89, 94].

5.4 COMPARISON OF RESULTS

This section presents the results obtained with the different methods described and compares them.

The different outputs obtained for each of these studies have been categorized as follows:

1. Recognition of pigment network
2. Recognition of atypical pigment network
3. Other

As can be observed in the explanation of these methods, recognition of pigment network (differentiating between absent and present) and recognition of atypical pigment network (differentiating between absent, typical, and atypical) are the main outputs of automated reticular pattern detection. There are methods that center solely on obtaining the pigment network structure, without offering results for the problem of pattern recognition (pigment network or atypical pigment network), presenting other types of quantitative results, or even not showing any (having been included in this chapter due to their interesting design and techniques used). In any case, most of the methods center on the pattern recognition problems.

The quantitative information is usually shown as data on sensitivity, specificity, and accuracy for a previously labeled database. Moreover, as we have mentioned, other types of quantitative information are sometimes reported, and even many of the studies do not contribute quantitative results.

As for the reliability of the results obtained, there are variables other than numerical data that must be taken into account. One of the most important is the number of images used. The number of images used varies in these studies. An algorithm is obviously more reliable when it is has been tested with more images.

Other important variables are the number of image sources and how difficult they are. Firstly, if the images are extracted from different sources, with different features, this implies greater robustness as opposed to those acquired in other conditions. Secondly, when the images selected to test a method are more difficult, this makes the results more reliable and robust. Regarding the number of sources, none of the studies specifies a number of sources (only in the case of [68] are two different atlases used for the tests, but they are obtained from the same source of data, so we can consider them a single source), and these data will therefore not be taken into account in the analysis. The difficulty of the images is certainly not easy to judge, and since this is barely mentioned in these studies, it will not be taken into account here either.

Table 5.2 includes a summary of the results obtained in the studies describing the state of the art, which are very diverse.

As can be observed, some works do not give numerical results [16, 35, 62, 69]. They have been included in this study because they propose innovative algorithms that are of interest to the state of the art. Nevertheless, the fact that they do not present quantitative results means that their reliability and robustness have not been assured.

Some results are not specifically about reticular or atypical reticular pattern recognition. In [37], the study focuses on finding the features of reticular structures (obtaining the mean line width and mean hole area as the most significant) and how to use these features to discriminate between nevus and melanoma. In [41], typical and atypical pigment networks are distinguished, although we do not place the study in the category of atypical reticular pattern recognition because there are no images without pigment network. The studies [50, 59, 80, 84, 89] discriminate between different patterns (homogeneous, reticular, and globular in [50]; reticular, globular, cobblestone, homogeneous, and parallel in [59]; reticular, globular, cobblestone, homogeneous, parallel ridge, and starbust in [80]; reticular, globular, cobblestone, homogeneous, parallel ridge, starbust, and multicomponent in [84]; and reticular, globular, and homogeneous in [89]), using in [50, 59, 84] image tiles with these patterns and in [80, 89] complete images. Finally, studies [43, 63] obtain the optimal texel measurements to detect pigment network using texture analysis, showing similar results in both works, using [43] image tiles and [63] image areas. Regarding

TABLE 5.2
Numerical Results Obtained in the Most Relevant Works

Proposed Work	Type	Output	N	Numerical Results
Fischer et al. 1996 [35]	No numerical results			
Fleming et al. 1999 [37]	OTH	Mean line width	69	Common nevi, 6.72; dysplastic nevi, 7.03; melanomas, 8.58
	OTH	Mean hole area	69	Common nevi, 251; dysplastic nevi, 308; melanomas, 345
	OTH	Discrimination between nevus and melanoma	69	80% ACC, using mean line width and mean hole area values
Caputo et al. 2002 [41]	OTH	Differentiation between typical and atypical pigment network	14	85.71% ACC, in the differentiation between 7 typical and 7 atypical
Anantha et al. 2004 [43]	OTH	Optimal texel size for the pigment network detection	155	10 pixels (0.22 mm, with the used image resolution)
	RPN	Detection of pigment network: discrimination between no-pigment network, partial, and full-pigment network	155	80% ACC in image tiles of size 64×64
Grana et al. 2007 [48]	RPN	Detection of pigment network	100	82% SE, 94% SP, 88% ACC
Tanaka et al. 2008 [50]	OTH	Discrimination between homogeneous, globular, and reticular patterns	852	94% ACC in 852 image tiles
Di Leo et al. 2008 [52]	RAPN	Detection of atypical pigment network	173	>85% SE, >85% SP
Serrano and Acha 2009 [59]	OTH	Discrimination between reticular, globular, cobblestone, homogeneous, and parallel patterns	100	86% ACC in 100 image tiles of size 40×40 (20 for each pattern)
	OTH	Discrimination between reticular and the others: globular, cobblestone, homogeneous, and parallel	100	90% ACC in 100 image tiles of size 40×40 (20 for each pattern)
Skrovseth et al. 2010 [62]	No numerical results			

(Continued)

TABLE 5.2 (*Continued*)
Numerical Results Obtained in the Most Relevant Works

Proposed Work	Type	Output	N	Numerical Results
Shrestha et al. 2010 [63]	OTH	Optimal size of GLCM	106	20 pixels (texel size of 0.2 mm, with the used image resolution, approximately 4–5 texels per mm)
	RAPN	Detection of atypical pigment network: discrimination between APN and non-APN areas	106	95.4% ACC in APN and non-APN areas marked in the images
Sadeghi et al. 2011 [66]	RPN	Detection of pigment network	500	94.3% ACC
Sadeghi et al. 2010 [68]	RPN	Detection of pigment network	436	93.3% ACC
	RAPN	Detection of atypical pigment network: discrimination between absent, typical, and atypical	436	82.3% ACC
Gola et al. 2011 [23]	RPN	Detection of pigment network	150	90% ACC (only 20 reticular images in the image database)
Wighton et al. 2011 [69]	No numerical results			
Barata et al. 2012 [75]	OTH	Detection of reticular pixels	200	57.6% SE, 85.4% SP, respect to the ground truths segmented by the experts
	RPN	Detection of pigment network	155	91.1% SE, 82.1% SP
Abbas et al. 2012 [80]	OTH	Discrimination between reticular and the other patterns: globular, cobblestone, homogeneous, parallel ridge, and starbust	100	90% SE, 93% SP, 0.94 AUC
Abbas et al. 2012 [84]	OTH	Discrimination between reticular and the other patterns: globular, cobblestone, homogeneous, parallel ridge, starbust, and multicomponent	350	87.11% SE, 97.96% SP, 0.981 AUC in 350 image tiles of size 450×450

(Continued)

TABLE 5.2 (*Continued*)

Numerical Results Obtained in the Most Relevant Works

Proposed Work	Type	Output	N	Numerical Results
Abbas et al. 2013 [16]	No numerical results			
Sáez et al. 2014 [89]	OTH	Discrimination between reticular, globular, and homogeneous patterns	90	78.44% ACC
	OTH	Discrimination between reticular and the others: globular and homogeneous	90	75.33% ACC
García et al. 2014 [94]	RPN	Detection of pigment network	220	86% SE, 81.67% SP, 83.64% ACC

Note: RPN, recognition of pigment network; RAPN, recognition of atypical pigment network; OTH, other; ACC, accuracy; SE, sensitivity; SP, specificity.

TABLE 5.3

Results of the Most Relevant Works in the Detection of Pigment Network

Works	# Images	Results
Anantha et al. 2004 [43]	155	80% ACC
Grana et al. 2007 [48]	100	82% SE, 94% SP, 88% ACC
Sadeghi et al. 2011 [66]	500	94.30% ACC
Sadeghi et al. 2010 [68]	436	93.30% ACC
Gola et al. 2011 [23]	150	90% ACC
Barata et al. 2012 [75]	200	91.1% SE, 82.1% SP
García et al. 2014 [94]	220	83.64% SE, 86% SP, 81.67% ACC

Note: ACC, accuracy; SE, sensitivity; SP, specificity.

the works focusing on reticular pattern recognition [23, 43, 48, 66, 68, 75, 94], in most cases the results are contrasted with complete images [23, 48, 66, 68, 75, 94] and with image tiles [43]. Table 5.3 presents a summary with the results of the studies on pigment network detection, in which we center our attention solely on the size of the image databases used and the results obtained to form a clear idea of the reliability of the various methods.

Taking into account the number of images and the numerical results obtained, we can consider that [66, 68, 75, 94] present the most reliable state-of-the-art methods. The high rates obtained and tests run on databases with a minimum of 200 complete images (not tiles as in [43]) are key aspects. The

TABLE 5.4

Results of the Most Relevant Works in the Detection of the Atypical Pigment Network

Works	# Images	Results
Di Leo et al. 2008 [52]	173	85% SE, 85% SP
Shrestha et al. 2010 [63]	106	95.4% ACC
Sadeghi et al. 2010 [68]	436	82.3% ACC

Note: ACC, accuracy; SE, sensitivity; SP, specificity.

principal problem of [23] is its low number of reticular images (20 images), and the problem of [48] is the number of images. In [75], the model was also contrasted with the ground truths segmented by experts, obtaining good results in the detection of reticular pixels.

As for works focusing on atypical reticular pattern recognition [52, 63, 68], in most cases the results are contrasted with complete images [52, 68], while in [63] this is performed on image areas. Table 5.4 presents a summary of the results of the works on atypical pigment network detection, in which we center our attention solely on the size of the image databases used and the results obtained to form a clear idea of the reliability of the various methods.

Taking into account the number of images and the numerical results obtained, we can consider that [52, 68] present the most reliable state-of-the-art methods. The high rates obtained and tests run on databases with a minimum of 173 complete images (not tiles as in [63]) are key aspects.

5.5 CONCLUSIONS

This chapter shows the most relevant works on reticular pattern recognition within the field of automated detection of melanoma in dermatoscopic images.

After a complete review of the state of the art, 20 studies were selected, together with another 19 works from the same research teams. The latter were either preliminary works or studies that covered a higher scope and included them for the purpose of pigment network detection. A detailed explanation of all of them is given, perhaps longer for the works that the authors consider to be most relevant, focusing on the image processing techniques used.

The numerical results obtained were analyzed in order to determine the reliability and robustness of the methods discussed, with special emphasis on the results obtained for reticular pattern and atypical reticular pattern recognition. All of the studies from the state of the art use a sole source of images and do not provide information on the difficulty of the images used. Therefore, a selection of the most relevant works was made, using the number of images and the numerical results for sensitivity, specificity, and accuracy as criteria.

Three main conclusions were reached.

Firstly, the problem of obtaining the pigment network structure and the consequences of reticular pattern recognition and atypical reticular pattern recognition are complex. This is due to their very nature, correct diagnosis of reticular pattern, and in the case of positive diagnoses, the difference between typical and atypical, is often even difficult for experts.

Secondly, there are several good methods that focus on these problems and have sometimes achieved good results. The approaches used in the different studies vary, with different algorithms, image processing techniques, and statistical and data mining models being used. After an analysis of all methods, four works were selected in reticular pattern recognition and two in atypical reticular pattern recognition.

Thirdly, this subject requires further study. In the state of the art, there is still no truly definitive work in terms of reliability and robustness that has been tested against a large number of images extracted from different sources, with different features and acquisition conditions and with a large sample of images having patterns that are difficult to recognize.

ACKNOWLEDGMENTS

This research was partially funded by the Basque Government Department of Education (eVIDA Certified Group IT579-13).

REFERENCES

1. World Cancer Research Fund International, Cancer statistics—Worldwide, http://www.wcrf.org/cancer _statistics/world_cancer_statistics.php (accessed June 11, 2014).

2. Skin Cancer Foundation, Skin cancer facts, http://www.skincancer.org/Skin-Cancer-Facts/ (accessed June 11, 2014).

3. J. Malvehy, S. Puig, G. Argenziano, A. A. Marghoob, and H. P. Soyer, Dermoscopy report: proposal for standardization. Results of a consensus meeting of the International Dermoscopy Society, *Journal of the American Academy of Dermatology*, vol. 57, pp. 84–95, 2007.

4. H. Pehamberger, A. Steiner, and K. Wolff, In vivo epiluminescence microscopy of pigmented skin lesions. I. Pattern analysis of pigmented skin lesions, *Journal of the American Academy of Dermatology*, vol. 17, pp. 571–583, 1987.

5. W. Stolz, A. Riemann, and A. Cognetta, ABCD rule of dermatoscopy: a new practical method for early recognition of malignant melanoma, *European Journal of Dermatology*, vol. 4, pp. 521–527, 1994.

6. S. W. Menzies, C. Ingvar, K. A. Crotty, and W. H. McCarthy, Frequency and morphologic characteristics of invasive melanomas lacking specific surface microscopic features, *Archives of Dermatology*, vol. 132, pp. 1178–1182, 1996.

7. G. Argenziano, G. Fabbrocini, P. Carli, V. De Giorgi, E. Sammarco, and M. Delfino, Epiluminescence microscopy for the diagnosis of doubtful melanocytic skin lesions. Comparison of the ABCD rule of dermatoscopy and a new

7-point checklist based on pattern analysis, *Archives of Dermatology*, vol. 134, pp. 1563–1570, 1998.

8. K. Korotkov and R. Garcia, Computerized analysis of pigmented skin lesions: A review, *Artificial Intelligence in Medicine*, vol. 56, pp. 69–90, 2012.

9. M. E. Celebi, W. V. Stoecker, and R. H. Moss, Advances in skin cancer image analysis, *Computerized Medical Imaging and Graphics*, vol. 35, no. 2, pp. 83–84, 2011.

10. J. Scharcanski and M. E. Celebi, eds., *Computer Vision Techniques for the Diagnosis of Skin Cancer*, Springer, Berlin, 2013.

11. H. Ganster, A. Pinz, R. Rohrer, E. Wildling, M. Binder, and H. Kittler, Automated melanoma recognition, *IEEE Transactions on Medical Imaging*, vol. 20, pp. 233–239, 2001.

12. M. E. Celebi, H. A. Kingravi, B. Uddin, H. Iyatomi, Y. A. Aslandogan, W. V. Stoecker, and R. H. Moss, A methodological approach to the classification of dermoscopy images, *Computerized Medical Imaging and Graphics*, vol. 31, pp. 362–373, 2007.

13. H. Iyatomi, H. Oka, M. E. Celebi, M. Hashimoto, M. Hagiwara, M. Tanaka, and K. Ogawa, An improved Internet-based melanoma screening system with dermatologist-like tumor area extraction algorithm, *Computerized Medical Imaging and Graphics*, vol. 32, pp. 566–579, 2008.

14. J. Fernandez Alcon, C. Ciuhu, W. Ten Kate, A. Heinrich, N. Uzunbajakava, G. Krekels, D. Siem, and G. De Haan, Automatic imaging system with decision support for inspection of pigmented skin lesions and melanoma diagnosis, *IEEE Journal of Selected Topics in Signal Processing*, vol. 3, pp. 14–25, 2009.

15. G. Di Leo, A. Paolillo, P. Sommella, and G. Fabbrocini, Automatic diagnosis of melanoma: a software system based on the 7-point check-list, in *2010 43rd Hawaii International Conference on System Sciences*, Honolulu, Hawai, pp. 1–10, 2010.

16. Q. Abbas, M. E. Celebi, I. Fondón, and W. Ahmad, Melanoma recognition framework based on expert definition of ABCD for dermoscopic images, *Skin Research and Technology*, vol. 19, no. 1, pp. e93–e102, 2013.

17. J. L. García Arroyo and B. García Zapirain, Automated detection of melanoma in dermoscopic images, in *Computer Vision Techniques for the Diagnosis of Skin Cancer* (J. Scharcanski and M. E. Celebi, eds.), pp. 139–192, Springer, Berlin, 2014.

18. H. Mirzaalian, T. K. Lee, and G. Hamarneh, Learning features for streak detection in dermoscopic color images using localized radial flux of principal intensity curvature, in *2012 IEEE Workshop on Mathematical Methods in Biomedical Image Analysis*, Breckenridge, CO, pp. 97–101, 2012.

19. M. Sadeghi, T. K. Lee, D. Mclean, H. Lui, and M. S. Atkins, Oriented pattern analysis for streak detection in dermoscopy images, in *Medical Image Computing and Computer-Assisted Intervention (MICCAI 2012)*, Nice, France, pp. 298–306, 2012.

20. M. Sadeghi, T. Lee, H. Lui, D. McLean, and S. Atkins, Detection and analysis of irregular streaks in dermoscopic images of skin lesions, *IEEE Transactions on Medical Imaging*, vol. 32, no. 5, pp. 849–861, 2013.

21. S. Yoshino, T. Tanaka, M. Tanaka, and H. Oka, Application of morphology for detection of dots in tumor, *SICE 2004 Annual Conference*, vol. 1, pp. 591–594, 2004.

22. J. Xu, K. Gupta, W. V. Stoecker, Y. Krishnamurthy, H. S. Rabinovitz, A. Bangert, D. Calcara et al., Analysis of globule types in malignant

melanoma, *Archives of Dermatology*, Sapporo, Japan, vol. 145, pp. 1245–1251, 2009.

23. A. Gola Isasi, B. García Zapirain, and A. Méndez Zorrilla, Melanomas non-invasive diagnosis application based on the ABCD rule and pattern recognition image processing algorithms, *Computers in Biology and Medicine*, vol. 41, pp. 742–755, 2011.

24. M. E. Celebi, H. Iyatomi, W. V. Stoecker, R. H. Moss, H. S. Rabinovitz, G. Argenziano, and H. P. Soyer, Automatic detection of blue-white veil and related structures in dermoscopy images, *Computerized Medical Imaging and Graphics*, vol. 32, pp. 670–677, 2008.

25. G. Di Leo, G. Fabbrocini, A. Paolillo, O. Rescigno, and P. Sommella, Towards an automatic diagnosis system for skin lesions: estimation of blue-whitish veil and regression structures, in *2009 6th International Multi-Conference on Systems, Signals and Devices*, Djerba, Tunisia, pp. 1–6, 2009.

26. J. L. García Arroyo, B. García Zapirain, and A. Mendez Zorrilla, Blue-white veil and dark-red patch of pigment pattern recognition in dermoscopic images using machine-learning techniques, in *2011 IEEE International Symposium on Signal Processing and Information Technology (ISSPIT)*, Bilbao, Spain, pp. 196–201, 2011.

27. A. Madooei, M. S. Drew, M. Sadeghi, and M. S. Atkins, Automatic detection of blue-white veil by discrete colour matching in dermoscopy images, in *Proceedings of the 16th International Conference on Medical Image Computing and Computer-Assisted Intervention (MICCAI 2013)*, Nagoya, Japan, pp. 453–460, 2013.

28. G. Betta, G. Di Leo, G. Fabbrocini, A. Paolillo, and P. Sommella, Dermoscopic image-analysis system: estimation of atypical pigment network and atypical vascular pattern, in *IEEE International Workshop on Medical Measurement and Applications*, Benevento, Italy, pp. 63–67, 2006.

29. W. V. Stoecker, K. Gupta, R. J. Stanley, R. H. Moss, and B. Shrestha, Detection of asymmetric blotches (asymmetric structureless areas) in dermoscopy images of malignant melanoma using relative color, *Skin Research and Technology*, vol. 11, pp. 179–184, 2005.

30. A. Khan, K. Gupta, R. J. Stanley, W. V. Stoecker, R. H. Moss, G. Argenziano, H. P. Soyer, H. S. Rabinovitz, and A. B. Cognetta, Fuzzy logic techniques for blotch feature evaluation in dermoscopy images, *Computerized Medical Imaging and Graphics*, vol. 33, pp. 50–57, 2009.

31. V. K. Madasu and B. C. Lovell, Blotch detection in pigmented skin lesions using fuzzy co-clustering and texture segmentation, in *2009 Digital Image Computing: Techniques and Applications*, Melbourne, Australia, pp. 25–31, 2009.

32. A. Dalal, R. H. Moss, R. J. Stanley, W. V. Stoecker, K. Gupta, D. A. Calcara, J. Xu et al., Concentric decile segmentation of white and hypopigmented areas in dermoscopy images of skin lesions allows discrimination of malignant melanoma, *Computerized Medical Imaging and Graphics*, vol. 35, pp. 148–154, 2011.

33. W. V. Stoecker, M. Wronkiewiecz, R. Chowdhury, R. J. Stanley, J. Xu, A. Bangert, B. Shrestha et al., Detection of granularity in dermoscopy images of malignant melanoma using color and texture features, *Computerized Medical Imaging and Graphics*, vol. 35, pp. 144–147, 2011.

34. H. Iyatomi, H. Oka, M. E. Celebi, K. Ogawa, G. Argenziano, H. P. Soyer, H. Koga, T. Saida, K. Ohara, and M. Tanaka, Computer-based classification

of dermoscopy images of melanocytic lesions on acral volar skin, *Journal of Investigative Dermatology*, vol. 128, pp. 2049–2054, 2008.

35. S. Fischer, P. Schmid, and J. Guillod, Analysis of skin lesions with pigmented networks, in *Proceedings of the International Conference on Image Processing, 1996*, Lausanne, Switzerland, vol. 1, pp. 323–326, 1996.

36. R. C. Gonzalez and R. E. Woods, *Digital Image Processing*, 3rd ed., Prentice Hall, Englewood Cliffs, NJ, 2008.

37. M. G. Fleming, C. Steger, A. B. Cognetta, and J. Zhang, Analysis of the network pattern in dermatoscopic images, *Skin Research and Technology*, vol. 5, no. 1, pp. 42–48, 1999.

38. C. Steger, An unbiased detector of curvilinear structures, *IEEE Transactions on Pattern Analysis and Machine Intelligence*, vol. 20, no. 2, pp. 113–125, 1998.

39. S. Lobregt and M. A. Viergever, A discrete dynamic contour model, *IEEE Transactions on Medical Imaging*, vol. 14, no. 1, pp. 12–24, 1995.

40. M. G. Fleming, C. Steger, J. Zhang, J. Gao, A. B. Cognetta, L. Pollak, and C. R. Dyer, Techniques for a structural analysis of dermatoscopic imagery, *Computerized Medical Imaging and Graphics*, vol. 22, pp. 375–389, 1998.

41. B. Caputo, V. Panichelli, and G. E. Gigante, Toward a quantitative analysis of skin lesion images, *Studies in Health Technology and Informatics*, vol. 90, pp. 509–513, 2002.

42. A. K. Jain, *Fundamentals of Digital Image Processing*, vol. 3, Prentice-Hall, Englewood Cliffs, NJ, 1989.

43. M. Anantha, R. H. Moss, and W. V. Stoecker, Detection of pigment network in dermatoscopy images using texture analysis, *Computerized Medical Imaging and Graphics*, vol. 28, pp. 225–234, 2004.

44. T. Lee, V. Ng, R. Gallagher, A. Coldman, and D. McLean, Dullrazor: a software approach to hair removal from images, *Computers in Biology and Medicine*, vol. 27, pp. 533–543, 1997.

45. K. I. Laws, Textured image segmentation, tech. rep., DTIC document, January 1980. http://www.dtic.mil/cgi-bin/GetTRDoc?Location=U2&doc=GetTRDoc.pdf&AD=ADA083283 (accessed June 11, 2014).

46. C. Sun and W. G. Wee, Neighboring gray level dependence matrix for texture classification, *Computer Vision, Graphics, and Image Processing*, vol. 23, no. 3, pp. 341–352, 1983.

47. A. Murali, W. V. Stoecker, and R. H. Moss, Detection of solid pigment in dermatoscopy images using texture analysis, *Skin Research and Technology*, vol. 6, no. 4, pp. 193–198, 2000.

48. C. Grana, V. Daniele, G. Pellacani, S. Seidenari, and R. Cucchiara, Network patterns recognition for automatic dermatologic images classification, in *Proceedings of the International Society for Optics and Photonics Medical Imaging Conference*, San Diego, CA, pp. 65124C–65124C, 2007.

49. C. Grana, R. Cucchiara, G. Pellacani, and S. Seidenari, Line detection and texture characterization of network patterns, in *18th International Conference on Pattern Recognition (ICPR '06)*, Hong Kong, China, vol. 2, pp. 275–278, 2006.

50. T. Tanaka, S. Torii, I. Kabuta, K. Shimizu, and M. Tanaka, Pattern classification of nevus with texture analysis, *IEEJ Transactions on Electrical and Electronic Engineering*, vol. 3, no. 1, pp. 143–150, 2008.

51. T. Tanaka, S. Torii, I. Kabuta, K. Shimizu, M. Tanaka, and H. Oka, Pattern classification of nevus with texture analysis, in *2004 Annual International*

Conference of the IEEE Engineering in Medicine and Biology Society (EMBC), San Francisco, CA, vol. 2, pp. 1459–1462, 2004.

52. G. Di Leo, C. Liguori, A. Paolillo, and P. Sommella, An improved procedure for the automatic detection of dermoscopic structures in digital ELM images of skin lesions, in *2008 IEEE Conference on Virtual Environments, Human-Computer Interfaces and Measurement Systems*, Istanbul, Turkey, pp. 190–194, 2008.

53. N. Otsu, A threshold selection method from gray-level histograms, *IEEE Transactions on Systems, Man, and Cybernetics*, vol. 9, no. 1, pp. 62–66, 1979.

54. J. R. Quinlan, *C4.5: Programs for Machine Learning*, vol. 1, Morgan Kaufmann, San Francisco, CA, 1993.

55. G. Di Leo, G. Fabbrocini, C. Liguori, A. Pietrosanto, and M. Sclavenzi, Elm image processing for melanocytic skin lesion diagnosis based on 7-point checklist: a preliminary discussion, in *Proceedings of the 13th International Symposium on Measurements for Research and Industry Applications, IMEKO*, Budapest, Hungary, pp. 474–479, 2004.

56. G. Betta, G. Di Leo, G. Fabbrocini, A. Paolillo, and M. Scalvenzi, Automated application of the "7-point checklist" diagnosis method for skin lesions: estimation of chromatic and shape parameters, in *Proceedings of the IEEE Instrumentation and Measurement Technology Conference (IMTC 2005)*, Ottawa, Canada, vol. 3, pp. 1818–1822, 2005.

57. G. Di Leo, A. Paolillo, P. Sommella, G. Fabbrocini, and O. Rescigno, A software tool for the diagnosis of melanomas, in *2010 IEEE Instrumentation and Measurement Technology Conference (I2MTC)*, Austin, TX, pp. 886–891, 2010.

58. G. Fabbrocini, V. D. Vita, S. Cacciapuoti, G. D. Leo, C. Liguori, A. Paolillo, A. Pietrosanto, and P. Sommella, Automatic diagnosis of melanoma based on the 7-point checklist, in *Computer Vision Techniques for the Diagnosis of Skin Cancer* (J. Scharcanski and M. E. Celebi, eds.), pp. 71–107, 2014.

59. C. Serrano and B. Acha, Pattern analysis of dermoscopic images based on Markov random fields, *Pattern Recognition*, vol. 42, no. 6, pp. 1052–1057, 2009.

60. S. Z. Li, *Markov Random Field Modeling in Image Analysis*, Springer, Berlin, 2001.

61. C. S. Mendoza, C. Serrano, and B. Acha, Pattern analysis of dermoscopic images based on FSCM color Markov random fields, in *Advanced Concepts for Intelligent Vision Systems*, pp. 676–685, 2009.

62. S. O. Skrovseth, T. R. Schopf, K. Thon, M. Zortea, M. Geilhufe, K. Mollersen, H. M. Kirchesch, and F. Godtliebsen, A computer aided diagnostic system for malignant melanomas, in *2010 3rd International Symposium on Applied Sciences in Biomedical and Communication Technologies (ISABEL 2010)*, Roma, Italy, pp. 1–5, 2010.

63. B. Shrestha, J. Bishop, K. Kam, X. Chen, R. H. Moss, W. V. Stoecker, S. Umbaugh et al., Detection of atypical texture features in early malignant melanoma, *Skin Research and Technology*, vol. 16, pp. 60–65, 2010.

64. R. M. Haralick, K. Shanmugam, and I. Dinstein, Textural features for image classification, *IEEE Transactions on Systems, Man, and Cybernetics*, vol. 3, pp. 610–621, 1973.

65. University of Waikato, WEKA: data mining software in Java, http://www.cs.waikato.ac.nz/ml/weka (accessed June 11, 2014).

66. M. Sadeghi, M. Razmara, T. K. Lee, and M. S. Atkins, A novel method for detection of pigment network in dermoscopic images using graphs, *Computerized Medical Imaging and Graphics*, vol. 35, pp. 137–143, 2011.

67. J. Kirk, Count loops in a graph, http://www.mathworks.com/matlabcentral/fileexchange/10722-count-loops-in-a-graph/content/run_loops.m (accessed June 11, 2014).

68. M. Sadeghi, M. Razmara, P. Wighton, T. K. Lee, and M. S. Atkins, Modeling the dermoscopic structure pigment network using a clinically inspired feature set, *Lecture Notes in Computer Science*, vol. 6326, pp. 467–474, 2010.

69. P. Wighton, T. K. Lee, H. Lui, D. I. McLean, and M. S. Atkins, Generalizing common tasks in automated skin lesion diagnosis, *IEEE Transactions on Information Technology in Biomedicine*, vol. 15, pp. 622–629, 2011.

70. M. Sadeghi, M. Razmara, M. Ester, T. Lee, and M. Atkins, Graph-based pigment network detection in skin images, in *Proceedings of the International Society for Optics and Photonics SPIE Medical Imaging Conference*, San Diego, CA, pp. 762312–762312, 2010.

71. M. Sadeghi, T. K. Lee, H. Lui, D. Mclean, and M. Atkins, Automated detection and analysis of dermoscopic structures on dermoscopy images, in *22nd World Congress of Dermatology*, Seoul, Korea, 2011.

72. M. Sadeghi, P. Wighton, T. K. Lee, D. McLean, H. Lui, and M. S. Atkins, Pigment network detection and analysis, in *Computer Vision Techniques for the Diagnosis of Skin Cancer* (J. Scharcanski and M. E. Celebi, eds.), pp. 1–22, Springer, Berlin, 2014.

73. J. Canny, A computational approach to edge detection, *IEEE Transactions on Pattern Analysis and Machine Intelligence*, no. 6, pp. 679–698, 1986.

74. A. Gola Isasi, B. García Zapirain, A. Méndez Zorrilla, and I. Ruiz Oleagordia, Automated diagnosis of melanomas based on globular and reticular pattern recognition algorithms for epiluminiscence images, in *18th European Signal Processing Conference (EUSIPCO-2010)*, Aalburg, Netherlands, pp. 264–268, 2010.

75. C. Barata, J. S. Marques, and J. Rozeira, A system for the detection of pigment network in dermoscopy images using directional filters, *IEEE Transactions on Biomedical Engineering*, vol. 59, pp. 2744–2754, 2012.

76. M. Silveira, J. C. Nascimento, J. S. Marques, A. R. Marçal, T. Mendonça, S. Yamauchi, J. Maeda, and J. Rozeira, Comparison of segmentation methods for melanoma diagnosis in dermoscopy images, *IEEE Journal of Selected Topics in Signal Processing*, vol. 3, no. 1, pp. 35–45, 2009.

77. C. Barata, J. S. Marques, and J. Rozeira, Detecting the pigment network in dermoscopy images: a directional approach, in *2011 Annual International Conference of the IEEE Engineering in Medicine and Biology Society (EMBC)*, Boston, MA, pp. 5120–5123, 2011.

78. C. Barata, Detection of Pigment Network in Dermoscopy Images, PhD thesis, Universidade Técnica de Lisboa, 2011.

79. C. Barata, J. S. Marques, and J. Rozeira, A system for the automatic detection of pigment network, in *2012 9th IEEE International Symposium on Biomedical Imaging (ISBI)*, Barcelona, Spain, pp. 1651–1654, 2012.

80. Q. Abbas, M. E. Celebi, and I. Fondón, Computer-aided pattern classification system for dermoscopy images, *Skin Research and Technology*, vol. 18, no. 3, pp. 278–289, 2012.

81. M. Unser, Texture classification and segmentation using wavelet frames, *IEEE Transactions on Image Processing*, vol. 4, no. 11, pp. 1549–1560, 1995.
82. T. Ojala, M. Pietikainen, and T. Maenpaa, Multiresolution gray-scale and rotation invariant texture classification with local binary patterns, *IEEE Transactions on Pattern Analysis and Machine Intelligence*, vol. 24, no. 7, pp. 971–987, 2002.
83. J. Weston and C. Watkins, Support vector machines for multi-class pattern recognition, in *Proceedings of the European Symposium on Artificial Neural Networks (ESANN 1999)*, Bruges, Belgium, pp. 219–224, 1999.
84. Q. Abbas, M. E. Celebi, C. Serrano, I. Fondón, and G. Ma, Pattern classification of dermoscopy images: a perceptually uniform model, *Pattern Recognition*, vol. 46, no. 1, pp. 86–97, 2012.
85. W. T. Freeman and E. H. Adelson, The design and use of steerable filters, *IEEE Transactions on Pattern Analysis and Machine Intelligence*, vol. 13, no. 9, pp. 891–906, 1991.
86. E. P. Simoncelli, W. T. Freeman, E. H. Adelson, and D. J. Heeger, Shiftable multiscale transforms, *IEEE Transactions on Information Theory*, vol. 38, no. 2, pp. 587–607, 1992.
87. R. E. Schapire and Y. Singer, Boostexter: a boosting-based system for text categorization, *Machine Learning*, vol. 39, no. 2–3, pp. 135–168, 2000.
88. R. Kumar, A. Vázquez-Reina, and H. Pfister, Radon-like features and their application to connectomics, in *2010 IEEE Computer Society Conference on Computer Vision and Pattern Recognition Workshops (CVPRW)*, San Francisco, CA, pp. 186–193, 2010.
89. A. Sáez, C. Serrano, and B. Acha, Model-based classification methods of global patterns in dermoscopic images, *IEEE Transactions on Medical Imaging*, vol. 33, pp. 1137–1147, 2014.
90. M. Sadeghi, T. K. Lee, D. McLean, H. Lui, and M. S. Atkins, Global pattern analysis and classification of dermoscopic images using textons, in *Proceedings of the SPIE Medical Imaging Conference*, San Diego, CA, vol. 8314, p. 83144X, 2012.
91. Y. Xia, D. Feng, and R. Zhao, Adaptive segmentation of textured images by using the coupled Markov random field model, *IEEE Transactions on Image Processing*, vol. 15, no. 11, pp. 3559–3566, 2006.
92. R. L. Kashyap and R. Chellappa, Estimation and choice of neighbors in spatial-interaction models of images, *IEEE Transactions on Information Theory*, vol. 29, no. 1, pp. 60–72, 1983.
93. G. Sfikas, C. Constantinopoulos, A. Likas, and N. P. Galatsanos, An analytic distance metric for Gaussian mixture models with application in image retrieval, in *Artificial Neural Networks: Formal Models and Their Applications (ICANN 2005)*, Warsaw, Poland, pp. 835–840, 2005.
94. J. L. García Arroyo and B. García Zapirain, Detection of pigment network in dermoscopy images using supervised machine learning and structural analysis, *Computers in Biology and Medicine*, vol. 44, pp. 144–157, 2014.

6 Global Pattern Classification in Dermoscopic Images

Aurora Sáez
University of Seville
Seville, Spain

Carmen Serrano
University of Seville
Seville, Spain

Begoña Acha
University of Seville
Seville, Spain

CONTENTS

183

6.1 INTRODUCTION

Dermoscopy (also known as dermatoscopy, epiluminescence microscopy, incident light microscopy, and skin-surface microscopy) is a noninvasive technique to examine pigmented anatomic structures of the epidermis, dermoepidermal junction, and superficial papillary dermis that are not visible to the naked eye [1]. The abnormal structural features of melanoma can be identified, borderline lesions may be closely observed, and benign lesions can be confidently diagnosed without the need for biopsy using dermoscopy. Dermoscopy has been shown to be more accurate than clinical examination for the diagnosis of melanoma in a pigmented skin lesion [2, 3].

There are two steps in the process of dermoscopic diagnosis of pigmented skin lesions [3, 4]. The first step is to decide whether the lesion is melanocytic or nonmelanocytic. Step 2 is the differentiation of benign melanocytic lesions from melanomas. In order to address this second step, there are four main diagnosis methods from dermoscopic images: ABCD rule [5], pattern analysis [4, 6], Menzies method [1], and 7-point checklist [7]. Pattern analysis is the method preferred by expert dermoscopists to diagnose melanocytic lesions [8], although this methodology is also able to classify nonmelanocytic lesions [9]. Indeed, this diagnosis method was deemed superior to the other algorithms in the 2000 Consensus Net Meeting on Dermoscopy (CNMD) [10]. It is a methodology first described by Pehamberger and colleagues [6], based on the analysis of more than 3000 pigmented skin lesions, and later revised by Argenziano et al. [4]. It is the most commonly used method for providing diagnostic accuracy for cutaneous melanoma [11] and it was demonstrated that it is the most reliable method to teach dermoscopy for residents (nonexperts) in dermatology [9].

Pattern analysis seeks to identify specific patterns, which may be local or global [12]. The melanocytic lesions are identified by their general dermoscopic features, defined global patterns, or specific dermoscopic criteria that determine their local patterns [11]. Thus, a lesion is categorized by a global pattern, although it can present more than one local pattern. Global features permit a broad classification of pigmented skin lesions, while a description of the local features provides more detailed information about a given lesion [13].

The utilization of computer vision techniques in the diagnosis of skin cancer cannot as yet provide a definitive diagnosis; however, they can be used to improve biopsy decision making as well as early melanoma detection [14]. In the literature we can find works that summarize the state of the art in this issue [14–16]. This chapter presents image analysis techniques to detect global features.

The chapter is organized as follows: First, the main global patterns are presented as well as their diagnostic significance. Then, the algorithmic methods published in the literature that address the global pattern detection are described. And finally, a discussion is given.

6.1.1 GLOBAL PATTERNS

The global features are presented as arrangements of textured patterns covering most of the lesion. They are determined by the predominantly dermatoscopic feature in the lesion that enable its diagnosis [11].

There are nine morphologically rather distinctive global features that allow a preliminary categorization of a given pigmented skin lesion [4]. However, the first seven patterns are the most common global characteristics to diagnose melanocytic lesions and to differentiate benign melanocytic lesions from malignant melanoma [8]. They are enumerated and described below:

- Reticular pattern
- Globular pattern
- Cobblestone pattern
- Homogeneous pattern
- Starbust pattern
- Parallel pattern
- Multicomponent pattern
- Lacunar pattern
- Unspecific pattern

The first seven patterns are the most common global characteristics to diagnose melanocytic lesions and differentiate benign melanocytic lesions from malignant melanoma [8].

The **reticular pattern**, or network pattern, is the most common global feature in melanocytic lesions. It is characterized by a pigment network covering most parts of a given lesion. The pigment network appears as a grid of thin, brown lines over a diffuse, light brown background. The reticular pattern represents the dermoscopic hallmark of benign acquired melanocytic nevi in general and of thin melanomas in particular. In Figure 6.1 different lesions with reticular pattern are shown.

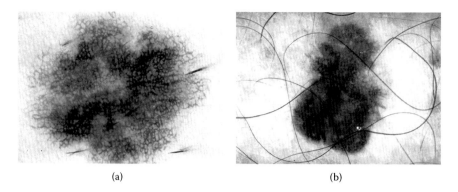

        (a)   (b)

FIGURE 6.1 (a) Clark nevus with reticular pattern. (b) Reticular pattern in melanoma. (Reprinted with permission from Argenziano, G. et al., *Dermoscopy: A Tutorial*, EDRA Medical Publishing and New Media, Milan, Italy, 2002.)

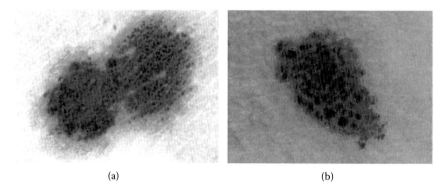

        (a)   (b)

FIGURE 6.2 (a), (b) Globular pattern in Clark nevi. (Reprinted with permission from Argenziano, G. et al., *Dermoscopy: A Tutorial*, EDRA Medical Publishing and New Media, Milan, Italy, 2002.)

The **globular pattern** is characterized by the presence of numerous, variously sized, round to oval structures with various shades of brown and gray–black coloration. Globular pattern is found in Clark nevi and also in Unna nevi, both belonging to the spectrum of acquired melanocytic nevi. Some examples can be seen in Figure 6.2.

The **cobblestone pattern** is very similar to the globular pattern but is composed of closer aggregated globules, which are somehow angulated, resembling cobblestones. The cobblestone pattern is found in dermal nevi (Unna nevus), in congenital nevi, and sometimes in the dermal part of compound Clark nevi (see Figure 6.3).

The **homogeneous pattern** appears as a diffuse, brown, gray–blue to gray–black, or reddish black pigmentation in the absence of pigment network

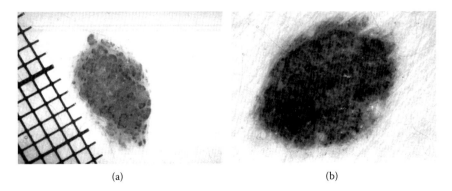

(a)   (b)

FIGURE 6.3   (a) Cobblestone pattern in a dermal nevus. (b) Clark nevus with cobblestone pattern. (Reprinted with permission from Argenziano, G. et al., *Dermoscopy: A Tutorial*, EDRA Medical Publishing and New Media, Milan, Italy, 2002.)

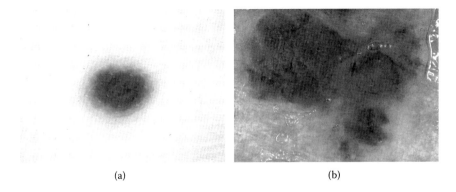

(a)   (b)

FIGURE 6.4   (a) Typical homogeneous pattern in a gray-blue nevus. (b) Homogeneous pattern in a melanoma. (Reprinted with permission from Argenziano, G. et al., *Dermoscopy: A Tutorial*, EDRA Medical Publishing and New Media, Milan, Italy, 2002.)

or other distinctive local features. This pattern, especially when bluish coloration is predominant, represents the morphologic hallmark of blue nevus. It may be present, however, also in Clark nevi, dermal nevi, and nodular and metastatic melanomas. Examples of a blue nevus and melanoma with homogeneous pattern are shown in Figure 6.4.

The so-called **starburst pattern** is characterized by the presence of streaks in a radial arrangement, which is visible at the periphery of the lesion. This pattern is commonly seen in Reed nevi or Spitz nevi (see Figure 6.5).

The **parallel pattern** is found exclusively in melanocytic lesions on palms and soles due to particular anatomic structures inherent to these sites. A parallel pattern in its various expressions is found in acral lesions (Figure 6.6).

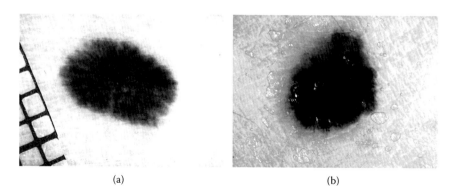

(a)   (b)

FIGURE 6.5 (a) Typical starburst pattern in a Reed nevus. (b) Starburst pattern in a melanoma. (Reprinted with permission from Argenziano, G. et al., *Dermoscopy: A Tutorial*, EDRA Medical Publishing and New Media, Milan, Italy, 2002.)

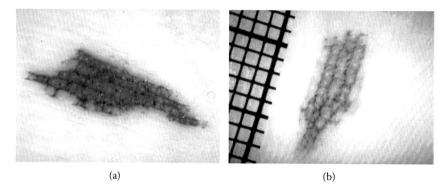

(a)   (b)

FIGURE 6.6 (a), (b) Parallel pattern in acral nevi. (Reprinted with permission from Argenziano, G. et al., *Dermoscopy: A Tutorial*, EDRA Medical Publishing and New Media, Milan, Italy, 2002.)

The combination of three or more distinctive dermoscopic structures within a given lesion is called **multicomponent pattern**. This pattern may be made up of zones of pigment network, clusters of dots/globules, and areas of diffuse hyper- or hypopigmentation. The multicomponent pattern is highly suggestive of melanoma (in Figure 6.7 some examples are shown) but it may also be frequently found in basal cell carcinoma.

The **lacunar pattern** is characterized by several to numerous smooth-bordered, round to oval, variously sized structures called red lacunas. The morphologic hallmark of these lacunar structures is their striking reddish, blue–purple, or black coloration (Figure 6.8).

When a pigmented lesion cannot be categorized into one of the above-listed global patterns, because its overall morphologic aspect does not fit into these patterns, the term **unspecific pattern** is used. Unspecific pattern may be a

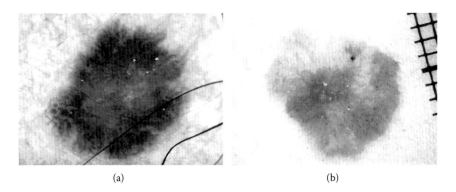

(a)   (b)

FIGURE 6.7 (a), (b) Multicomponent pattern in melanomas. (Reprinted with permission from Argenziano, G. et al., *Dermoscopy: A Tutorial*, EDRA Medical Publishing and New Media, Milan, Italy, 2002.)

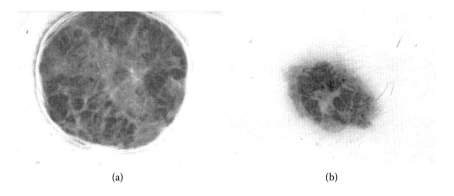

(a)   (b)

FIGURE 6.8 (a), (b) Lacunar pattern in vascular lesions with reddish coloration. (Reprinted with permission from Argenziano, G. et al., *Dermoscopy: A Tutorial*, EDRA Medical Publishing and New Media, Milan, Italy, 2002.)

clue for the diagnosis of the so-called featureless melanoma. Some examples are shown in Figure 6.9.

6.2 GLOBAL PATTERN DETECTION

In this section some algorithms published in the literature that address the global pattern detection are detailed.

6.2.1 TEXTURE ANALYSIS FOR GLOBAL PATTERN CLASSIFICATION BY TANAKA ET AL. [17, 18]

Tanaka et al. [17, 18] proposed an analysis of texture to classify a pattern into three categories: homogeneous, globular, and reticular. The analysis was

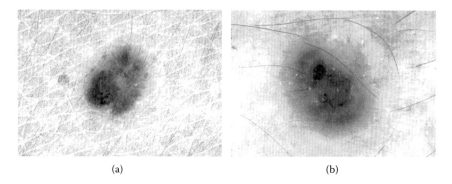

(a)   (b)

FIGURE 6.9   (a) Unspecific pattern in Clark nevus. (b) Unspecific pattern in basal cell carcinoma. (Reprinted with permission from Argenziano, G. et al., *Dermoscopy: A Tutorial*, EDRA Medical Publishing and New Media, Milan, Italy, 2002.)

carried out in grayscale images. The Y component image from the YIQ color space was used as grayscale image.

6.2.1.1   Segmentation

The lesion was segmented using a thresholding method, whose threshold was obtained using the Laplacian histogram method and discriminant analysis proposed in [19]. Then, each lesion area was divided into small regions of subimages.

6.2.1.2   Feature Extraction

Texture features are extracted from the subimages. In a first step, the authors extracted 7 features from the intensity histogram, 7 features from statistical difference, 14 features from the Fourier power spectrum, 5 features from the run-length matrix, and 13 features from the co-occurrence matrix. Then, 16 more features were extracted from the run-length matrix, but taking into account the intensity information, and 48 from the connected components obtained after a binarization of each subimage. The image resulting from average filtering is used as a threshold surface for the binarization with respect to each pixel. A total of 110 texture features of each subimage were calculated.

6.2.1.3   Feature Selection

To this end, a statistical analysis was performed, in which the following methods were used:

- F-test. It is used to compare the distributions of the 110 features for each pair of patterns: homogeneous and globular, globular and reticular, and reticular and homogeneous. The idea is to study if the

TABLE 6.1

Classification Results in [17] and [18] for 852 Regions Extracted from 44 Images

	Homogeneous	Globular	Reticular
Homogeneous	336 (95.5%)	10 (2.8%)	6 (1.7%)
Globular	5 (2.2%)	211 (93.4%)	10 (4.4%)
Homogeneous	5 (2.9%)	15 (5.5%)	254 (92.6%)

Note: Discriminant analysis using the 35 selected features.

variances of the distributions are equal. Finally, the authors removed all the texture features that were not valid for the discrimination of the three patterns under analysis.

- t-test. It is used to test whether each pattern displays differences in feature value, computed for the features selected from the result of the F-test. The idea is to study if the mean value of each texture feature is different for two different patterns. If this difference is not significant, the feature is removed.
- Stepwise method. The idea is to search the minimal number of discriminative features from the features selected in the previous methods. A principal component analysis is used to reduce the dimension of the feature vector.

As a result, 35 features were selected.

6.2.1.4 Classification

Pattern classification is performed using the discriminant method.

Forty-four pigmented lesion images from the *Interactive Atlas of Dermoscopy* [4] with homogeneous, globular, or reticular pattern were used for the study. Each image, therefore, was classified into one of these three patterns. The lesions belonged to blue nevi, Clark nevi, and dermal nevi. Eight hundred fifty-two subimages were extracted from these 44 images. The classification results of the discriminant method are shown in Table 6.1.

6.2.2 PARALLEL PATTERN DETECTION BY IYATOMI ET AL. [20]

Iyatomi et al.'s work [20] is only focused on the detection of parallel patterns motivated by the fact that in non-white populations, melanoma is frequently seen on acral skin [21]. The authors reported that the parallel ridge pattern is the most typical characteristic of acral volar melanoma and the parallel furrow pattern is usually seen in melanocytic nevi. The proposed method describes an automated system for the classification of acral volar melanomas, which parametrizes the lesions objectively and evaluates them instead of detecting the ridges or furrows in the images directly.

The authors developed an acral melanoma nevus classifier and three detectors for typical patterns of acral volar lesions: parallel ridge pattern, parallel furrow pattern, and fibrillar pattern.

6.2.2.1 Segmentation

The lesion area was extracted using a methodology previously proposed by the same authors [22].

6.2.2.2 Feature Extraction

Four hundred twenty-eight image features were extracted, which included color-related features, symmetry features, border-related features, and texture features.

6.2.2.3 Feature Selection

The extracted features were transformed into 198 orthogonal principal components (PCs) using a principal component analysis (PCA). For each classifier and detector, the first 10 more discriminative PCs were selected by an incremental stepwise method with a hypothesis test of Wilk's lambda [23]. This method searched appropriate input parameters one after the other according to the statistical rule. In each step, a statistical F-test was performed and the parameter with the highest partial correlation coefficient under $p < 0.05$ was selected. During this selection step, inefficient (statistically negligible; $p > 0.10$) parameters were rejected from already selected parameters, if they exist. For each classifier and detector, this process was repeated until no further input satisfied the above-mentioned criteria.

6.2.2.4 Classification

The authors focused more on finding effective input features rather than searching for the optimal classification model. Therefore, they proposed classifiers developed by a linear model that enabled them examine the relationship between input parameters and each class more clearly.

A total of 199 acral volar dermoscopy images from four Japanese hospitals and two European university hospitals as part of the *Interactive Atlas of Dermoscopy* [4] were used. The classifiers' performance was evaluated using leave-one-out cross-validation. The sensitivity (SE) and specificity (SP) measures and the area under the receiver operating characteristic (ROC) curve (AUC) [24] were used. The AUC ranges from 0 to 1, and the greater its value, the higher is the classification accuracy. The achieved results are shown in Table 6.2.

TABLE 6.2

Classification Results from [20]

Classifier	SE(%)	SP(%)	AUC
Melanoma	100	95.9	0.993
Parallel ridge pattern	93.1	97.7	0.985
Parallel furrow pattern	90.4	85.9	0.931
Fibrillar pattern	88	77.9	0.89

Note: SE, sensitivity; SP, specificity; AUC, area under the receiver operating characteristic (ROC) curve.

6.2.3 COLOR AND TEXTURE ANALYSIS FOR GLOBAL PATTERN CLASSIFICATION BY ABBAS ET AL. [25]

This work aims to measure the color, architectural order, symmetry of a pattern, and homogeneity (CASH) to classify a lesion into seven global patterns: reticular pattern, globular pattern, cobblestone pattern, homogeneous pattern, parallel pattern, starburst pattern, and multicomponent pattern.

6.2.3.1 Segmentation

The authors proposed to extract a region of interest (ROI), which consisted of a region of size 450×450 pixels, automatically selected from the center of each dermoscopic image of 768×512 pixels.

6.2.3.2 Feature Extraction

Both color and texture features were extracted. The color-related features were extracted using JCh (lightness, chroma, and hue) uniform color space from the CIECAM02 color appearance model. First, six shades of dominant colors and their percentages of occurrence were computed following the work proposed in [26]. Then, to find out color symmetry, the perceived color differences among the set of six dominant colors were computed using the $\triangle E_{02-opt}$ formula. Consequently, the color percentage and symmetric distance differences were utilized for the definition of color features.

For texture feature analysis, the local and global statistical properties were extracted using the multiscale steerable pyramid transform (SPT) technique. The SPT [27, 28] decomposition algorithm is a multiscale and multidirectional representation of frequency transform with interesting translation and rotation invariance properties. First, an input J plane image of size (450×450) pixels is divided into eight rectangular blocks of size (32×32) pixels. The J plane input is decomposed into high-pass and low-pass band images by using steerable high- and low-pass filters [28]. Next, a low-pass image is decomposed into subband images by using four orientation band-pass filters. Mean,

TABLE 6.3

Classification Results from [25]

Pattern	SE (%)	SP (%)	AUC
Reticular	87.11	97.96	0.981
Globular	86.25	97.21	0.997
Cobblestone	87.76	93.23	0.990
Homogeneous	90.47	95.10	0.996
Parallel	85.25	89.50	0.989
Starburst	89.62	90.14	0.966
Multicomponent	98.50	93.11	0.989

Note: SE, sensitivity; SP, specificity; AUC, area under the receiver operating characteristic (ROC) curve.

standard deviation, and skewness texture characteristics are extracted from low-pass, high-pass, and every sub-band-oriented image for each rectangular block. In order to minimize the prediction error of the classification model, the authors applied a principal component analysis (PCA) method to the attributes extracted from the four subband images to select 24 diagonal eigenvalues. Finally, a texture feature vector based on statistical properties of the high- and low-pass subband images was created.

6.2.3.3   Classification

For dermoscopy pattern discrimination a multiclass input boosting algorithm (AdaBoost.MH) [29] was adopted, which is extended to multiclass output by using maximum a posterior (MAP) and robust ranking principles, obtaining the so-called AdaBoost.MC classifier. The color–texture feature vector constructed is finally learned by this AdaBoost.MC multilabel classifier to distinguish between different pattern classes.

A total of 350 dermoscopic images (50 per class) from the *Interactive Atlas of Dermoscopy* [4] were used. Twenty percent of each class was used for testing and 80% for training. To evaluate the diagnostic performance of the proposed model, the area under the curve (AUC) [24] of the receiver operating characteristic (ROC), the sensitivity (SE), and specificity (SP) were used. Results are summarized in Table 6.3.

6.2.4   TEXTONS FOR GLOBAL PATTERN ANALYSIS BY SADEGHI ET AL. [30]

In this work [30] five classes of global lesion patterns (reticular, globular, cobblestone, homogeneous, and parallel) were classified. The proposed approach is based on texton classification [31] where texture features are modeled by the joint probability distribution of filter responses. This distribution is represented by texton (cluster center) frequencies, and textons are learned from training images. The classification of an unseen image proceeds by mapping the image to a texton distribution and comparing this distribution to the learned models.

6.2.4.1 Segmentation

This method only classified patches of 81×81 pixels extracted from a lesion.

6.2.4.2 Classification Method

The texton-based classification procedure was divided into a learning step and a classification step.

6.2.4.2.1 Learning Stage

- A set of 81×81 pixel images representing the five patterns were assembled.
- Training images were convolved with a filter bank to generate filter responses.
- Exemplar filter responses were chosen as textons (via K-means clustering) and were used to label each filter response in the training images.
- The histogram of texton frequencies was used to form models corresponding to the training images.

6.2.4.2.2 Classification Stage

- The same procedure as in the learning stage was followed to build the histogram corresponding to the unseen image.
- This histogram was then compared with the models of the texton dictionary.
- A nearest-neighbor classifier was used and the chi-square statistic was employed to measure distances.

The authors proposed a filter bank composed of $18 + 18 + 2$ filters to detect average intensity, edges, spots, wave, meshes, and ripples of dermatoscopic structures. This set of filters was compared with seven other filter sets: Leung and Malik (ML) [32], Root Filter Set (RFS), Maximum Response filters (MR8) [33], filters proposed by Laws [34] and Schmid [35], texture-specific filters learned by the Convolutional Restricted Boltzmann Machine (CRBM) [36], intensity filters band (JDI) [31], and with color components (JDC). Three hundred and seventy-five patches of 81×81 pixels from 325 dermoscopic images were used, and a three-fold cross-validation was used to evaluate the texton method.

The algorithm that obtained the most satisfactory results was the one based on JDC in $L^*a^*b^*$ space, with a success rate of 86.8%.

6.2.5 GLOBAL PATTERN DETECTION BASED ON MARKOV RANDOM FIELDS BY SERRANO AND ACHA [37]

Serrano and Acha [37] were pioneers in the classification of global patterns following a model-based technique. In the model-based methods, image classification is treated as an incomplete data problem, where the value of each pixel is known and the label, which designated the texture pattern the pixel belongs to, is missing. The authors proposed a method to automatically classify five types of global patterns (reticular, globular, cobblestone, homogeneous, and parallel), in which Markov random field–based texture modeling was performed.

6.2.5.1 Segmentation

This method only classified 40×40 image samples extracted from a lesion.

6.2.5.2 Image Model and Feature Extraction

Following Xia et al.'s model [38], in [37] an image was considered a random field G, defined on a $W \times H$ rectangular lattice, where W and H represented the image dimensions. The lattice was denoted by $S = \{(i,j) : 1 \leq i \leq W, 1 \leq j \leq H\}$, which was indexed by the coordinate (i,j). The color values were represented by $G = \{\mathbf{G_s} = \mathbf{g_s} : \mathbf{s} \in \mathbf{S}\}$, where $s = (i,j)$ denoted a specific site and the random variable $\mathbf{G_s}$ represented a color pixel in the $L^*a^*b^*$ color space. An observed image was an instance of G. It could be described by a finite symmetric conditional model (FSCM) [39] as follows:

$$\mathbf{g}_s = \mu_s + \sum_{t \in v_g} \beta_{s,t}[(\mathbf{g}_{s+t} - \mu_{s+t}) + (\mathbf{g}_{s-t} - \mu_{s-t})] + \mathbf{e}_s \qquad (6.1)$$

where $v_g = \{t_1, t_2, t_3, t_4\} = \{(0,1), (1,0), (1,1), (-1,1)\}$ is the set of shift vectors corresponding to the second-order neighborhood system, $\mu_s = [\mu_L, \mu_a, \mu_b]^T$ is the mean of the color pixels in a window centered in site s, $\{\beta_{s,t} : t \in v_g\}$ is the set of correlation coefficients associated with the set of translations from the central site s, and $\{\mathbf{e}_s\}$ is a stationary Gaussian noise color sequence with a diagonal covariance matrix Σ as

$$\Sigma = \begin{bmatrix} \sigma_L^2 & 0 & 0 \\ 0 & \sigma_a^2 & 0 \\ 0 & 0 & \sigma_a^2 \end{bmatrix} \qquad (6.2)$$

Thus, an 18-component feature vector characterized the random field G:

$$\mathbf{f} = (\mu_L, \mu_a, \mu_b, \sigma_L^2, \sigma_a^2, \sigma_b^2, \beta_{L,t}, \beta_{a,t}, \beta_{b,t} : t \in v_g) \qquad (6.3)$$

In order to estimate the parameter vector $\mathbf{f}$, the least-squares estimation method proposed by Manjunath and Chellappa [40] was applied. Consider a region $N \times N$ (patch) containing a single texture. Let Ω be the set of all the sites belonging to the patch under consideration and Ω_I be the interior of the region of Ω, that is, $\Omega_I = \Omega - \Omega_B$, $\Omega_B = \{s = (s_i, s_j), s \in \Omega, \text{ and } s \pm t \notin \Omega \text{ for at least some } t \in v_g\}$:

$$\hat{\beta} = \left[\sum_{\Omega_I} Q_s Q_s^T\right]^{-1} \left[\sum_{\Omega_I} Q_s g_s\right] \tag{6.4}$$

$$\hat{\sigma}^2 = \frac{1}{N^2} \sum_{\Omega_I} \left[g_s - \hat{\beta}^T Q_s\right]^2 \tag{6.5}$$

$$\mu = \frac{1}{N^2} \sum_{\Omega} g_s \tag{6.6}$$

where Q_s is defined by $Q_s = [g_{s+t} + g_{s-t} : t \in v_g]$. Because we are processing color images, the dimensions of the parameters are $(4 \times 1 \times 3)$ for $\hat{\beta}$, that is, a column vector for each color channel, (1×3) for $\hat{\sigma}^2$ and (1×3) for μ.

6.2.5.3 Classification

Features of images belonging to each class were supposed to follow a multivariate normal distribution, with a different mean vector and covariance matrix for each different global pattern. In other words, if λ represents the pattern class, features will follow the distribution

$$N(\mathbf{M}_\lambda, \Sigma_\lambda) = \frac{1}{\sqrt{(2\pi)^n |\Sigma_\lambda|}} \exp\left(-\frac{1}{2}(\mathbf{f} - \mathbf{M}_\lambda)^T \Sigma_\lambda^{-1} (\mathbf{f} - \mathbf{M}_\lambda)\right) \tag{6.7}$$

In order to find the optimum label the pattern belongs to, the *maximum a posteriori* (MAP) criterion was applied together with the assumption that the five possible global patterns (reticular, cobblestone, homogeneous, parallel, and globular) were equally probable, which resulted in the *maximum likelihood* (ML) criterion. Then

$$\hat{\lambda} = \arg\max_{\lambda \in \Lambda} P(\mathbf{F} = \mathbf{f} | \lambda) \tag{6.8}$$

This ML problem can then be solved by minimizing the following energy:

$$\hat{\lambda} = \min_{\lambda \in \Lambda} E_G(\mathbf{f}, \lambda) = \min_{\lambda \in \Lambda} \{((\mathbf{f} - \mathbf{M}_\lambda)^T \Sigma_\lambda^{-1} (\mathbf{f} - \mathbf{M}_\lambda)) + \ln\left((2\pi)^{18} |\Sigma_\lambda|\right)\} \tag{6.9}$$

The proposed algorithm was tested on a database containing a hundred 40×40 image samples of the five types of patterns. For each type, 20 images were used. Tenfold cross-validation was performed: 90% of the total set of images was used to train (90 images) and 10% to validate (10 images). The total set was divided into 10 groups for the testing. Each time, one different testing group was employed to validate the algorithm. In this way, 18 images of each pattern were used to train and 2 images of each type were used to validate. The authors compared different color spaces obtaining the success classification percentages described in Table 6.4. Although satisfactory results were obtained for the four color spaces, the algorithm with $L^*a^*b^*$ outperforms the others.

Later, Mendoza et al. [41] considered a lesion divided by overlapping patches. Each patch was classified following the mentioned method [37]. The final classification of the whole lesion was determined by a polling process. The aim was to classify whole lesions into one of the following patterns: reticular, globular, cobblestone, and homogeneous. Nine dermatoscopic images of each pattern were employed for the evaluation. The images were extracted from a private database. As training, the authors used fifty 50×50 different patches for each of the four possible textures. Considering the small size of the available database, five patches were extracted from every lesion. For the classification of the patches inside a lesion, only patches from the other lesions were used for training. Each test image was analyzed in 50×50 overlapping patches. In Table 6.5 the results presented by the authors are shown. The success rate of the classification was measured using the percentage of lesions assigned to the correct global pattern. The robustness measurement in this

TABLE 6.4

Percentage of Success Classification in Five Global Patterns for Different Color Spaces

	Reticular	Globular	Cobblestone	Homogeneous	Parallel	Average
RGB	85	85	50	95	85	80
YIQ	75	90	70	95	70	80
HSV	70	80	65	95	95	81
$L^*a^*b^*$	90	80	80	90	90	86

Note: RGB (Red, Green, Blue); YIQ (Luma information, Orange-blue range, Purple-green range); and HSV (Hue, Saturation, Value).

TABLE 6.5

Classification Results from [41]

Pattern	Success Rate	Robustness
Reticular	1.00	0.65
Globular	1.00	0.84
Cobblestone	0.89	0.82
Homogeneous	0.56	0.80

table takes into account the percentage of properly classified patches inside the globally successfully classified lesion.

6.2.6 MODEL-BASED GLOBAL PATTERN CLASSIFICATION BY SÁEZ ET AL. [42]

This work [42] proposed to identify the global pattern that a lesion presents by modeling in different ways. First, an image was modeled as a Markov random field in $L^*a^*b^*$ color space to obtain texture features. In turn, these texture features were supposed to follow different models along the lesion: Gaussian model, Gaussian mixture model, and a bag-of-visual-words histogram model. Different distance metrics between distributions and between histograms were analyzed. A k-nearest-neighbor algorithm based on these distance metrics was then applied, assigning to the test image the global pattern of the closest training image.

The main aim of this paper was the classification of an entire pigmented lesion into a reticular pattern, globular pattern, or homogeneous pattern by texture analysis. However, also presented was further evaluation where the multicomponent pattern was analyzed. There were different reasons behind this decision to instead address the classification of the seven main global patterns. Globules are also predominant in the cobblestone pattern; however, they are larger and more closely aggregated than in the globular pattern, for what can be considered a special case of globular pattern. Consequently, in the database used in this work, images belonging to cobblestone pattern were included in the globular class. Regarding the parallel pattern, its automatic detection does not have a significant interest for the clinical community because lesions with this pattern are only located in the palm or sole. The starburst pattern is characterized by the presence of pigmented streaks at the edge of a given lesion. As the objective was the texture analysis of an entire lesion, this type of lesion escaped from the study.

6.2.6.1 Segmentation

An edge-based level set technique [43] was proposed as a segmentation method. In this technique, the level set formulation proposed by Li et al. [44] was used, in which the edge information was modified by using a color vector gradient implemented in $L^*a^*b^*$ and using the CIE94 color difference equation proposed in [43]. A method to automatically find the initial contour required to begin the process was also proposed.

6.2.6.2 Feature Extraction

The feature extraction step is the same one proposed in the previous work presented by Serrano and Acha [37]. An image was described by a finite symmetric conditional model (FSCM), and the estimated parameters from this model were considered texture features. As a result, an 18-component feature vector characterized an observed image.

6.2.6.3   Model-Based Classification

The classification method proposed in this work was based on the study of the distribution of the features within a lesion. A distribution of features was supposed that follows different models along the lesion: a Gaussian model (GM), a Gaussian mixture model (GMM), and a bag-of-features histogram model (BoF). The results concluded that the Gaussian mixture model–based method outperformed the rest [42]. This method will be presented in this chapter.

For the GMM method, two different scenarios regarding the training set were considered, that is, two different training sets of images were used. Complete lesions composed the first data-set, whereas the second set was constituted by individual patches, each patch extracted from a different lesion of the first data-set. The extraction of these patches was performed randomly. The test set was always constituted by complete lesions. None of the lesions included in the test data-set were included in the training data-set.

In order to analyze a whole lesion, the lesion was divided into overlapping patches. After testing different sizes, the patch size was fixed to 81×81 pixels, achieving a trade-off between computational cost and size, which should be large enough to distinguish and detect different textures. A displacement equal to nine rows or nine columns on the lesion was applied to obtain the next sample. Only the patches without background or with a background area of up to 10% sample area were taken into account.

In this GMM approach, the features extracted from patches constituting a test lesion were supposed to follow a Gaussian mixture model. This model represents a probability density function (PDF) as

$$p(f) = \sum_{j=1}^{K} \pi_j N(M_j, \Sigma_j) \tag{6.10}$$

where M_j and Σ_j are the mean vectors and the covariance matrices of Gaussian kernel j and π_j are the mixing weights. These parameters and weights were estimated iteratively from the input features using the expectation–maximization (EM) algorithm [45]. K stands for the number of Gaussian kernels mixed. After different tests, the best classification results were obtained with a three-component Gaussian mixture model.

Based on this assumption, other two scenarios regarding to the training set were considered:

1. GMM1: Individual patches constituted the training set. The features extracted from the individual training patches belonging to each class followed a Gaussian mixture distribution.

$$p_\lambda(f) = \sum_{i_\lambda=1}^{K} \pi_{i_\lambda} N(M_{i_\lambda}, \Sigma_{i_\lambda}) \tag{6.11}$$

where λ represents each global pattern, K stands for the number of Gaussian kernels mixed for each pattern, M_{i_λ} and Σ_{i_λ} are the mean vectors and covariance matrices of Gaussian kernel i_λ, and π_{i_λ} are the mixing weights.

2. GMM2: The training set consisted of full lesions that were supposed to follow a Gaussian mixture distribution.

$$p'(f) = \sum_{i=1}^{K} \pi'_i N(M'_i, \Sigma'_i) \qquad (6.12)$$

The idea was to compare the Gaussian mixture model of a test lesion with the mixture distribution corresponding to the training sets. To this purpose, different distance metrics between Gaussian mixture models were used: the symmetric Kullback Leibler divergence [46], the Bhattacharyya-based distance metric [46], earth mover's distance (EMD) [47], and a distance metric proposed by Sfikas et al. [46].

The computation of the Kullback Leibler divergence between two GMM distributions is not direct. In fact, there is no analytical solution, and it is necessary to resort to Monte Carlo methods or numerical approximations. Thus, in this work the approximation proposed by [46] was used:

$$SKL(p, p') = \left| \frac{1}{2N} \sum_{f \sim p} lnp(f) - \frac{1}{2N} \sum_{f \sim p} lnp'(f) + \right.$$

$$\left. + \frac{1}{2N} \sum_{f \sim p'} lnp(f) - \frac{1}{2N} \sum_{f \sim p'} lnp'(f) \right| \qquad (6.13)$$

where N is the number of data samples generated from the $p(f)$ and $p'(f)$, and $p(f)$ and $p'(f)$ are estimated iteratively with EM [46].

The Bhattacharyya-based distance metric was computed as

$$BhGMM(p, p') = \sum_{i=1}^{L} \sum_{j=1}^{K} \pi_j \pi'_i B(p_j, p'_i) \qquad (6.14)$$

where p, p' are Gaussian mixture models consisting of K and L kernels, respectively. p_j, p'_i denote the kernel parameters, and π_j, π'_i are the mixing weights. B denotes the Bhattacharyya distance between two Gaussian kernels, defined as

$$B(F_i, F_t) = \frac{1}{8} u^T \left(\frac{\Sigma_i + \Sigma_t}{2} \right)^{-1} u + \frac{1}{2} ln \left[\frac{\left| \frac{\Sigma_i + \Sigma_t}{2} \right|}{\sqrt{|\Sigma_i||\Sigma_t|}} \right] \qquad (6.15)$$

where $u = (M_i - M_t)$.

The EMD for GMMs was computed as

$$EMD(p, p') = \frac{\sum_{i=1}^{L} \sum_{j=1}^{K} f_{ij} Fr(p_j, p_i')}{\sum_{i=1}^{L} \sum_{j=1}^{K} f_{ij}} \tag{6.16}$$

$$\sum_{i=1}^{L} \sum_{j=1}^{K} f_{ij} = min\left(\sum_{j=1}^{K} \pi_j, \sum_{i=1}^{L} \pi_i'\right) \tag{6.17}$$

where $Fr(p_j, p_i')$ is the Frechet distance [48] between p_j and p_i':

$$Fr(F_i, F_t) = \sqrt{\left(u^T u + tr(\Sigma_i + \Sigma_t - 2\sqrt{\Sigma_i \Sigma_t})\right)} \tag{6.18}$$

The distance metric proposed by Sfikas et al. [46] to compare Gaussian mixtures is computed as

$$C2(p, p') = -log$$

$$\left[\frac{2 \sum_{i,j} \pi_i \pi_j' \sqrt{\frac{|V_{ij}|}{e^{k_{ij}} |\Sigma_i||\Sigma_j'|}}}{\sum_{i,j} \left\{ \pi_i \pi_j \sqrt{\frac{|V_{ij}|}{e^{k_{ij}} |\Sigma_i||\Sigma_j|}} \right\} + \sum_{i,j} \left\{ \pi_i' \pi_j' \sqrt{\frac{|V_{ij}|}{e^{k_{ij}} |\Sigma_i'||\Sigma_j'|}} \right\}} \right] \tag{6.19}$$

$$V_{ij} = \left(\Sigma_i^{-1} + \Sigma_j'^{-1} \right)^{-1} \tag{6.20}$$

$$k_{ij} = M_i^T \Sigma_i^{-1}(M_i - M_j') + M_j'^T \Sigma_j'^{-1}(M_j' - M_i) \tag{6.21}$$

π, π' are the mixing weights, i and j are indexes on the Gaussian kernels, and M, Σ and M', Σ' are the mean and covariance matrices for the kernels of Gaussian mixtures $p(f)$ and $p'(f)$, respectively.

In order to classify a lesion, in the first case, a test image is identified with the closest pattern according to the four distances proposed above, and in the second case, the test image is assigned to the pattern of the closest training image. The complete process is presented in Figure 6.10.

The image database used in this work was formed by 30 images of each type of pattern, a total of 90 images. These 30 images from each global pattern were randomly chosen. As the cobblestone pattern was considered a special case of globular pattern, 8 images out of the 30 categorized as globular pattern belonged to the cobblestone pattern. All images were extracted from the *Interactive Atlas of Dermoscopy*, published by EDRA Medical Publishing and New Media [4].

A 20-times three-fold cross-validation was used to evaluate the performance of the proposed methods.

The success classification rate achieved for the three distance metrics proposed in the two methods based on the multivariate Gaussian mixture model is presented in Figure 6.11. The C2 distance proposed in [46] outperformed

Method	Training set	Test set	Classifier	Result
GMM1	→ GMM_{glo} → GMM_{hom} → GMM_{ret}	→ GMM_{test}	Dist (GMM_{ci}, GMM_{test})	Closest pattern
GMM2	→ GMM_{train}	→ GMM_{test}	Dist $(GMM_{train}, GMM_{test})$	Pattern of the closest training image

FIGURE 6.10 (**See color insert.**) Classification methods based on Gaussian mixture model.

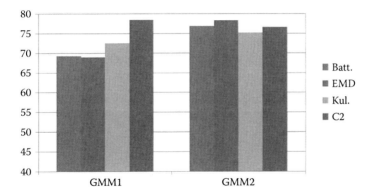

FIGURE 6.11 Performance of the methods proposed based on Gaussian mixture model (GMM1 and GMM2) when using different distance metrics: Bhattacharyya based (Batt.), earth mover's distance (EMD), Kullback Leibler divergence (Kul.), and C2 distance [46]. y-Axis shows the classification success rate of the classification methods.

the rest in the first scenario, whereas in the second case, EMD outperformed the rest of the distances.

Table 6.6 shows the classification success rate for the distances that provided the highest classification rate obtained. In addition, the classification success rate obtained in the identification of each global pattern is shown.

A further evaluation, in which the multicomponent pattern was included, was performed. Thirty images of melanomas with multicomponent pattern were chosen randomly from the *Interactive Atlas of Dermoscopy* [4]. Table 6.7 presents the results.

TABLE 6.6

Classification Results for the Methods Based on Gaussian Mixture Model

Method	Globular	Homogeneous	Reticular	Average
GMM1 (C2)	62.00%	98.00%	75.33%	78.44%
GMM2 (EMD)	66.50%	99.67%	69.00%	78.38%

TABLE 6.7

Classification Results when the Multicomponent Pattern Was Included

Method	Globular	Homogeneous	Reticular	Multicomponent	Average
GMM2 (EMD)	64.33%	95.83%	67.00%	64.5%	72.91%

The homogeneous pattern is identified with a success rate of more than 95% in all cases, decreasing this rate for globular and reticular pattern identification. However, the overall result is considerably good, with a classification success rate of 78%. The inclusion of the multicomponent pattern in the classification procedure reduces the success rate by only 5.53%. These promising results show the potential of this system for early melanoma diagnosis.

6.3 DISCUSSION

Assessing skin lesions by dermoscopy basically includes three main steps [49]. First, the overview of the lesion gives indications on the global pattern of the lesion. The second step is the definition of the melanocytic or nonmelanocytic nature of the lesion itself, thanks to the recognition of specific dermoscopic structures. Dermoscopic criteria suggestive of melanocytic lesions are pigment network, dots, globules (larger than dots), streaks/pseudopods, blotches, structureless areas, regression pattern, and blue–white veil [10]. Once the melanocytic nature is defined, the further step is to study the characteristics and the organization of such dermoscopic structures by applying a dermoscopic algorithm in order to achieve a correct diagnosis between benign and malignant melanocytic lesions. The pattern analysis method, which is based on a qualitative analysis of the global and local features, allows the highest rates of diagnostic accuracy. Therefore, identification of global patterns covers several crucial steps to reach a diagnosis on pigmented lesions.

Global patterns allow a quick preliminary categorization of a given pigmented skin lesion. The detection of these global features is the first step carried out in the diagnostic algorithm called pattern analysis. This methodology defines both global and local dermoscopic patterns. A pigmented lesion is identified by a global pattern and by one or more than one local patterns. Pattern analysis not only allows dermatologists to distinguish between benign and malignant growth features, but it also determines the type of lesion. Each diagnostic category within the realm of pigmented skin lesions is characterized by few global patterns and a rather distinctive combination of specific local features.

However, despite its importance, automatic detection of global patterns has been addressed in only few works. The authors consider that the main cause is the difficulty in the classification, which may be due to the following reasons:

- Considering that the global pattern is determined by the dermato-scopic feature predominant in the lesion, its automated classification becomes hard due to the possible presence of different local patterns in the same lesion.
- Intraclass variability: Lesions belonging to the same global pattern can present a very different appearance
- Interclass similarity: Lesions belonging to the different global patterns can present a certain similar appearance.

There are nine global patterns (reticular, globular, cobblestone, homogeneous, parallel, starbust, multicomponent, lacunar, and unspecific); however, the lacunar pattern is not used to diagnose melanoma because it is characteristic of nonmelanocitic lesions [4]. The term *unspecific pattern* is used when a pigmented lesion cannot be categorized into one of the rest of the global patterns. Therefore, we can consider that there are seven main global features. Abbas et al. [25] classified the seven patterns using only color and texture features. However, the evaluation does not seem very exhaustive; 80% of images were taken as a training set without cross-validation.

A common characteristic among the rest of the works is that none detects the starbust pattern due to the fact it is only characterized by the presence of streaks at the periphery of the lesion. However, there are works devoted exclusively to the detection of streaks [50–52]. A review is presented in [12].

On the contrary, all works (except Iyatomi et al. [20], which only detects parallel patterns) address the detection of reticular, globular, and homogeneous patterns—probably because of being some of the most common global patterns in melanocitic lesions [53]. However, the multicomponent pattern, which is the most suggestive of melanoma, is only detected by Abbas et al. [25] and our work [42]. The authors think that more effort in detecting this pattern should be made.

As it has been mentioned, Iyatomi et al. [20] only focused on the detection of the different existing types of parallel pattern. Since this pattern is only found on palms and soles, we think that this option is more interesting than the parallel pattern that is distinguished from other global patterns.

Regarding the methodology, we can observe that some of the works presented in this chapter are based on the classic approach of pattern recognition

[18, 20, 25], feature extraction from the region of interest, and use of a classifier with supervised learning [54], whereas other works focus on modeling each texture [30, 37, 42].

Another highlight is what type of image is under study. In this sense, the classification of entire lesions is interestingly addressed in our work [42], in contrast to the rest of the works that classify only patches or subimages extracted from a lesion.

Finally, we conclude that the automatic detection of global patterns is a growing research field, since this detection is essential to developing a system that emulates the method of pattern analysis, together with the detection of local patterns.

REFERENCES

1. S. Menzies, C. Ingvar, K. Crotty, and W. McCarthy, Frequency and morphologic characteristics of invasive melanomas lacking specific surface microscopic features, *Archives of Dermatology*, vol. 132, no. 10, pp. 1178–1182, 1996.

2. M. L. Bafounta, A. Beauchet, P. Aegerter, and P. Saiag, Is dermoscopy (epiluminescence microscopy) useful for the diagnosis of melanoma? Results of a meta-analysis using techniques adapted to the evaluation of diagnostic tests, *Archives of Dermatology*, vol. 137, no. 10, pp. 1343–1350, 2001.

3. R. Braun, H. Rabinovitz, M. Oliviero, A. Kopf, and J. Saurat, Pattern analysis: A two-step procedure for the dermoscopic diagnosis of melanoma, *Clinics in Dermatology*, vol. 20, no. 3, pp. 236–239, 2002.

4. G. Argenziano, H. Soyer, V. De Giorgio, D. Piccolo, P. Carli, M. Delfino, and A. Ferrari, *Interactive Atlas of Dermoscopy*, EDRA-Medical Publishing and New Media, Milan, Italy, 2000.

5. F. Nachbar, W. Stolz, T. Merkle, A. Cognetta, T. Vogt, M. Landthaler, P. Bilek, O. Braun-Falco, and G. Plewig, The ABCD rule of dermatoscopy, *Journal of the American Academy of Dermatology*, vol. 30, no. 4, pp. 551–559, 1994.

6. H. Pehamberger, A. Steiner, and K. Wolff, In vivo epiluminescence microscopy of pigmented skin lesions. I. Pattern analysis of pigmented skin lesions, *Journal of the American Academy of Dermatology*, vol. 17, no. 4, pp. 571–583, 1987.

7. G. Argenziano, G. Fabbrocini, P. Carli, V. De Giorgi, E. Sammarco, and M. Delfino, Epiluminescence microscopy for the diagnosis of doubtful melanocytic skin lesions: Comparison of the ABCD rule of dermatoscopy and a new 7-point checklist based on pattern analysis, *Archives of Dermatology*, vol. 134, no. 12, pp. 1563–1570, 1998.

8. DermNet NZ, Pattern analysis, http://www.dermnetnz.org/doctors/dermoscopy-course/pattern-analysis.html.

9. P. Carli, E. Quercioli, S. Sestini, M. Stante, L. Ricci, G. Brunasso, and V. De Giorgi, Pattern analysis, not simplified algorithms, is the most reliable method for teaching dermoscopy for melanoma diagnosis to residents in dermatology, *British Journal of Dermatology*, vol. 148, no. 5, pp. 981–984, 2003.

10. G. Argenziano, H. P. Soyer, S. Chimenti, R. Talamini, R. Corona, F. Sera, and M. Binder, Dermoscopy of pigmented skin lesions: Results of a consensus meeting via the internet. *Journal of the American Academy of Dermatology*, vol. 81, no. 3, pp. 261–268, 2006.

11. G. Rezze, B. De S, and R. Neves, Dermoscopy: The pattern analysis, *Anais Brasileiros de Dermatologia*, vol. 81, no. 3, pp. 261–268, 2006.

12. A. Sáez, B. Acha, and C. Serrano, Pattern analysis in dermoscopic images, in *Computer Vision Techniques for the Diagnosis of Skin Cancer* (J. Scharcanski and M. E. Celebi, eds.), Series in BioEngineering, pp. 23–48, Springer, 2013.

13. H. Soyer, G. Argenziano, V. Ruocco, and S. Chimenti, Dermoscopy of pigmented skin lesions (part II), *European Journal of Dermatology*, vol. 11, no. 5, pp. 483–498, 2001.

14. J. Scharcanski and M. E. Celebi, *Computer Vision Techniques for the Diagnosis of Skin Cancer*, Springer, 2013.

15. K. Korotkov and R. Garcia, Computerized analysis of pigmented skin lesions: A review, *Artificial Intelligence in Medicine*, vol. 56, no. 2, pp. 69–90, 2012.

16. M. E. Celebi, W. V. Stoecker, and R. H. Moss, Advances in skin cancer image analysis, *Computer Medical Imaging and Graphics*, vol. 35, no. 2, pp. 83–84, 2011.

17. T. Tanaka, S. Torii, I. Kabuta, K. Shimizu, M. Tanaka, and H. Oka, Pattern classification of nevus with texture analysis, in *Proceedings of the Annual International Conference of IEEE Engineering in Medicine and Biology*, San Francisco, CA, vol. 26 II, pp. 1459–1462, 2004.

18. T. Tanaka, S. Torii, I. Kabuta, K. Shimizu, and M. Tanaka, Pattern classification of nevus with texture analysis, *IEEJ Transactions on Electrical and Electronic Engineering*, vol. 3, no. 1, pp. 143–150, 2008.

19. N. Otsu, An automatic threshold selection method based on discriminate and least squares criteria, *Transactions of the Institute of Electronics and Communication Engineering of Japan*, vol. J63-D, no. 4, pp. 349–356, 1980.

20. H. Iyatomi, H. Oka, M. E. Celebi, K. Ogawa, G. Argenziano, H. Soyer, H. Koga, T. Saida, K. Ohara, and M. Tanaka, Computer-based classification of dermoscopy images of melanocytic lesions on acral volar skin, *Journal of Investigative Dermatology*, vol. 128, no. 8, pp. 2049–2054, 2008.

21. T. Saida, S. Oguchi, and A. Miyazaki, Dermoscopy for acral pigmented skin lesions, *Clinics in Dermatology*, vol. 20, no. 3, pp. 279–285, 2002.

22. H. Iyatomi, H. Oka, M. Saito, A. Miyake, M. Kimoto, J. Yamagami, S. Kobayashi et al., Quantitative assessment of tumour extraction from dermoscopy images and evaluation of computer-based extraction methods for an automatic melanoma diagnostic system, *Melanoma Research*, vol. 16, no. 2, pp. 183–190, 2006.

23. B. Everitt, G. G. Dunn, and B. Everitt, *Applied Multivariate Data Analysis*, London: E. Arnold New York, 1991. Rev. ed. of *Advanced Methods of Data Exploration and Modelling*, 1983.

24. A. Bradley, The use of the area under the ROC curve in the evaluation of machine learning algorithms, *Pattern Recognition*, vol. 30, no. 7, pp. 1145–1159, 1997.

25. Q. Abbas, M. E. Celebi, C. Serrano, I. F. Garcia, and G. Ma, Pattern classification of dermoscopy images: A perceptually uniform model, *Pattern Recognition*, vol. 46, no. 1, pp. 86–97, 2013.

26. J. Chen, T. Pappas, A. Mojsilovic, and B. Rogowitz, Adaptive perceptual color-texture image segmentation, *IEEE Transactions on Image Processing*, vol. 14, no. 10, pp. 1524–1536, 2005.

27. W. T. Freeman and E. H. Adelson, The design and use of steerable filters, *IEEE Transactions on Pattern Analysis and Machine Intelligence*, vol. 13, no. 9, pp. 891–906, 1991.

28. E. P. Simoncelli, W. T. Freeman, E. H. Adelson, and D. J. Heeger, Shiftable multiscale transforms, *IEEE Transactions on Information Theory*, vol. 38, no. 2, pp. 587–607, 1992.

29. R. Schapire and Y. Singer, Boostexter: A boosting-based system for text categorization, *Machine Learning*, vol. 39, no. 2, pp. 135–168, 2000.

30. M. Sadeghi, T. Lee, D. McLean, H. Lui, and M. Atkins, Global pattern analysis and classification of dermoscopic images using textons, in *Progress in Biomedical Optics and Imaging—Proceedings of SPIE*, vol. 8314, 2012.

31. M. Varma and A. Zisserman, Texture classification: Are filter banks necessary? in *Proceedings of the IEEE Computer Society Conference on Computer Vision and Pattern Recognition*, Portland, ON, vol. 2, pp. II/691–II/698, 2003.

32. T. Leung and J. Malik, Representing and recognizing the visual appearance of materials using three-dimensional textons, *International Journal of Computer Vision*, vol. 43, no. 1, pp. 29–44, 2001.

33. M. Varma and A. Zisserman, A statistical approach to texture classification from single images, *International Journal of Computer Vision*, vol. 62, no. 1–2, pp. 61–81, 2005.

34. M. Anantha, R. Moss, and W. Stoecker, Detection of pigment network in dermatoscopy images using texture analysis, *Computerized Medical Imaging and Graphics*, vol. 28, no. 5, pp. 225–234, 2004.

35. P. Schmid, Segmentation of digitized dermatoscopic images by two-dimensional color clustering, *IEEE Transactions on Medical Imaging*, vol. 18, no. 2, pp. 164–171, 1999.

36. M. Norouzi, M. Ranjbar, and G. Mori, Stacks of convolutional restricted Boltzmann machines for shift-invariant feature learning, in *2009 IEEE Computer Society Conference on Computer Vision and Pattern Recognition Workshops, CVPR Workshops 2009*, Miami, Florida, pp. 2735–2742, 2009.

37. C. Serrano and B. Acha, Pattern analysis of dermoscopic images based on Markov random fields, *Pattern Recognition*, vol. 42, no. 6, pp. 1052–1057, 2009.

38. Y. Xia, D. Feng, and R. Zhao, Adaptive segmentation of textured images by using the coupled Markov random field model, *IEEE Transactions on Image Processing*, vol. 15, no. 11, pp. 3559–3566, 2006.

39. R. L. Kashyap and R. Chellappa, Estimation and choice of neighbors in spatial-interaction models of images, *IEEE Transactions on Information Theory*, vol. IT-29, no. 1, pp. 60–72, 1983.

40. B. Manjunath and R. Chellappa, Unsupervised texture segmentation using Markov random field models, *IEEE Transactions on Pattern Analysis and Machine Intelligence*, vol. 13, no. 5, pp. 478–482, 1991.

41. C. Mendoza, C. Serrano, and B. Acha, Pattern analysis of dermoscopic images based on FSCM color Markov random fields, *Lecture Notes in Computer Science*, Bordeaux, France, vol. 5807, pp. 676–685, 2009.

42. A. Sáez, C. Serrano, and B. Acha, Model-based classification methods of global patterns in dermoscopic images, *IEEE Transactions on Medical Imaging*, vol. 33, no. 5, pp. 1137–1147, 2014.

43. A. Sáez, C. S. Mendoza, B. Acha, and C. Serrano, Development and evaluation of perceptually adapted colour gradients, *IET Image Processing*, vol. 7, no. 4, pp. 355–363, 2013.

44. C. Li, C. Xu, C. Gui, and M. Fox, Level set evolution without re-initialization: A new variational formulation, in *Proceedings of the IEEE Computer Society Conference on Computer Vision and Pattern Recognition*, San Diego, CA, vol. 1, pp. 430–436, 2005.

45. G. Mclachlan and D. Peel, *Finite Mixture Models*, 1st ed., Wiley Series in Probability and Statistics, Wiley-Interscience, 2000.

46. G. Sfikas, C. Constantinopoulos, A. Likas, and N. Galatsanos, An analytic distance metric for Gaussian mixture models with application in image retrieval, *Lecture Notes in Computer Science* (including subseries *Lecture Notes in Artificial Intelligence* and *Lecture Notes in Bioinformatics*), vol. 3697, pp. 835–840, 2005.

47. H. Greenspan, G. Dvir, and Y. Rubner, Context-dependent segmentation and matching in image databases, *Computer Vision and Image Understanding*, vol. 93, no. 1, pp. 86–109, 2004.

48. D. Dowson and B. Landau, The Frechet distance between multivariate normal distributions, *Journal of Multivariate Analysis*, vol. 12, no. 3, pp. 450–455, 1982.

49. A. Gulia, A. M. G. Brunasso, and C. Massone, Dermoscopy: Distinguishing malignant tumors from benign, *Expert Review of Dermatology*, vol. 7, no. 5, pp. 439–458, 2012.

50. H. Mirzaalian, T. Lee, and G. Hamarneh, Learning features for streak detection in dermoscopic color images using localized radial flux of principal intensity curvature, in *Proceedings of the Workshop on Mathematical Methods in Biomedical Image Analysis*, Breckenridge, CO, pp. 97–101, 2012.

51. M. Sadeghi, T. Lee, D. McLean, H. Lui, and M. Atkins, Detection and analysis of irregular streaks in dermoscopic images of skin lesions, *IEEE Transactions on Medical Imaging*, vol. 32, no. 5, pp. 849–861, 2013.

52. G. Fabbrocini, G. Betta, G. D. Leo, C. Liguori, A. Paolillo, A. Pietrosanto, P. Sommella et al., Epiluminescence image processing for melanocytic skin lesion diagnosis based on 7-point check-list: A preliminary discussion on three parameters, *Open Dermatology Journal*, vol. 4, pp. 110–115, 2010.

53. B. Amorim and T. Mendonca, Database system for clinical and computer assisted diagnosis of dermoscopy images, in *Topics in Medical Image Processing and Computational Vision* (J. M. R. Tavares and R. M. Natal Jorge, eds.), vol. 8 of *Lecture Notes in Computational Vision and Biomechanics*, pp. 261–274, Springer, 2013.

54. M. E. Celebi, H. A. Kingravi, B. Uddin, H. Iyatomi, Y. A. Aslandogan, W. V. Stoecker, and R. H. Moss, A methodological approach to the classification of dermoscopy images, *Computer Medical Imaging and Graphics*, vol. 31, no. 6, pp. 362–373, 2007.

7 Streak Detection in Dermoscopic Color Images Using Localized Radial Flux of Principal Intensity Curvature

Hengameh Mirzaalian
Simon Fraser University
British Columbia, Canada

Tim K. Lee
University of British Columbia
and
Vancouver Coastal Health Research Institute
and
British Columbia Cancer Agency
British Columbia, Canada

Ghassan Hamarneh
Simon Fraser University
British Columbia, Canada

CONTENTS

7.1   INTRODUCTION

Malignant melanoma (MM) is one of the common cancers among the white population [1]. Dermoscopy, a noninvasive method for early recognition of MM, allows a clear visualization of skin internal structures, which are often analyzed by a dermoscopic algorithm, such as the ABCD rule of dermoscopy or the 7-point checklist [2]. These methods utilize different dermoscopic features for diagnosing pigmented melanocytic lesions; for example, ABCD analyzes the weighted features of asymmetry (A), border (B), color (C), and differential structures (D). On the other hand, the 7-point checklist looks for the presence of seven different patterns (atypical pigment network, blue–white veil, atypical vascular pattern, irregular streaks, irregular dots/globules, irregular blotches, regression structures). Depending on the presence or absence of each of these patterns, a weight score is assigned to a pigmented lesion. These scores are added up and used for the diagnosis of melanoma. Studies showed that these dermoscopic algorithms can improve the diagnostic accuracy of melanoma.

Interpreting dermoscopic features requires a steep learning curve. Without proper training, these complex visual features could confuse even experienced dermatologists. Recently, a considerable amount of research has focused on automating the feature extraction and classification of dermoscopic images with the aim of developing a computer-aided diagnostic technique for early melanoma detection. A review of the existing computerized methods to analyze images of pigmented skin lesions utilizing dermoscopy has been recently reported in [3–6].

Among the dermoscopic features, streaks are important. Although streaks in children are likely to be benign, adults with streaks should be examined carefully [7]. Irregular streaks are often associated with melanomas. In this chapter, we present a fully automated method for streak detection based on a machine learning approach, which is useful for a computer-aided diagnosis (CAD) system for pigmented skin lesions. In the following paragraphs, the typical pipeline for a CAD system is described.

7.1.1   ARTIFACT REMOVAL

The first step of a CAD system for dermoscopic images is *artifact removal* as a preprocessing step; dermoscopic images are often degraded by artifacts such as black frames, rulers, air bubbles, and hairs (Figure 7.1). In particular, hairs are the most common artifacts. The existence of such artifacts complicates lesion segmentation, feature detection, and classification tasks. Although artifact removal has been investigated extensively [8–13], the problem has not been fully solved. One of the problems is the lack of validation

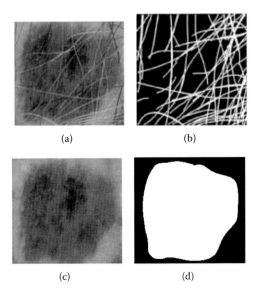

(a)   (b)

(c)   (d)

FIGURE 7.1 (a) Example of real hair-occluded image. (b) Hair masks of the image in (a). (c) Hair-free image of (a); generated by applying the in-painting approach in [8]. (d) Mask of the segmented lesions in (c). (Reprinted with permission from Argenziano, G. et al., *Dermoscopy: A Tutorial*, EDRA Medical Publishing and New Media, Milan, Italy, 2002.)

tools. For example, since hairs are very thin with spatially varying width, preparing a ground truth manually for a large number of hair pixels would be exorbitantly tedious, let alone for a large number of images. In order to assist validation and benchmarking of hair enhancement and segmentation, we developed a simulation, HairSim, which is available publicly at www.cs.sfu.ca/~hamarneh/software/hairsim. An example of a simulated hair-occluded image generated by HairSim is shown in Figure 7.2a.

7.1.2 IN-PAINTING

After identifying artifacts, the next step is to replace the pixels comprising the artifact with new values by estimating the underlying color of the scene. In computer vision, the technique of reconstructing the lost or deteriorated part of an image is called in-painting. There exist limited works on in-painting on dermoscopic images, for example, using color [14] and texture [15] diffusion. An example in-painted (hair-disoccluded) image is shown in Figure 7.1c.

7.1.3 LESION SEGMENTATION

The next step in the traditional pipeline is lesion segmentation, on which there exist considerable amounts of work, mostly using color clustering [9, 16, 17], region growing [18–21], active contours [22–25], and graph labeling [26–28]

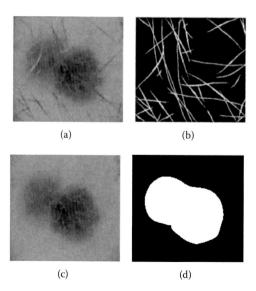

(a)   (b)

(c)   (d)

FIGURE 7.2 (a) Example of simulated hair-occluded image. (b) Hair masks of the image in (a). (c) Hair-free image of (a); the original skin image processed by HairSim software to generate the simulated hair-occluded images in (a). (d) Mask of the segmented lesion in (c). (Reprinted with permission from Argenziano, G. et al., *Dermoscopy: A Tutorial*, EDRA Medical Publishing and New Media, Milan, Italy, 2002.)

approaches (recent surveys: [29, 30]). Examples of lesion segmentation masks are shown in Figures 7.1 and 7.2.

7.1.4 FEATURE EXTRACTION AND CLASSIFICATION

The last step of a CAD system is feature extraction and classification. A notable number of methods have been proposed to this end. In general, we classify the existing feature descriptors in three major groups:

- Color-based features, which are simple statistics of pixel intensities, such as means and variances in different color spaces (e.g., RGB, HSI, and Luv) [31–34].
- Statistical texture descriptors, which measure texture properties such as smoothness, coarseness, and regularity of the lesion, for example, intensity distribution descriptors [16, 35, 36], wavelet-based (WT) descriptors* [34, 37, 38], SIFT descriptors [38], and gray-level dependence matrix (GLDM)† [35].

---

* WT-based descriptors are set as the mean and variance of the WT coefficients of the different subbands.
† GLDM-based descriptors are rotation invariant, which consider the relation between a pixel and all its neighbors.

- Geometric-based features, which describe the shape or the spatial relationship of a lesion mainly with respect to the segmented border, for example, elongation or border irregularity [31–33, 39, 40]. Recently, a set of geometric-based information was extracted from lesions for orientation analysis of structures, for example, by considering a histogram of oriented gradients [26] and detecting cyclic subgraphs corresponding to skin texture structures [41].

In this chapter, we focus on the extraction of a new geometric-based feature for streak detection. Streaks, also referred to as radial streamings, appear as linear structures located at the periphery of a lesion and are classified as either regular or irregular depending on the appearance of their intensity, texture, and color distribution [42]. Examples of dermoscopic images in the absence and presence of streaks are shown in Figures 7.3 through 7.5. We notice that

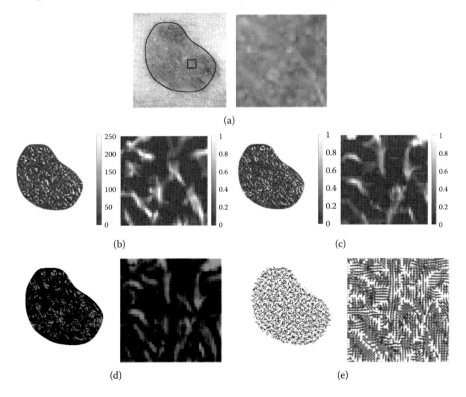

FIGURE 7.3 (a) Dermoscopic image in the absence of streaks. The image is overlaid with a segmented border of the lesion. A close-up of the region inside the blue box is shown on the right side of the image. (b, c) Frangi filter responses ν^+ (b) and ν^- (c) Equation 7.7, which are encoded to the red and green channels (light gray) in (d). (e) Direction of the minimum intensity curvature. (Reprinted with permission from Argenziano, G. et al., *Dermoscopy: A Tutorial*, EDRA Medical Publishing and New Media, Milan, Italy, 2002.)

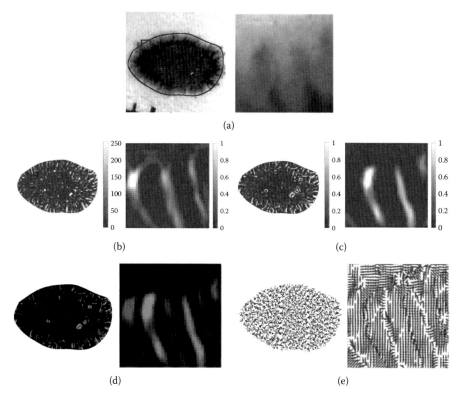

FIGURE 7.4 (a) Dermoscopic image in the presence of regular streaks. The image is overlaid with a segmented border of the lesion. A close-up of the region inside the blue box is shown on the right side of the image. (b, c) Frangi filter responses v^+ (b) and v^- (c) Equation 7.7, which are encoded to the red and green channels (light gray) in (d). (e) Direction of the minimum intensity curvature. (Reprinted with permission from Argenziano, G. et al., *Dermoscopy: A Tutorial*, EDRA Medical Publishing and New Media, Milan, Italy, 2002.)

the appearance of vasculature in biomedical images resembles to some degree the appearance of streaks in dermoscopic images. Despite notable differences (e.g., vessel images are typically single channel, whereas dermoscopic images are colored), methods for dermoscopic image analysis stand to benefit from methods for the detection and analysis of tubular structures, as has been witnessed in state-of-the-art research on vascular image analysis. In the following, we describe our streak detection approach, which is based on our earlier work [43].

We extract orientation information of streaks through the use of eigenvalue decomposition of the Hessian matrix (Section 7.2.4). After estimating tubularness and streak direction, we define a vector field in order to quantify the

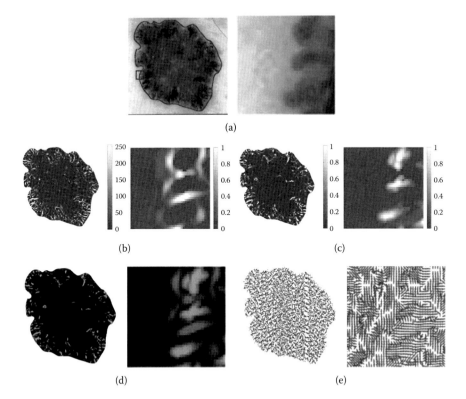

FIGURE 7.5 (a) Dermoscopic image in the presence of irregular streaks. The image is overlaid with a segmented border of the lesion. A close-up of the region inside the blue box is shown on the right side of the image. (b, c) Frangi filter responses v^+ (b) and v^- (c) Equation 7.7, which are encoded to the red and green channels (light gray) in (d). (e) Direction of the minimum intensity curvature. (Reprinted with permission from Argenziano, G. et al., *Dermoscopy: A Tutorial*, EDRA Medical Publishing and New Media, Milan, Italy, 2002.)

radial component of the streak pattern. In particular, we compute the amount of flux of calculated vector field passing through isodistance lesion contours. We construct our appearance descriptor based on the mean and variance of this flux through different concentric bands of the lesion, which in turn allows for more localized features without the prerequisite of explicitly calculating a point-to-point correspondence between the lesion shapes (Section 7.2.5). We validate the classification performance of a support vector machine (SVM) classifier based on our extracted features (Section 7.3). Our results on 99 dermoscopic images show that we obtain improved classification, by up to 9% in terms of area under the receiver operating characteristic (ROC) curves, compared to the state of the art (Section 7.4).

7.2 METHODS

We start by having a short introduction on the Hessian matrix (Section 7.2.1), followed by introducing Frangi filter tubularness (Section 7.2.2), quaternion color curvature (Section 7.2.3), and our proposed feature descriptor for streak detection (Section 7.2.5).

7.2.1 IMAGE HESSIAN MATRIX

Local shape characteristics of an image can be analyzed using the Hessian matrix of the image. In the presence of lines (i.e., straight or nearly straight curvilinear features) and edges, a low curvature is measured via the Hessian in the direction of the lines and edges, where there is little change in image intensities and a high curvature in the orthogonal direction of them. For a two-dimensional (2D) scalar image I, its 2×2 Hessian is a matrix of the second derivatives of the image

$$H(\mathbf{x}, s) = \begin{bmatrix} I_{xx}(\mathbf{x}, s) & I_{xy}(\mathbf{x}, s) \\ I_{xy}(\mathbf{x}, s) & I_{yy}(\mathbf{x}, s) \end{bmatrix} \tag{7.1}$$

$I_{xx}(\mathbf{x})$, $I_{xy}(\mathbf{x})$, and $I_{yy}(\mathbf{x})$ are the second-order partial derivatives of the scalar image I evaluated at pixel $\mathbf{x} = <x_1, x_2>$, and s is the scale of Gaussian functions convolved with the image to compute the partial derivatives:

$$I_{xx}(\mathbf{x}, s) = I(\mathbf{x}) * G_{xx}(\mathbf{x}, s)$$
$$I_{xy}(\mathbf{x}, s) = I(\mathbf{x}) * G_{xy}(\mathbf{x}, s) \tag{7.2}$$
$$I_{yy}(\mathbf{x}, s) = I(\mathbf{x}) * G_{yy}(\mathbf{x}, s)$$

where $*$ is the convolution operator:

$$I(\mathbf{x}) * G_{xx}(\mathbf{x}, s) = \sum_{m=-3s}^{3s} \sum_{n=-3s}^{3s} I(\mathbf{x}_1 - m, \mathbf{x}_2 - n)G_{xx}(m, n, s)$$

$$I(\mathbf{x}) * G_{xy}(\mathbf{x}, s) = \sum_{m=-3s}^{3s} \sum_{n=-3s}^{3s} I(\mathbf{x}_1 - m, \mathbf{x}_2 - n)G_{xy}(m, n, s) \tag{7.3}$$

$$I(\mathbf{x}) * G_{yy}(\mathbf{x}, s) = \sum_{m=-3s}^{3s} \sum_{n=-3s}^{3s} I(\mathbf{x}_1 - m, \mathbf{x}_2 - n)G_{yy}(m, n, s)$$

In the above equations, G_{xx}, G_{xy}, and G_{yy} are second derivatives of a 2D Gaussian function computed as

$$G(x_1, x_2, s) = \exp^{-\frac{x_1^2 + x_2^2}{2s^2}}$$

$$G_{xx}(x_1, x_2, s) = \frac{x_1 - s^2}{s^4} \exp^{-\frac{x_1^2 + x_2^2}{2s^2}}$$

$$G_{xy}(x_1, x_2, s) = \frac{x_1 x_2}{s^4} \exp^{-\frac{x_1^2 + x_2^2}{2s^2}} \tag{7.4}$$

$$G_{yy}(x_1, x_2, s) = \frac{x_2 - s^2}{s^4} \exp^{-\frac{x_1^2 + x_2^2}{2s^2}}$$

The eigenvalues of $H(\mathbf{x}, s)$ in Equation 7.1 are called principal curvatures and are computed as

$$H(\mathbf{x}, s)\mathbf{e}_i(\mathbf{x}, s) = \lambda_i(\mathbf{x}, s)\mathbf{e}_i(\mathbf{x}, s) \tag{7.5}$$

where λ_i represents the eigenvalue corresponding to the ith normalized eigenvector $\mathbf{e}_i$. Given $\lambda_1 \leq \lambda_2$, the ordered eigenvalues of H, the eigenvectors $\mathbf{e}_1$ and $\mathbf{e}_2$ define an orthogonal coordinate system aligned with the direction of the minimum and maximum curvatures, respectively.

7.2.2 TUBULARNESS FILTER FOR STREAK ENHANCEMENT

Given the image I and its computed eigenvalues λ_i in Equation 7.5 resulting from singular value decomposition (SVD) of the Hessian matrix at scale s, Frangi et al. [44] proposed to measure the tubularness $v(\mathbf{x}, s)$ at pixel $\mathbf{x} = <x_1, x_2>$ using

$$v(\mathbf{x}, s) = e^{-\frac{R^2(\mathbf{x}, s)}{2\beta^2}} \left(1 - e^{\left(-\frac{S^2(\mathbf{x}, s)}{2c^2} \right)} \right)$$

$$R(\mathbf{x}, s) = \frac{\lambda_1(\mathbf{x}, s)}{\lambda_2(\mathbf{x}, s)} \tag{7.6}$$

$$S(\mathbf{x}, s) = \sqrt{\sum_{i \leq 2} \lambda_i^2(\mathbf{x}, s)}$$

R and S are measures of blobness and second-order structureness, respectively. β and c are parameters that control the sensitivity of the filter to the measures R and S.

Since the sign of the largest eigenvalue is an indicator of the brightness or darkness of the pixels (i.e., dark on bright vs. bright on dark), the following sign tests are used to determine the tubularness of the light, v^-, and dark, v^+, structures [44]*:

$$v^-(\mathbf{x}, s) = \begin{cases} 0 & \text{if } \lambda_2(\mathbf{x}, s) > 0 \\ v(\mathbf{x}, s) & \text{if } \lambda_2(\mathbf{x}, s) < 0 \end{cases}$$
$$v^+(\mathbf{x}, s) = \begin{cases} 0 & \text{if } \lambda_2(\mathbf{x}, s) < 0 \\ v(\mathbf{x}, s) & \text{if } \lambda_2(\mathbf{x}, s) > 0 \end{cases} \tag{7.7}$$

Note that $v(\mathbf{x}, s) = v^-(\mathbf{x}, s) + v^+(\mathbf{x}, s)$. Figures 7.3 through 7.5c and d show examples of the computed v^- and v^+ for dermoscopic images of the different types: in the absence, presence of regular, and presence of irregular streaks, denoted by ABS, REG, and IRG, respectively.

7.2.3   QUATERNION TUBULARNESS

To measure vesselness in color images, Shi et al. [45] use quaternion curvature to derive vesselness. In the quaternion representation of an RGB image, the intensity of each pixel $\mathbf{x}$ is represented by a quaternion number:

$$I(\mathbf{x}) = I^r(\mathbf{x})i + I^g(\mathbf{x})j + I^b(\mathbf{x})k \tag{7.8}$$

where I^r, I^g, and I^b represent the intensities of the red, green, and blue channels, and i, j, and k are three imaginary bases. The quaternion Hessian matrix H_Q of the image is defined as

$$H_Q(\mathbf{x}, s) = \begin{bmatrix} I^r_{xx}(\mathbf{x}) & I^r_{xy}(\mathbf{x}) \\ I^r_{xy}(\mathbf{x}) & I^r_{yy}(\mathbf{x}) \end{bmatrix} i + \begin{bmatrix} I^g_{xx}(\mathbf{x}) & I^g_{xy}(\mathbf{x}) \\ I^g_{xy}(\mathbf{x}) & I^g_{yy}(\mathbf{x}) \end{bmatrix} j + \begin{bmatrix} I^b_{xx}(\mathbf{x}) & I^b_{xy}(\mathbf{x}) \\ I^b_{xy}(\mathbf{x}) & I^b_{yy}(\mathbf{x}) \end{bmatrix} k \tag{7.9}$$

The eigenvalues and eigenvectors of H_Q can be computed by applying quaternion singular value decomposition (QSVD), which is a generalization algorithm of SVD. As shown in Section 7.4, considering quaternion tubularness using QSVD leads to a better lesion classification than applying tubularness using SVD.

7.2.4   FLUX ANALYSIS OF THE STREAKS' PRINCIPAL CURVATURE VECTORS

While computing tubularness of the streaks using Equation 7.7, we make an estimation of the streak direction $\phi(\mathbf{x}, s)$. It is computed as the angle between the x-axis and the eigenvector corresponding to $\lambda_1(\mathbf{x}, s)$, which points along

---

* Superscripts − and + indicate the sign of the largest eigenvalue of the pixels inside the light and dark tubular objects, respectively.

the direction of the minimum intensity curvature. Given ϕ and v, we define a streak vector field as

$$\vec{E}^+ = (v^+ \cos(\phi), v^+ \sin(\phi))$$
$$\vec{E}^- = (v^- \cos(\phi), v^- \sin(\phi)) \tag{7.10}$$

To quantify a radial streaming pattern of the vector field with respect to a lesion contour C_o, we measure the amount of the flow of $\vec{E}$ parallel and perpendicular to C_o, denoted by $\psi_\parallel$ and $\psi_\perp$, respectively, using

$$\psi_\parallel^+(\vec{E}^+, C_o) = \oint_{C_o} \| \vec{E}^+ \times \vec{n} \| \ dc$$

$$\psi_\parallel^-(\vec{E}^-, C_o) = \oint_{C_o} \| \vec{E}^- \times \vec{n} \| \ dc$$

$$\psi_\perp^+(\vec{E}^+, C_o) = \oint_{C_o} |<\vec{E}^+ . \vec{n}>| \ dc \tag{7.11}$$

$$\psi_\perp^-(\vec{E}^-, C_o) = \oint_{C_o} |<\vec{E}^- . \vec{n}>| \ dc$$

where $\vec{n}$ is the normal vector to C_o, $\times$ and $<.>$ denote cross and dot products between the vectors, and $\| . \|$ and $|.|$ measure the L_2 norm of the vector and the absolute value of the scalar, respectively.

By computing Equation 7.11, we state our hypothesis as follows: in the presence of streaks on the contour C_o, $\psi_\parallel$ and $\psi_\perp$ take low and high values, respectively, capturing the known radial characteristic of the streaks. In Section 7.2.5, we discuss how to utilize the measured flux to construct a feature vector for streak detection.

Note that in our implementation, we make an initial estimation of C_o by applying a binary graph cut segmentation [46], where the data term and regularization terms are set using the distribution of the pixel intensities and the Pott's model, respectively [47]. The intensity distributions of the foreground and background are estimated by clustering, in color space, the image pixels into two distinct clusters.

7.2.5 STREAK DETECTION FEATURES

We measure $\psi_\parallel$ and $\psi_\perp$ according to Equation 7.11 over isodistance contours of the lesion, where each contour is the loci of the pixels that have equal distance from the outer lesion contour C_o. We calculate the distance transform (DT) of the lesion mask to extract the isodistance contours, denoted by C_d, where d represents the distance between C_d and C_o. Figure 7.6 shows an example of the computed DT of a lesion mask and the isodistance contours C_d.

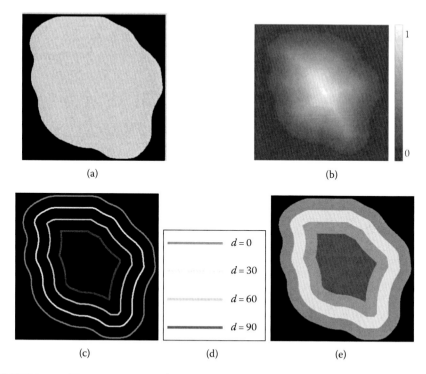

(a)   (b)

(c)   (d)   (e)

FIGURE 7.6 (**See color insert.**) The isodistance contours and subbands of a lesion. (a) Lesion mask. (b) Distance transform of (a). (c) Isodistance contours C_d of the lesion, where d represents the distance between C_d and the lesion border in (a). (e) Bands of the lesion defined according to Equation 7.12 between the contours in (d).

We compute the mean and variance of the flux of the different bands of the lesion, where the Kth band of thickness Δ, $B_{K,\Delta}$, is defined as the region limited between the contours $C_{K\Delta}$ and $C_{(K-1)\Delta}$ and is given by

$$B_{K,\Delta}(\mathbf{x}) = \chi(C_{K\Delta}(\mathbf{x})) \cap (1 - \chi(C_{(K-1)\Delta}(\mathbf{x}))) \tag{7.12}$$

where $\chi(C)$ is the region inside contour C. Therefore, the mean and variance of the flux over band $B_{K,\Delta}$ are given by

$$\mu_{K,\parallel}^{+} = \sum_{d=(K-1)\Delta}^{K\Delta} \psi_{\parallel}^{+}(C_d) \Big/ \int_{\mathbf{x}\in\Omega} B_{K,\Delta}(\mathbf{x})\, d\mathbf{x}$$

$$\mu_{K,\parallel}^{-} = \sum_{d=(K-1)\Delta}^{K\Delta} \psi_{\parallel}^{-}(C_d) \Big/ \int_{\mathbf{x}\in\Omega} B_{K,\Delta}(\mathbf{x})\, d\mathbf{x}$$

$$\sigma^+_{K,\|} = \sqrt{\sum_{d=(K-1)\Delta}^{K\Delta} (\psi^+_\|(C_d) - \mu^+_{K,\|})^2 / \int_{\mathbf{x}\in\Omega} B_{K,\Delta}(\mathbf{x})\, d\mathbf{x}}$$

$$\sigma^-_{K,\|} = \sqrt{\sum_{d=(K-1)\Delta}^{K\Delta} (\psi^-_\|(C_d) - \mu^-_{K,\|})^2 / \int_{\mathbf{x}\in\Omega} B_{K,\Delta}(\mathbf{x})\, d\mathbf{x}} \tag{7.13}$$

$$\mu^+_{K,\perp} = \sum_{d=(K-1)\Delta}^{K\Delta} \psi^+_\perp(C_d) / \int_{\mathbf{x}\in\Omega} B_{K,\Delta}(\mathbf{x})\, d\mathbf{x}$$

$$\mu^-_{K,\perp} = \sum_{d=(K-1)\Delta}^{K\Delta} \psi^-_\perp(C_d) / \int_{\mathbf{x}\in\Omega} B_{K,\Delta}(\mathbf{x})\, d\mathbf{x}$$

$$\sigma^+_{K,\perp} = \sqrt{\sum_{d=(K-1)\Delta}^{K\Delta} (\psi^+_\perp(C_d) - \mu^+_{K,\perp})^2 / \int_{\mathbf{x}\in\Omega} B_{K,\Delta}(\mathbf{x})\, d\mathbf{x}}$$

$$\sigma^-_{K,\perp} = \sqrt{\sum_{d=(K-1)\Delta}^{K\Delta} (\psi^-_\perp(C_d) - \mu^-_{K,\perp})^2 / \int_{\mathbf{x}\in\Omega} B_{K,\Delta}(\mathbf{x})\, d\mathbf{x}} \tag{7.14}$$

where Ω is the image domain. Note that the denominator in Equation 7.14 corresponds to the area of the Kth band, which is used to normalize the extracted features. After computing μ and σ of the flux of the N different bands ($K = \{1, 2, \ldots, N\}$), our SVD flux-based feature vector, denoted by SVD-FLX, is constructed by concatenating the measurements of the different bands and is given by

$$\text{SVD-FLX} = [\mu^+_{1,\|}\ \mu^-_{1,\|}\ \sigma^+_{1,\|}\ \sigma^-_{1,\|}\ \mu^+_{1,\perp}\ \mu^-_{1,\perp}\ \sigma^+_{1,\perp}\ \sigma^-_{1,\perp} \cdots$$
$$\mu^+_{N,\|}\ \mu^-_{N,\|}\ \sigma^+_{N,\|}\ \sigma^-_{N,\|}\ \sigma^+_{N,\perp}\ \sigma^-_{N,\perp}\ \mu^+_{N,\perp}\ \mu^-_{N,\perp}] \tag{7.15}$$

Note that to make use of color information in the computed tubularness in Equation 7.6, the tubularness is measured using the eigenvalues of the quaternion Hessian matrix of the color image [45]. We denote the feature vector utilizing the quaternion Hessian matrix by QSVD-FLX and provide a comparison between the classification accuracies of SVD-FLX and QSVD-FLX in Section 7.4.

7.3 MACHINE LEARNING FOR STREAK CLASSIFICATION

The final step in our approach is to learn how the extracted descriptors can best distinguish the three different classes: the absence (ABS), presence of regular (REG), or presence of irregular (IRG) streaks in the dermoscopic images. The three-class classification task is realized using an efficient pairwise classification. The pairwise classification is based on a nonlinear SVM, trained and then validated according to a leave-one-out scheme [48].

The nonlinear SVM classifier requires the setting of two parameters: ξ, which assigns a penalty to errors, and γ, which defines the width of a radial basis function [49]. We compute the false positive (FP) and true positive (TP) rates of the classifier for different values of ξ and γ in a logarithmic grid search (from 2^{-8} to 2^8) to create a ROC curve. Therefore, each pair of the parameters (ξ_i, γ_j) would generate a point (FP_{ij}, TP_{ij}) in the graph. The ROC curve is constructed by selecting the set of optimal operating points. Point (FP_{ij}, TP_{ij}) is optimal if there is no other point (FP_{mn}, TP_{mn}) such that $FP_{mn} \leq FP_{ij}$ and $TP_{mn} \geq TP_{ij}$. We use the area under the generated ROC curves obtained from classification involving different descriptors to compare their discriminatory power.

7.4 RESULTS

The proposed algorithm has been tested on ninety-nine 768×512 pixel dermoscopic images obtained from Argenziano et al.'s atlas of dermoscopy [42], including 33 images with no streak (ABS), 33 images with regular streaks (REG), and 33 images with irregular streaks (IRG). Note that the entire dataset [42] consists of 527 images of different resolutions, ranging from 0.033 to 0.5 mm/pixel. However, only the lesions occupying more than 10% of the image were selected, because these images were large enough for texture analysis.

Figure 7.7 and Table 7.1 compare the classification performances of the different descriptors in terms of the ROC curves and the areas under them, where GLOB, WT, SVD-FLX, and QSVD-FLX denote the global descriptors used in [32],* WT-based descriptors used in [34],† and our flux-based descriptors using the eigenvalues of the luminance and RGB images in Equation 7.6, respectively. In the last row of Table 7.1, we report the multiclass classification performances as the geometric mean of the pairwise classifiers, as suggested in [50].

The results indicate that, averaged over all the groups (the last row of Table 7.1), we achieved a mean AUC = 92.66% for QSVD-FLX, a 9% increase in terms of area under ROC curves compared with GLOB and WT. Furthermore, it can be noticed that QSVD-FLX, which is obtained by considering the color information, results in an average of 2.5% improvement over the SVD-FLX.

---

* GLOB is constructed using the mean and variance of pixel intensities in different color spaces (RGB, HSI, and Luv) and the border irregularities, where the latter is measured via the change in the lesion contour pixels' coordinates relative to the lesion's centroid and the ratio between the lesion contour length and the maximum axis of the contour's convex hull (details in [32]).

† The WT-based descriptors are constructed by concatenating the mean and variance of the WT coefficients of the different subbands of the WT using Haar wavelets and three decomposition levels (details in [34]).

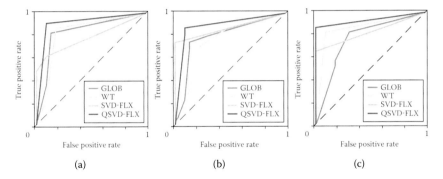

(a)   (b)   (c)

FIGURE 7.7 (See color insert.) ROC curves of the pairwise classifiers resulting from using the different descriptors. Areas under the ROC curves are reported in Table 7.1. (a, b, c) represent binary classification results for ABS vs REG (a), ABS vs IRG (b), REG vs IRG (c).

TABLE 7.1
Area under the ROC Curves in Figure 7.7

Group 1 vs. Group 2	Area under the ROC Curves				Selected Descriptor(s)
	GLOB	**WT**	**SVD-FLX**	**QSVD-FLX**	
ABS × REG	0.8913	0.9130	0.9130	**0.9565**	SVD-FLX
ABS × IRG	0.8091	0.8478	0.8478	**0.8696**	QSVD-FLX
REG × IRG	0.8781	0.7439	**0.9783**	0.9565	SVD-FLX
Geometric mean	0.8587	0.8319	0.9115	**0.9266**	QSVD-FLX

Note: The last column shows the descriptor(s) that generated the highest AUC. Note that we report multiclass classification performances in terms of geometric mean (GM) of the pairwise classifiers (as suggested by [50]) in the last row.

7.5 SUMMARY

In this chapter, we reviewed the general pipeline for a CAD system of dermoscopic images, and described our streak descriptor. Streaks usually appear at the periphery bands. We model them by localized radial fluxes of a set of lesion bands. Using the leave-one-out validation of a nonlinear SVM classifier, our experimental results showed that the color version of the flux-based descriptor QSVD-FLX achieved the best performance compared with the grayscale version, SVD-FLX, and the state-of-the-art global and wavelet transfer-based descriptors. We plan to extend our method to detect and classify the presence of other dermoscopic features (e.g., pigment network, dots, vascular structures), moving us an important step forward toward a machine learning—based computer-aided diagnosis system for early detection of MM.

ACKNOWLEDGMENTS

This work was supported in part by a scholarship from the Canadian Institutes of Health Research (CIHR) Skin Research Training Centre and by grants from the Natural Sciences and Engineering Research Council of Canada (NSERC) and the Canadian Dermatology Foundation.

REFERENCES

1. Canadian Cancer Society's Steering Committee, Canadian cancer statistics, Toronto, Canada, 2009.
2. G. Argenziano, G. Fabbrocini, P. Carli, V. Giorgi, E. Sammarco, and M. Delfino, Epiluminescence microscopy for the diagnosis of doubtful melanocytic skin lesions comparison of the ABCD rule of dermatoscopy and a new 7-point checklist based on pattern analysis, *Archives of Dermatology*, vol. 134, no. 7, pp. 1563–1570, 1998.
3. K. Korotkov and R. Garcia, Computerized analysis of pigmented skin lesions: A review, *Artificial Intelligence in Medicine*, vol. 56, pp. 69–90, 2012.
4. I. Maglogiannis and C. Doukas, Overview of advanced computer vision systems for skin lesions characterization, *IEEE Journal of Biomedical and Health Informatics*, vol. 13, no. 5, pp. 721–733, 2009.
5. J. Scharcanski and M. E. Celebi, eds., *Computer Vision Techniques for the Diagnosis of Skin Cancer*, Springer, Berlin, 2013.
6. M. E. Celebi, W. V. Stoecker, and R. H. Moss, Advances in skin cancer image analysis, *Computerized Medical Imaging and Graphics*, vol. 35, no. 2, pp. 83–84, 2011.
7. S. Menzies, C. Ingvar, and W. McCarthy, A sensitivity and specificity analysis of the surface microscopy features of invasive melanoma, *Melanoma Research*, vol. 6, no. 1, pp. 55–62, 1996.
8. T. Lee, V. Ng, R. Gallagher, A. Coldman, and D. McLean, DullRazor: A software approach to hair removal from images, *Computers in Biology and Medicine*, vol. 27, no. 3, pp. 533–543, 1997.
9. P. Schmid-Saugeon, J. Guillod, and J. Thiran, Towards a computer-aided diagnosis system for pigmented skin lesions, *Computerized Medical Imaging and Graphics*, vol. 27, no. 1, pp. 65–78, 2003.
10. F. Xie, S. Qin, Z. Jiang, and R. Meng, PDE-based unsupervised repair of hair-occluded information in dermoscopy images of melanoma, *Computerized Medical Imaging and Graphics*, vol. 33, no. 4, pp. 275–282, 2009.
11. M. Fiorese, E. Peserico, and A. Silletti, Virtualshave: Automated hair removal from digital dermatoscopic images, in *Proceedings of the Annual Conference of the IEEE Engineering in Medicine and Biology Society*, Boston, MA, pp. 4378–4381, 2011.
12. A. Afonso and M. Silveira, Hair detection in dermoscopic images using percolation, in *Proceedings of the Annual Conference of the IEEE Engineering in Medicine and Biology Society*, San Diego, CA, pp. 4378–4381, 2012.
13. Q. Abbas, M. E. Celebi, and I. F. Garcia, Hair removal methods: A comparative study for dermoscopy images, *Biomedical Signal Processing and Control*, vol. 6, pp. 395–404, 2011.

14. P. Wighton, T. Lee, and S. Atkins, Dermascopic hair disocclusion using inpainting, in *Proceedings of the SPIE Medical Imaging Conference*, pp. 1–8, 2008.

15. H. Zhou, M. Chen, R. Gass, and J. M. Rehg, Feature-preserving artifact removal from dermoscopy images, in *Proceedings of the SPIE Medical Imaging Conference*, vol. 6914, pp. 1–9, 2008.

16. M. E. Celebi, Q. Wen, S. Hwang, H. Iyatomia, and G. Schaefer, Lesion border detection in dermoscopy images using ensembles of thresholding methods, *Skin Research and Technology*, vol. 19, no. 1, pp. 252–258, 2013.

17. H. Zhou, G. Schaefer, A. Sadka, and M. E. Celebi, Anisotropic mean shift based fuzzy c-means segmentation of dermoscopy images, *IEEE Journal of Selected Topics in Signal Processing*, vol. 3, no. 1, pp. 26–34, 2009.

18. H. Iyatomi, H. Oka, M. E. Celebi, M. Hashimoto, M. Hagiwara, M. Tanaka, and K. Ogawa., An improved Internet-based melanoma screening system with dermatologist-like tumor area extraction algorithm, *Computerized Medical Imaging and Graphics*, vol. 32, no. 7, 2008.

19. M. E. Celebi, H. Kingravi, H. Iyatomi, Y. Aslandogan, W. V. Stoecker, R. Moss, J. Malters, J. Grichnik, A. Marghoob, and H. Rabinovitz, Border detection in dermoscopy images using statistical region merging, *Skin Research and Technology*, vol. 14, no. 3, pp. 347–353, 2008.

20. M. E. Celebi, Y. Aslandogan, W. V. Stoecker, H. Iyatomi, H. Oka, and X. Chen, Unsupervised border detection in dermoscopy images, *Skin Research and Technology*, vol. 13, no. 4, pp. 454–462, 2007.

21. M. E. Celebi, H. Kingravi, B. Uddin, H. Iyatomi, Y. Aslandogan, W. V. Stoecker, and R. Moss, A methodological approach to the classification of dermoscopy images, *Computerized Medical Imaging and Graphics*, vol. 31, no. 6, pp. 362–373, 2007.

22. B. Erkol, R. Moss, R. Joe, W. V. Stoecker, and E. Hvatum, Automatic lesion boundary detection in dermoscopy images using gradient vector flow snakes, *Skin Research and Technology*, vol. 11, no. 1, pp. 17–26, 2005.

23. H. Zhou, X. Li, G. Schaefer, M. E. Celebi, and P. Miller, Mean shift based gradient vector flow for image segmentation, *Computer Vision and Image Understanding*, vol. 117, no. 9, pp. 1004–1016, 2013.

24. Q. Abbas, M. E. Celebi, and I. F. Garcia, A novel perceptually-oriented approach for skin tumor segmentation, *International Journal of Innovative Computing, Information and Control*, vol. 8, no. 3, pp. 1837–1848, 2012.

25. H. Zhou, G. Schaefer, M. E. Celebi, F. Lin, and T. Liu, Gradient vector flow with mean shift for skin lesion segmentation, *Computerized Medical Imaging and Graphics*, vol. 35, no. 2, pp. 121–127, 2011.

26. P. Wighton, T. K. Lee, H. Lui, D. I. McLean, and M. S. Atkins, Generalizing common tasks in automated skin lesion diagnosis, *IEEE Transactions on Information Technology in Biomedicine*, vol. 15, no. 4, pp. 622–629, 2011.

27. P. Wighton, T. Lee, G. Mori, H. Lui, D. McLean, and M. Atkins, Conditional random fields and supervised learning in automated skin lesion diagnosis, *International Journal of Biomedical Imaging*, vol. 2011, no. 8, pp. 11–21, 2011.

28. P. Wighton, M. Sadeghi, T. K. Lee, and M. S. Atkins, A fully automatic random walker segmentation for skin lesions in a supervised setting, in *Proceedings of the 12th International Conference on Medical Image Computing and Computer Assisted Intervention*, London, UK, pp. 1108–1115, 2009.

29. M. E. Celebi, H. Iyatomi, G. Schaefer, and W. V. Stoecker, Lesion border detection in dermoscopy images, *Computerized Medical Imaging and Graphics*, vol. 33, no. 2, pp. 148–153, 2009.

30. M. Silveira, J. Nascimento, J. Marques, A. Marcal, T. Mendonca, S. Yamauchi, J. Maeda, and J. Rozeira, Comparison of segmentation methods for melanoma diagnosis in dermoscopy images, *IEEE Journal of Selected Topics in Signal Processing*, vol. 3, no. 1, pp. 35–45, 2009.

31. G. Betta, G. D. Leo, G. Fabbrocini, A. Paolillo, and M. Scalvenzi, Automated application of the 7-point checklist diagnosis method for skin lesions: Estimation of chromatic and shape parameters, in *Instrumentation and Measurement Technology Conference*, Ottawa, CA, vol. 3, pp. 1818–1822, 2005.

32. G. Fabbrocini, G. Betta, G. Leo, C. Liguori, A. Paolillo, A. Pietrosanto, P. Sommella et al., Epiluminescence image processing for melanocytic skin lesion diagnosis based on 7-point check-list: A preliminary discussion on three parameters, *The Open Dermatology Journal*, vol. 4, pp. 110–115, 2010.

33. A. Tenenhaus, A. Nkengne, J. Horn, C. Serruys, A. Giron, and B. Fertil, Detection of melanoma from dermoscopic images of naevi acquired under uncontrolled conditions, *Skin Research and Technology*, vol. 16, no. 1, pp. 85–97, 2009.

34. G. Surowka and K. Grzesiak-Kopec, Different learning paradigms for the classification of melanoid skin lesions using wavelets, in *Proceedings of the 29th Annual International Conference of the IEEE Engineering in Medicine and Biology Society*, Lyon, France, pp. 3136–3139, 2007.

35. M. Anantha, R. H. Moss, and W. V. Stoecker, Detection of pigment network in dermatoscopy images using texture analysis, *Computerized Medical Imaging and Graphics*, vol. 28, no. 5, pp. 225–234, 2004.

36. H. Iyatomi, K. Norton, M. E. Celebi, G. Schaefer, M. Tanaka, and K. Ogawa, Classification of melanocytic skin lesions from non-melanocytic lesions, in *Proceedings of the 32nd Annual International Conference of the IEEE Engineering in Medicine and Biology Society*, Buenos Aires, Argentina, pp. 540–544, 2010.

37. M. Elbaum, A. Kopf, H. Rabinovitz, R. Langley, H. Kamino, M. Mihm, A. Sober et al., Automatic differentiation of melanoma from melanocytic nevi with multispectral digital dermoscopy: A feasibility study, *Journal of the American Academy of Dermatology*, vol. 44, no. 2, pp. 207–218, 2001.

38. N. Situ, T. Wadhawan, X. Yuan, and G. Zouridakis, Modeling spatial relation in skin lesion images by the graph walk kernel, in *Proceedings of the 32nd Annual International Conference of the IEEE Engineering in Medicine and Biology Society*, Buenos Aires, Argentina, pp. 613–616, 2010.

39. T. K. Lee, D. McLean, and S. Atkins, Irregularity index: A new border irregularity measure for cutaneous melanocytic lesions, *Medical Image Analysis*, vol. 7, no. 1, pp. 47–64, 2003.

40. V. Ng, B. Fung, and T. Lee, Determining the asymmetry of skin lesion with fuzzy borders, *Computers in Biology and Medicine*, vol. 35, no. 2, pp. 103–120, 2005.

41. M. Sadeghi, T. Lee, D. McLean, H. Lui, and S. Atkins, Detection and analysis of irregular streaks in dermoscopic images of skin lesions, *IEEE Transactions on Medical Imaging*, vol. 32, no. 5, pp. 849–861, 2013.

42. G. Argenziano, H. Soyer, V. Giorgio, D. Piccolo, P. Carli, M. D. A. Ferrari, R. Hofmann et al., *Interactive Atlas of Dermoscopy*, EDRA Medical Publishing and New Media, Milan, Italy, 2000.

43. H. Mirzaalian, T. Lee, and G. Hamarneh, Learning features for streak detection in dermoscopic color images using localized radial flux of principal intensity curvature, in *2012 IEEE Workshop on Mathematical Methods in Biomedical Image Analysis*, Breckenridge, CO, pp. 97–101, 2012.

44. A. Frangi, W. J. Niessen, K. L. Vincken, and M. A. Viergever, Multiscale vessel enhancement filtering, in *Proceedings of the International Conference on Medical Image Computing and Computer Assisted Intervention*, Cambridge, MA, pp. 130–137, 1998.

45. L. Shi, B. Funt, and G. Hamarneh, Quaternion color curvature, in *Proceedings of the IS&T Sixteenth Color Imaging Conference*, Portland, OR, pp. 338–341, 2008.

46. Y. Boykov and G. Funka-Lea, Graph cuts and efficient N-D image segmentation, *International Journal of Computer Vision*, vol. 70, pp. 109–131, 2006.

47. Y. Boykov, O. Veksler, and R. Zabih, Fast approximate energy minimization via graph cuts, *IEEE Transactions on Pattern Analysis and Machine Intelligence*, vol. 23, p. 2001, 1999.

48. S. Park and J. Furnkranz, Efficient pairwise classification, in *Proceedings of the European Conference on Machine Learning*, vol. 4701, pp. 658–665, 2007.

49. V. Vapnik, *Statistical Learning Theory*, Wiley, 1998.

50. Y. Sun, M. Kamel, and Y. Wang, Boosting for learning multiple classes with imbalanced class distribution, in *Proceedings of the IEEE International Conference on Data Mining*, Hong Kong, China, pp. 592–602, 2006.

8 Dermoscopy Image Assessment Based on Perceptible Color Regions

Gunwoo Lee
Korea University Medical Center
Seoul, Korea

Onseok Lee
Gimcheon University
Gimcheon, Korea

Jaeyoung Kim
Korea University Medical Center
Seoul, Korea

Jongsub Moon
Korea University
Seoul, Korea

Chilhwan Oh
Korea University Medical Center
and
Korea University College of Medicine
Seoul, Korea

CONTENTS

8.1 INTRODUCTION

Malignant melanoma is one of the most serious skin cancers. Hence, early diagnosis is very important because early-stage melanoma can often be cured by simple excision, significantly increasing the chance of patient survival. Therefore, dermatologists strive to diagnose malignant melanoma as early as possible [1].

Dermoscopy is frequently used as an initial diagnostic modality in dermatology. It can assist dermatologists in the diagnosis of melanoma. The practical use of dermoscopy raises the diagnostic accuracy for malignant melanoma compared to traditional diagnosis with the naked eye [2]. Dermoscopy images provide more detail in terms of color, surface, and subsurface structures than can be seen with the naked eye [3–11]. However, dermoscopy does not assist a novice dermatologist in diagnosing melanoma. Training is needed to make effective use of this information for diagnosis because the observed information is often extremely complex and subjective; this could decrease the diagnostic accuracy of inexperienced dermatologists. In some surveys on the usefulness of dermoscopy, respondents indicated that extensive training was required for using dermoscopy, though it was effective in reducing patient anxiety and helped in the early detection of melanoma [5–8].

Color information is one of very important diagnostic factors for malignant melanoma. In many diagnostic methods such as the ABCD rule, the Menzies method, and the seven-point rule, color information is considered an important factor in melanoma detection. However, dermoscopic diagnosis based on color is sometimes difficult because of the resulting poor color perception. Therefore, visual assessment of lesion color can be very subjective.

In this chapter, we present an effective color assessment method to assist in the diagnosis of malignant melanoma using 27 perceptible color regions.

8.2 IMPORTANCE OF COLOR INFORMATION FOR MELANOMA DIAGNOSIS

Color assessment is an essential step in the diagnosis of malignant melanoma. Most melanocytic lesions, including melanoma in dermoscopy images, are described by colors, typically dark, that differ from that of the surrounding skin owing to the proliferation of melanin-containing cells (melanocytes). These lesions contain various colors that mainly result from the presence of hemoglobin (vasculature) and melanin, and vary with the thickness of the stratum corneum. In dermoscopy images, vasculature appears red or red–blue. The color of melanin in dermoscopy images depends on its depth, appearing black at the stratum corneum, dark brown at the epidermis, brown at the dermoepidermal junction, and gray or blue at the dermis [4, 11].

With the ABCD rules, the Menzies scoring method, and the seven-point checklist, which are all well-known melanoma diagnosis methods, color features such as multiple colors or bluish colors are considered important factors for melanoma diagnosis [4, 11–18]. In the ABCD rules, the total number of colors in the melanocytic lesion contributes to approximately 30% of the final diagnostic score [14]. According to the Menzies scoring method, the presence of multiple colors (five or six colors) represents a positive feature, whereas the presence of only a single color is considered a negative feature. With this method, a blue–white veil is also considered a positive feature, regardless of the color count [15]. The seven-point checklist considers a blue–white color to be the major diagnostic criterion [16]. However, many colors in dermoscopy images are only slightly different from each other. These imperceptible color differences can hinder the feature assessment of the lesions. During lesion extraction, these color differences prevent the clear identification of the lesion border, which can lead to inaccurate lesion extraction by an inexperienced dermatologist [19]. Sometimes this lack of clarity can even lead to extraction errors by experienced dermatologists. Often, the most difficult aspect of the image assessment, as a result of these slight color differences, lies in determining the number of colors in a lesion. Many melanomas exhibit a variety of colors. However, inexperienced dermatologists cannot easily assess or discern them within the lesions. While dermoscopy provides more detailed information, it makes it difficult to perceive the different colors and can lead to a subjective diagnosis. Therefore, it is important for dermatologists to identify lesions on the basis of perceptible color differences using an objective and quantitative method.

Because of the diagnostic importance of color information, many color analysis methods have been studied for assessing dermoscopy images. Simplifying the color information is one of the most common approaches, including such methods as color palette comprising the representative colors in a melanocytic lesion, uniform color clustering by subdividing the color space, K-means clustering, and color quantization by the median cut algorithm [13, 20–25].

8.3 COLOR ASSESSMENT FOR MELANOMA DIAGNOSIS

8.3.1 DMB SYSTEM

Twenty-four-bit color images have thousands of colors, making it difficult to clearly distinguish each color. In particular, many melanomas in dermoscopy images have neighbor colors, which are slightly different from each other. Slightly different neighbor colors hinder an objective color assessment. Therefore, it is necessary to reduce the amount of color information based on the concept of perception.

We presented a new method for the color assessment of melanocytic lesions that is based on perceptible color regions. To simplify the color information, we constructed perceptible color regions using a stack of red (R), green (G), and blue (B) channel images, which were classified into three degrees of brightness by the multithresholding method. The three degrees of brightness in each color channel produced a maximum of 27 perceptible color regions, consisting of a stack of three channels. We refer to the 27 perceptible color regions as the dark–middle–bright (DMB) system.

This DMB system simplifies the color information in dermoscopy images. The three degrees represent lesions, suspicious areas, and the skin surrounding the lesion for each color channel. It is often difficult to clearly distinguish between a lesion and the surrounding skin with the naked eye due to slightly differing neighbor colors. The three degrees of brightness, including the middle degree as a suspicious area, make color differences more perceptible to the naked eye. The three degrees of brightness in each color channel form the DMB system, and they are divided into dark, middle, and bright color intensities. The approximate colors of each region were determined by averaging the contribution of each color in the region and were used to represent separate regions in the dermoscopy image.

The DMB system is an effective method for assessing color information because it is constructed by three degrees of brightness, including the middle degree as a suspicious area. This suspicious area is one of the factors that produces the diverse colors in dermoscopy images. If the lesion and surrounding skin contain only one color and the lesion is clearly separated from the surrounding skin, same-size lesions are detected in each channel. The dermoscopy image is then represented as two colors, one corresponding to the lesion and another corresponding to the skin. However, in general, dermoscopy images contain different-size lesions in each color channel, and this leads to suspicious areas between the lesion and the skin. Eventually, diverse colors are produced in the dermoscopy images by combining the three degrees of brightness in each channel.

Furthermore, the DMB system is less sensitive to illumination conditions because it is not constructed from the absolute color in each channel. Many color assessment methods are based on absolute color. The measurement of absolute color is dependent on the acquisition technique and the imaging device. For example, the RGB color space is device dependent, and therefore, color calibration is required for color assessment using absolute color.

8.3.2 ESTABLISHMENT OF DMB COLOR REGIONS

To obtain the three degrees of brightness in each color channel, we used the multithresholding method extended from Otsu's thresholding method [26, 27]. Each RGB channel has an intensity function with L intensity levels. The number of pixels with intensity level i is denoted by n_i, and the total number of pixels is denoted by N. The intensity-level histogram is normalized and regarded as a probability of the intensity level.

$$p_i = \frac{n_i}{N}, \quad p_i \geq 0, \quad \sum_{i=1}^{L} p_i = 1 \qquad (8.1)$$

In three-level thresholding of an intensity image, three classes, ($C_1 = [1, 2, \ldots, t_1], C_2 = [t_{1+1}, \ldots, t_2]$, and $C_3 = [t_2 + 1, \ldots, L]$), in an intensity image are divided by two thresholds, $\{t_1, t_2\}$. The optimal thresholds $\{t_1^*, t_2^*\}$ are determined by maximizing σ_B^2 such that

$$\{t_1^*, t_2^*\} = Arg \max_{1 \leq t_1 < t_2 < L} \{\sigma_B^2(t_1, t_2)\} \tag{8.2}$$

where

$$\sigma_B^2 = \sum_{k=1}^{3} \omega_k (\mu_k - \mu_T)^2$$

$$\omega_k = \sum_{i \in C_k} p_i$$

$$\mu_k = \sum_{i \in C_k} i \cdot \frac{p_i}{\omega_k} = \frac{\mu(k)}{\omega_k}$$

and

$$\mu(k) = \sum_{i \in C_k} i \cdot p_i$$

In these equations, ω_k and μ_k are the zero- and first-order cumulative moments, respectively, of the kth class (C_k). The between-class variance can be rewritten using the following relations for any choice of two thresholds:

$$\sum_{k=1}^{3} \omega_k = 1 \tag{8.3}$$

$$\mu_T = \sum_{k=1}^{3} \omega_k \mu_k \tag{8.4}$$

and

$$\sigma_B^2(t_1, t_2) = \sum_{k=1}^{3} \omega_k \mu_k^2 - \mu_T^2 \tag{8.5}$$

Because the second term (μ_T^2) of Equation 8.5 is regardless of the choice of optimal thresholds, it can be omitted. Therefore, Equation 8.5 can be modified as follows:

$$(\sigma_B')^2 = \sum_{k=1}^{M} \omega_k \mu_k^2 \tag{8.6}$$

Each DMB color region in the dermoscopy images was established from a stack of R, G, and B channel images that were classified into three degrees of brightness by using Equation 8.6. The representative colors of the DMB color regions were expressed as approximate colors determined by averaging the contribution of each color in the region.

8.3.3   LESION SEGMENTATION-BASED DMB SYSTEM

We segmented the lesions in the dermoscopy images using the average color distance ratio for each representative color of the DMB color region. The representative colors of the DMB color regions were expressed as approximate colors determined by averaging the contribution of each color in the region. The average color distance ratio D_i of the ith DMB color region is defined as

$$D_i = \frac{1}{N-2} \sum_{\substack{j=1 \\ j \neq i}}^{N-1} \frac{d(C_i, C_j)}{d(C_i, C_S)} \tag{8.7}$$

where the total number of color regions $N = 27$ and $d(C_i, C_j)$ is the Euclidean distance between C_i and C_j. The skin color (C_S) is the intersection of the brightest areas in the R, G, and B channels, which mainly corresponds to the skin surrounding the lesion. The average color distance ratio D_i is the ratio between the average distance and the other DMB color regions and the distance to the skin color. When D_i is greater than 1.0, C_i is closer to the lesion than the surrounding skin. Conversely, when D_i is less than 1.0, C_i is closer to the surrounding skin than the lesion.

Many dermoscopy images have only slight variations in color. If there is a slight color difference between the lesion and the surrounding skin, it may induce the incorrect lesion segmentation. When D_i is approximately 1.0, the images contain color regions that are roughly equidistant to both the lesion and the surrounding skin. These color regions disrupt accurate lesion segmentation. To prevent this, we defined the skin surrounding the lesion as having $D_i \geq 1.2$ and set $D_i < 1.2$ to be the lesion area.

$$D_i = \begin{cases} \textit{Surrounding Skin} & \text{if } D_i \geq 1.2 \\ \textit{Lesion} & \text{otherwise} \end{cases}$$

To obtain the final lesion image, morphological postprocessing was applied to fill any holes and to select the largest connected component in the binary image consisting of the lesion and the surrounding skin (Figure 8.1).

8.3.4   COLOR ASSESSMENT BASED ON DMB SYSTEM

Color assessment was performed on the DMB system constructing dark, middle, and bright degrees in each color channel image using the multithresholding method. The different color regions were named based on the brightness levels (dark—d, middle—m, or bright—b) of the R, G, and B channels, respectively. For example, mbd is composed of the middle level in the red channel, the bright level in the green channel, and the dark level in the blue channel. Table 8.1 shows the DMB system color region results for malignant melanoma and benign pigmented lesions. We only considered color regions containing more than 1% of the total lesion area because those less than 1% lacked clinical relevance.

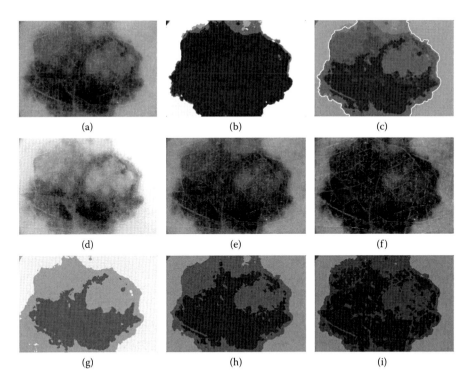

FIGURE 8.1 (See color insert.) An example of the DMB system and lesion segmentation. (a) The original image. (b) The average color distance ratio image for determining the region of interest (ROI). (c) The result of automated segmentation for the pigmented lesion, where the lesion border is shown by the white line. (d–f) The red, green, blue channel images, respectively. (g–i) Three degrees of brightness images from d–f, respectively. (From Lee, G. et al., *Skin Research and Technology*, vol. 18, pp. 462–470, 2012.)

After identifying the lesion, three diagnostic parameters were measured: the dominant color regions (DCRs), the bluish dominant regions (BDRs), and the number of minor color regions (MCRs) on 150 dermoscopy images, including 75 malignant melanomas and 75 benign pigmented lesions. With the DMB system, 9 color regions (*ddd, ddm, dmm, mdd, mdm, mmd, mmm, bmd,* and *bmm*) were present in more than 1% of dermoscopy images, whereas 18 color regions (*ddb, dmd, dmb, dbd, dbm, dbb, mdb, mmb, mbd, mbm, mbb, bdd, bdm, bdb, bmb, bbd, bbm,* and *bbb*) were detected under 1% in both malignant melanoma and benign pigmented lesion images [28].

The *ddd, mdd, mmd, mmm,* and *bmm* regions were present in more than 70% of all images selected as five DCRs (5-DCRs) because they were so common. The percentage lesion area occupied by 5-DCRs is shown in Figure 8.2. The 5-DCRs made up a larger percentage of the total lesion region

TABLE 8.1

Presence Rate and Occupying Rate of DMB System in Malignant Melanoma and Benign Pigmented Lesions on 150 Dermoscopy Images Comprising 75 Malignant Melanomas and 75 Benign Pigmented Lesions

DMB Color Region	Presence Rate (%)		Occupying Rate (%)	
	Malignant Melanoma	Benign Pigmented Lesion	Malignant Melanoma	Benign Pigmented Lesion
ddd	100	100	33.5	41.4
ddm	53.3	2.67	3.25	0.32
ddb	0	0	0	0
dmd	2.67	13.3	0.18	0.47
dmm	18.7	6.67	1.2	0.24
dmb	1.33	0	0.03	0
dbd	0	0	0	0
dbm	0	0	0	0
dbb	0	0	0	0
mdd	100	96	16.6	16.5
mdm	40	2.67	1.66	0.17
mdb	0	0	0	0
mmd	100	98.7	11.8	15.4
mmm	97.3	85.3	17.6	15.8
mmb	14.7	0	0.36	0.04
mbd	0	0	0	0
mbm	1.33	9.33	0.08	0.29
mbb	0	0	0.05	0.03
bdd	1.33	0	0.09	0.02
bdm	1.33	0	0.05	0
bdb	0	0	0	0
bmd	44	34.7	2.01	1.13
bmm	88	78.7	9.65	7.14
bmb	10.7	0	0.3	0.02
bbd	0	0	0	0
bbm	24	26.7	0.99	0.88
bbb	14.7	1.33	0.55	0.15

Note: The DMB group incidences in each lesion were calculated if they occupied more than 1% of the total ROI area.

of interest (ROI) for the benign pigmented lesions than for the malignant melanomas. The 5-DCRs occupied more than 90% of the ROI area in 93.33% of the benign pigmented lesions. In contrast, the 5-DCRs comprised more than 90% of the area in 52.0% of the malignant melanoma lesions. 5-DCRs were commonly present in both malignant melanoma and benign pigmented lesions, and most benign lesions consisted of 5-DCRs. However, the occupying rate of melanoma was less than that of the benign pigmented lesion because a number of colors were considered as one of important factors in melanoma diagnosis.

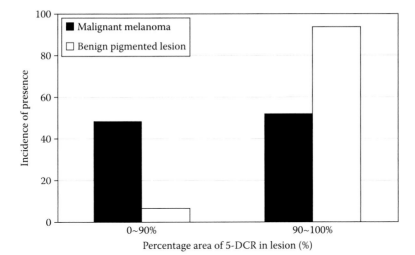

FIGURE 8.2   The percentage of 5-DCRs occupying lesions in each malignant melanoma (black bar) and benign pigmented lesion (white bar).

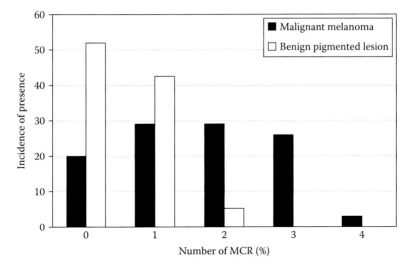

FIGURE 8.3   The number of MCRs in each malignant melanoma (black bar) and benign pigmented lesion (white bar).

In nine color regions which that present in more than 1% of dermoscopy images, five color regions (*ddd*, *mdd*, *mmd*, *mmm*, and *bmm*) were selected as 5-DCRs, which are commonly presented in lesions The remaining four color regions (*ddm*, *dmm*, *mdm*, and *bmd*) were defined as minor color regions (MCRs). The number of MCRs in lesions is shown in Figure 8.3. Less than one MCR was detected in 94.67% of the benign pigmented lesion group, and

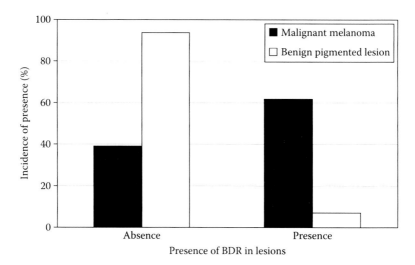

FIGURE 8.4 The incidence of BDRs in malignant melanoma (black bars) and benign pigmented lesions (white bar).

52% was not detected. In contrast, more than two MCRs were detected in 58.46% of the malignant melanoma group.

Bluish colors such as blue–white veil are another important color feature in melanoma diagnosis, and these colors are expressed when the B channel is higher in RGB color space. We defined the BDRs (*ddm*, *ddb*, *dmb*, *mdb*, and *mmb*) as regions having higher brightness in the B channel than in the R and G channels. The *ddb* and *mdb* were not detected in any images, and therefore only the *ddm*, *dmb*, and *mmb* were included as BDRs in this study (Table 8.1). The ratio of BDRs in the lesions is shown in Figure 8.4. The BDRs were present (at more than 1% of the lesion) in only 6.67% of the benign pigmented lesion group, compared to 61.33% of the malignant melanoma group.

The diagnostic accuracy was calculated using three diagnostic parameters derived from the 5-DCRs, BDRs, and the number of MCRs. The DCR diagnostic parameter was considered positive when the DCRs occupied less than 80% of the lesion. The BDR diagnostic parameter was considered positive when the area of the BDRs was detected in the lesion area. The number of MCRs diagnostic parameter was considered positive when the lesion contained more than two. A positive melanoma diagnosis resulted from each of these three diagnostic parameters being positive.

The diagnostic accuracy using the three diagnostic parameters was calculated in terms of sensitivity and specificity (Table 8.2). In the case of one positive diagnostic parameter, the sensitivity was 73.33% and specificity was 92.00%. In the case of two positive diagnostic parameters, the sensitivity was 53.33% and specificity was 96.00%. In the case of three positive diagnostic parameters, the sensitivity was 30.67% and specificity was 98.67%.

TABLE 8.2

Diagnostic Accuracy of Melanoma Based on the Three Diagnostic Parameters

	Diagnostic Accuracy by Three Diagnostic Parameters		
	Positive in Single Parameter	**Positive in Two Parameters**	**Positive in Three Parameters**
Sensitivity	73.33%	53.33%	30.67%
Specificity	92.00%	96%	98.67%

Note: The sensitivity and specificity were calculated for combinations of the diagnostic parameters derived from 5-DCRs, BDRs, and the number of MCRs.

8.3.5 PERCEPTIBLE COLOR DIFFERENCE

The colors of the color regions are based on the three gray levels in each channel. These colors are different from the colors observed in the original image. Hence, we approximated the color regions to the color of the original image by using the average color of each color region.

In order to assess the number of colors, every color for the assessment is required to have a perceptible color difference from the other colors. If two colors have a slight difference or an imperceptible difference, these two colors have to be considered one color. We used the National Bureau of Standards (NBS) unit to calculate the color difference of the approximated colors. The NBS unit was established to better approximate human color perception, and it has a close relation with the value of human color perception [29]. However, the NBS unit is based on the CIE 1994 color difference model (ΔE_{94}^*) calculated using the CIE L*a*b* color space. Therefore, a color space conversion is required.

The definition of CIE L*a*b* is based on the CIEXYZ color space, which is derived from the RGB color space as follows:

$$\begin{bmatrix} X \\ Y \\ Z \end{bmatrix} = \begin{bmatrix} 0.4124564 & 0.3575761 & 0.1804375 \\ 0.2126729 & 0.7151522 & 0.0721750 \\ 0.0193339 & 0.1191920 & 0.9503041 \end{bmatrix} \begin{bmatrix} R \\ G \\ B \end{bmatrix} \quad (8.8)$$

Then, the XYZ color space is transformed into L*a*b* using the CIE L*a*b* formula given in Equation 8.9.

$$\begin{cases} L^* = 116 f\left(\dfrac{Y}{100}\right) - 16 \\ a^* = 500\left[f\left(\dfrac{X}{95.05}\right) - f\left(\dfrac{Y}{100}\right)\right] \\ b^* = 200\left[f\left(\dfrac{Y}{100}\right) - f\left(\dfrac{Z}{108.88}\right)\right] \end{cases} \quad (8.9)$$

with

$$f(q) = \begin{cases} q^{\frac{1}{3}}, & \text{if } q > 0.008856 \\ 7.787q + \dfrac{16}{116}, & \text{otherwise} \end{cases} \tag{8.10}$$

In this study we set the white reference as D65 for the two transformations.

In the CIE L*a*b* color space, L* correlates with the perceived lightness, and a* and b* correlate approximately with the red–green and yellow–blue chroma perceptions. a* and b* in this color space can also be represented in terms of C_{ab}^* (chroma) and H_{ab}^* (hue) as expressed in Equations 8.11 and 8.12, respectively [30].

$$C_{ab}^* = \sqrt{a* + b*} \tag{8.11}$$

$$H_{ab}^* = \tan^{-1}\left(\frac{b*}{a*}\right) \tag{8.12}$$

In the transformed color space CIE L*a*b*, the CIE 1994 color difference model with the symbol ΔE_{94}^* is calculated using Equations 8.13 and 8.14

$$\Delta E_{94}^* = \left[\left(\frac{\Delta L^*}{k_L S_L}\right)^2 + \left(\frac{\Delta C_{ab}^*}{k_C S_C}\right)^2 + \left(\frac{\Delta H_{ab}^*}{k_H S_H}\right)^2 \right] \tag{8.13}$$

$$S_L = 1, \quad S_C = 1 + 0.045 C_{ab}^*, \quad S_H = 1 + 0.015 C_{ab}^* \tag{8.14}$$

The parametric factors, k_L, k_C, and k_H, are used for adjusting the relative weighting of the lightness, chroma, and hue, respectively, of the color difference for various experimental conditions [30]. In order to calculate ΔE_{94}^*, these three parametric factors are set as follows:

$$K_L = K_C = K_H = 1 \tag{8.15}$$

The NBS unit is used as the unit representing the color difference, and it has one when $\Delta E^* = 1$. The NBS unit can be roughly classified into five levels according to the degrees of color difference perceived by humans as given in Table 8.3. From the table, the NBS unit indicates that the color difference is almost the same or slightly different when the NBS unit is smaller than 3.0 and is remarkably different when the NBS unit is between 3.0 and 6.0. In this study, we define color difference to be imperceptibly the same for three grades (NBS unit: less than 3, 4.5, and 6) and the color regions that the color difference is less than each grade are merged.

8.3.6   COLOR ASSESSMENT BASED ON PERCEPTIBLE GRADE

Imperceptible colors are determined on the basis of three NBS units (3, 4.5, and 6), and the number of colors is assessed by the number of perceptible colors in the lesion. Table 8.4 shows the sensitivity, specificity, and diagnosis accuracy values obtained by using the three NBS units. In the case of three NBS units,

TABLE 8.3

Correspondence between the Human Color Perception and the NBS Unit

NBS Unit	Human Perception
0–1.5	Almost the same
1.5–3.0	Slightly different
3.0–6.0	Remarkably different
6.0–12.0	Very different
12.0–	Different color

TABLE 8.4

Sensitivity (SE), Specificity (SP), and Diagnostic Accuracy (ACC) Values at Three Grades of NBS Unit

	3 NBS Units			4.5 NBS Units			6 NBS Units		
	SE (%)	SP (%)	ACC (%)	SE (%)	SP (%)	ACC (%)	SE (%)	SP (%)	ACC (%)
More than 2 colors ≥ 2	100.00	2.67	51.33	100.00	2.67	51.33	100.00	2.67	51.33
≥ 3	100.00	18.97	59.33	100.00	22.67	61.33	100.00	33.33	66.67
≥ 4	100.00	42.67	71.33	100.00	53.33	76.67	97.33	69.33	83.33
≥ 5	96.00	60	78.00	92.00	77.33	84.67	82.67	94.67	88.67
≥ 6	92.00	93.33	92.67	78.67	96.00	87.33	52.00	98.67	75.33
≥ 7	64.00	98.67	81.33	48.00	100.00	74.00	29.33	98.67	64.00

the highest diagnosis accuracy of 92.67% with 92.00% sensitivity and 93.33% specificity is obtained at more than six colors. In the case of 4.5 NBS units, the highest diagnosis accuracy of 87.33% with 78.67% sensitivity and 96.00% specificity is obtained at more than six colors. In the case of six NBS units, the highest diagnosis accuracy of 88.67% with 82.67% sensitivity and 94.67% specificity is obtained at more than five colors.

In the color assessment, each color region is formed by three discernable gray levels in each channel. The three gray levels are regarded as the lesion, the doubtful area, and the surrounding skin from the perspective of extraction. They are also regarded as dark, middle, and bright from the perspective of color. Therefore, each color region refers to a distinct region constructed by a perceptible classification, and the approximated colors of color regions by means of each color region can be expressed as the representative colors in the dermoscopic image. However, the number of representative colors is not equal to the number of colors in a lesion because some representative colors can be slightly different. The number of colors is estimated by counting the number of different perceptible colors. The NBS unit is useful for judging the perceptible color difference. This unit is based on the CIE 1994 color difference model and is closely related to the value of human color perception. The NBS unit indicates that the colors are almost the same or slightly different when its value is less than 3, remarkably different when the value is between 3 and 6, and very different when the value is more than 6. In this study, we defined the imperceptible color difference on the basis of three grades (3, 4.5, and 6 NBS units) in a remarkably different range and counted the number of colors in the lesion. The number of colors is assessed from the sensitivity, specificity, and diagnosis accuracy. In the case of three NBS units, the highest diagnosis accuracy of 92.67% with 92.00% sensitivity and 93.33% specificity is obtained at more than six colors. In the case of 4.5 NBS units, the highest diagnosis accuracy of 87.33% with 78.67% sensitivity and 96.00% specificity was obtained at more than six colors. In the case of six NBS units, the highest diagnosis accuracy of 88.67% with 82.67% sensitivity and 94.67% specificity was obtained at more than five colors. The highest diagnosis accuracy was obtained in the three NBS units.

8.4   CONCLUSION

In this chapter, we have presented a new method for color assessment in melanocytic lesions based on 27 color regions called the DMB system, simplifying the color information in dermoscopy images. We classified each color channel into three degrees of brightness using the multithresholding method. We performed the color assessment as based on the DMB system, which is constructed by perceptible three degrees of brightness in each RGB channel. Five dominant color regions (5-DCR), bluish dominant regions (BDRs), and the number of minor color regions (MCRs) were calculated as diagnostic parameters, and diagnostic accuracy was calculated according to the number of positive parameters.

ACKNOWLEDGMENT

This work was supported by the Ministry of Commerce, Industry and Energy by a grant from the Strategic Nation R&D Program (Grant 10028284), a Korea University grant (K0717401), and the National Research Foundation of Korea (NRF) (Grant 2012R1A1A2006556). Also, the Seoul Research and Business Development Program supported this study financially (Grant 10574).

REFERENCES

1. A. A. Marghoob and A. Scope, The complexity of diagnosing melanoma, *Journal of Investigative Dermatology*, vol. 129, pp. 11–13, 2009.

2. H. Kittler, H. Pehamberger, K. Wolff, and M. Binder, Diagnostic accuracy of dermoscopy, *Lancet Oncology*, vol. 3, pp. 159–165, 2002.
3. M. E. Vestergaard, P. Macaskill, P. E. Holt, and S. W. Menzies, Dermoscopy compared with naked eye examination for the diagnosis of primary melanoma: a meta-analysis of studies performed in a clinical setting, *British Journal of Dermatology*, vol. 159, pp. 669–676, 2008.
4. S. W. Menzies, K. A. Crotty, C. Ingvar, and W. J. McCarthy, *An Atlas of Surface Microscopy of Pigmented Skin Lesions: Dermoscopy.* McGraw-Hill, Roseville, 2003.
5. O. Noor, A. Nanda, and B. K. Rao, A dermoscopy survey to assess who is using it and why it is or is not being used, *International Journal of Dermatology*, vol. 48, pp. 951–952, 2009.
6. J. Scharcanski and M. E. Celebi, eds., *Computer Vision Techniques for the Diagnosis of Skin Cancer*, Springer-Verlag, Berlin, Heidelberg, 2013.
7. K. Korotkov and R. Garcia, Computerized analysis of pigmented skin lesions: a review, *Artificial Intelligence in Medicine*, vol. 56, pp. 69–90, 2012.
8. M. E. Celebi, W. V. Stoecker, and R. H. Moss, Advances in skin cancer image analysis, *Computerized Medical Imaging and Graphics*, vol. 35, pp. 83–84, 2011.
9. G. Argenziano, G. Ferrara, S. Francione, K. Di Nola, A. Martino, and I. Zalaudek, Dermoscopy: the ultimate tool for melanoma diagnosis, *Seminars in Cutaneous Medicine and Surgery*, vol. 28, pp. 142–148, 2009.
10. G. Campos-do-Carmo and M. R. E. Silva, Dermoscopy: basic concepts, *International Journal of Dermatology*, vol. 47, pp. 712–719, 2008.
11. W. Stolz, O. Braun-Falco, P. Bilek, M. Landthaler, W. H. C. Burgforf, and A. B. Cognetta, *Color Atlas of Dermatoscopy*, 2nd ed., Blackwell Publishing, Hoboken, NJ, 2002.
12. R. H. Johr, Dermoscopy: alternative melanocytic algorithms—the ABCD rule of dermatoscopy, Menzies scoring method, and 7-point checklist, *Clinics in Dermatology*, vol. 20, pp. 240–247, 2002.
13. S. Seidenari, G. Pellacani, and C. Grana, Computer description of colours in dermoscopic melanocytic lesion images reproducing clinical assessment, *British Journal of Dermatology*, vol. 149, pp. 523–529, 2003.
14. W. Stolz, A. Riemann, A. B. Cognetta, L. Pillet, W. Abmayr, D. Holzel, P. Bilek, F. Nachbar, M. Landthaler, and O. Braunfalco, ABCD rule of dermatoscopy: a new practical method for early recognition of malignant-melanoma, *European Journal of Dermatology*, vol. 4, pp. 521–527, 1994.
15. S. W. Menzies, C. Ingvar, K. A. Crotty, and W. H. McCarthy, Frequency and morphologic characteristics of invasive melanomas lacking specific surface microscopic features, *Archives of Dermatology*, vol. 132, pp. 1178–1182, 1996.
16. G. Argenziano, G. Fabbrocini, P. Carli, V. De Giorgi, E. Sammarco, and M. Delfino, Epiluminescence microscopy for the diagnosis of doubtful melanocytic skin lesions: comparison of the ABCD rule of dermatoscopy and a new 7-point checklist based on pattern analysis, *Archives of Dermatology*, vol. 134, pp. 1563–1570, 1998.
17. M. E. Celebi and A. Zornberg, Automated quantification of clinically significant colors in dermoscopy images and its application to skin lesion classification, *IEEE Systems Journal*, vol. 8, pp. 980–984, 2014.

18. M. E. Celebi, Q. Wen, S. Hwang, and G. Schaefer, Color quantization of dermoscopy images using the K-means clustering algorithm, in *Color Medical Image Analysis* (M. E. Celebi and G. Schaefer, eds.), Springer, Netherlands, 2012, pp. 87–107.

19. M. E. Celebi, H. Iyatomi, G. Schaefer, and W. V. Stoecker, Lesion border detection in dermoscopy images, *Computerized Medical Imaging and Graphics*, vol. 33, pp. 148–153, 2009.

20. H. Ganster, A. Pinz, R. Rohrer, E. Wildling, M. Binder, and H. Kittler, Automated melanoma recognition, *IEEE Transactions on Medical Imaging*, vol. 20, pp. 233–239, 2001.

21. S. Seidenari, C. Grana, and G. Pellacani, Colour clusters for computer diagnosis of melanocytic lesions, *Dermatology*, vol. 214, pp. 137–143, 2007.

22. G. Pellacani, C. Grana, and S. Seidenari, Automated description of colours in polarized-light surface microscopy images of melanocytic lesions, *Melanoma Research*, vol. 14, pp. 125–130, 2004.

23. A. Tenenhaus, A. Nkengne, J. F. Horn, C. Serruys, A. Giron, and B. Fertil, Detection of melanoma from dermoscopic images of naevi acquired under uncontrolled conditions, *Skin Research and Technology*, vol. 16, pp. 85–97, 2010.

24. R. J. Stanley, W. V. Stoecker, and R. H. Moss, A relative color approach to color discrimination for malignant melanoma detection in dermoscopy images, *Skin Research and Technology*, vol. 13, pp. 62–72, 2007.

25. G. Lee, S. Park, S. Ha, G. Park, O. Lee, J. Moon, M. Kim, and C. Oh, Differential diagnosis between malignant melanoma and non-melanoma using image analysis, in *Stratum Corneum V*, Cardiff, UK, 2007.

26. N. Otsu, Threshold selection method from gray-level histograms, *IEEE Transactions on Systems Man and Cybernetics*, vol. 9, pp. 62–66, 1979.

27. P. S. Liao, T. S. Chew, and P. C. Chung, A fast algorithm for multilevel thresholding, *Journal of Information Science and Engineering*, vol. 17, pp. 713–727, 2001.

28. G. Lee, O. Lee, S. Park, J. Moon, and C. Oh, Quantitative color assessment of dermoscopy images using perceptible color regions, *Skin Research and Technology*, vol. 18, pp. 462–470, 2012.

29. H. Yan, Z. Wang, and S. Guo, String extraction based on statistical analysis method in color space, in *Graphics Recognition. Ten Years Review and Future Perspectives*, Springer, Berlin, Heidelberg, pp. 173–181, 2006.

30. M. D. Fairchild, *Color Appearance Models*, 2nd ed., Wiley-IS&T, Hoboken, NJ, 2005.

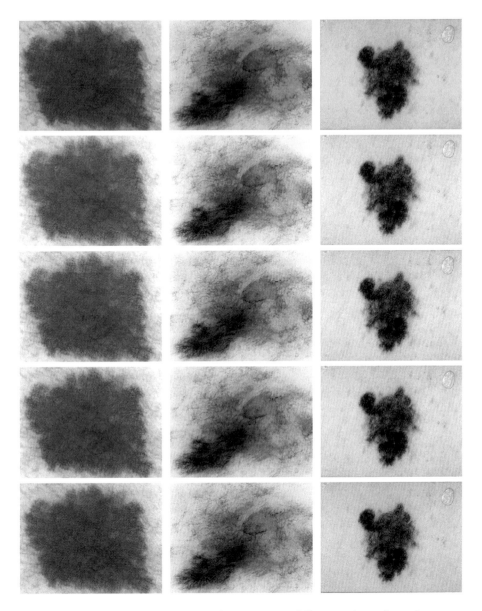

FIGURE 1.5 Examples of color normalization using different values of p melanomas. From top row to bottom: original image, $p = 1$, $p = 3$, $p = 6$, and $p = \infty$. (Reprinted with permission from Argenziano, G. et al., *Dermoscopy: A Tutorial*, EDRA Medical Publishing and New Media, Milan, Italy, 2002.)

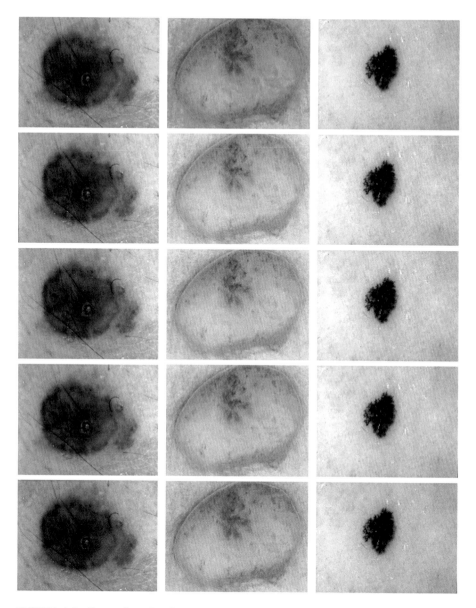

FIGURE 1.6 Examples of color normalization using different values of p benign. From top row to bottom: original image, $p = 1$, $p = 3$, $p = 6$, and $p = \infty$. (Reprinted with permission from Argenziano, G. et al., *Dermoscopy: A Tutorial*, EDRA Medical Publishing and New Media, Milan, Italy, 2002.)

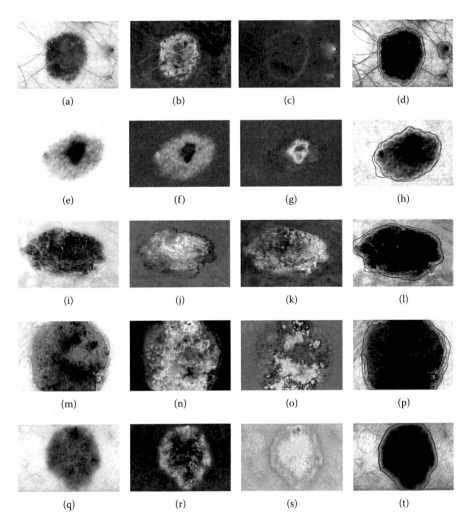

(a) (b) (c) (d)

(e) (f) (g) (h)

(i) (j) (k) (l)

(m) (n) (o) (p)

(q) (r) (s) (t)

FIGURE 2.16 Benign lesions. On geo-mean image, the blue border shows expert segmentation, whereas the red border is our segmentation boundary produced by applying Algorithm 2.4. The first column is input image followed by melanin, hemoglobin, and geo-mean channels in the following columns.

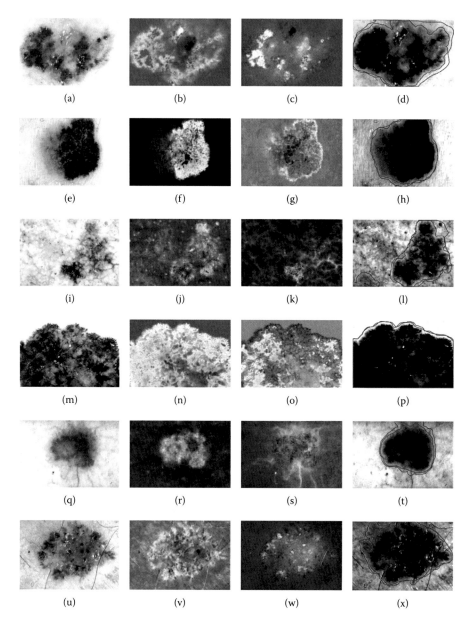

FIGURE 2.17 Malignant lesions. The first column is input image followed by melanin, hemoglobin, and geo-mean channels in the following columns.

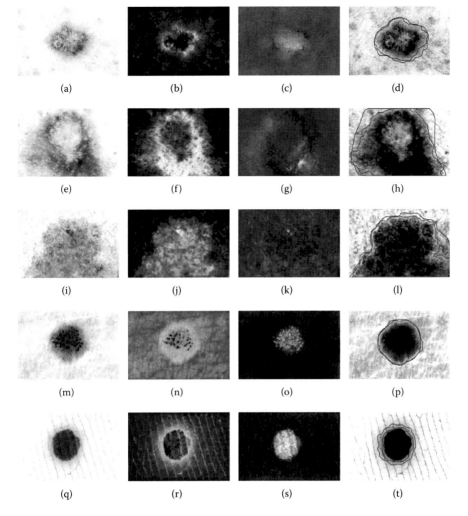

(a)	(b)	(c)	(d)
(e)	(f)	(g)	(h)
(i)	(j)	(k)	(l)
(m)	(n)	(o)	(p)
(q)	(r)	(s)	(t)

FIGURE 2.18 Some more benign lesions. The first column is input image followed by melanin, hemoglobin, and geo-mean channels in the following columns.

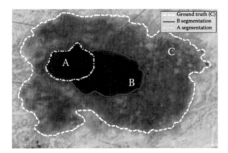

FIGURE 3.4 An example of the counterintuitive behavior of NPRI. Even though segmentation B is in greater agreement than segmentation A with the reference segmentation C, it achieves a lower (i.e., worse) PRI equal to 0.5 (vs. 0.52 of A). NPRI, being simply a linear rescaling of PRI, maintains the anomaly. (Reprinted from *Pattern Recognition Letters*, 31, E. Peserico and A. Silletti, Is (N)PRI suitable for evaluating automated segmentation of skin lesions? 2464–2467, Copyright 2010, with permission from Elsevier.)

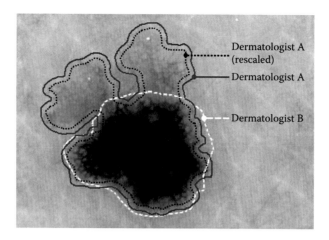

FIGURE 3.5 Compensation for systematic bias in border drawing, as performed in [20]. All lesions according to dermatologist A are rescaled (in this case tightened) by the same factor, so as to make lesion size identical to that of dermatologist B on average. (Belloni Fortina, A. et al.: Where's the Naevus? Inter-Operator Variability in the Localization of Melanocytic Lesion Border. *Skin Research and Technology*, 2011. 18. 311–315. Copyright Wiley-VCH Verlag GmbH & Co. KGaA. Reproduced with permission.)

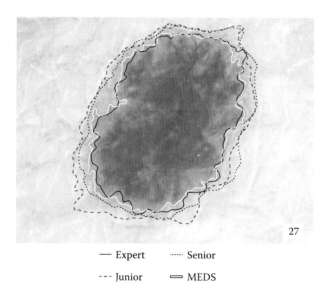

FIGURE 3.9 Melanocytic lesion segmentation performed by human dermatologists and MEDS. (Reprinted from Peruch, F. et al., Simple, fast, accurate melanocytic lesion segmentation in 1-D color space, in *Proceedings of VISAPP 2013*, pp. 191–200, 2013, Barcelona, Spain. Copyright 2013, with permission from INSTICC/SciTePress.)

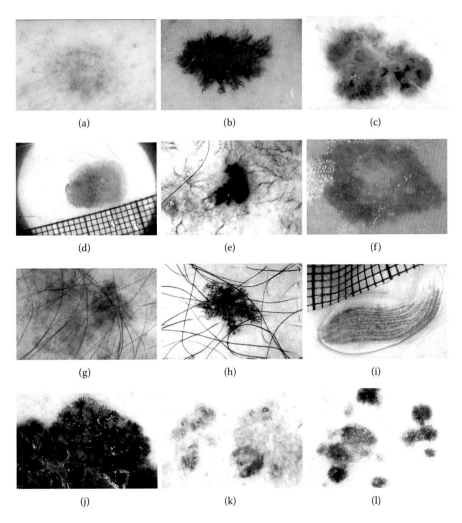

FIGURE 4.1 Factors that complicate border detection. (a) Low contrast [3]. (b) Irregular border [3]. (c) Fuzzy border [2]. (d) Black frame [2]. (e) Blood vessels. (f) Bubbles [2]. (g) Thin hairs [3]. (h) Thick hairs [2]. (i) Distortion [2]. (j) Variegated coloring [2]. (k) Regression [2]. (l) Multiple lesions [2]. (Reprinted with permission from Argenziano, G. et al., *Dermoscopy: A Tutorial*, EDRA Medical Publishing and New Media, Milan, Italy, 2002.)

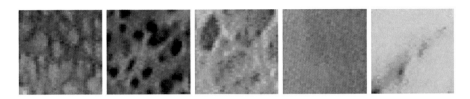

FIGURE 5.10 In Serrano and Acha's method, five dermoscopic 40×40 image samples of each type of pattern to classify: reticular, globular, cobblestone, homogeneous, and parallel. (Reprinted with permission from Serrano, C. and Acha, B., *Pattern Recognition*, vol. 42, no. 6, pp. 1052–1057, 2009.)

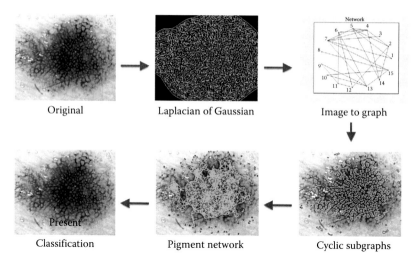

FIGURE 5.12 Overview of the algorithm proposed by Sadeghi et al.: work 1. (Reprinted with permission from Sadeghi, M. et al., *Computerized Medical Imaging and Graphics*, vol. 35, pp. 137–143, 2011.)

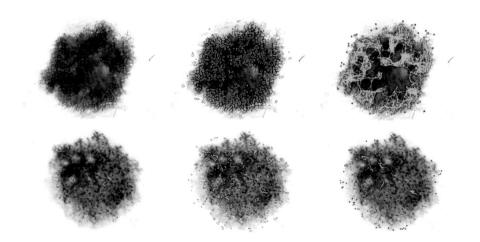

FIGURE 5.13 Two examples with the algorithm proposed by Sadeghi et al.: work 1. Firstly, the original images; in the second place, the cyclic subgraphs; and thirdly, the diagnosis (present in the first lesion and absent in the second one). (Reprinted with permission from Sadeghi, M. et al., *Computerized Medical Imaging and Graphics*, vol. 35, pp. 137–143, 2011.)

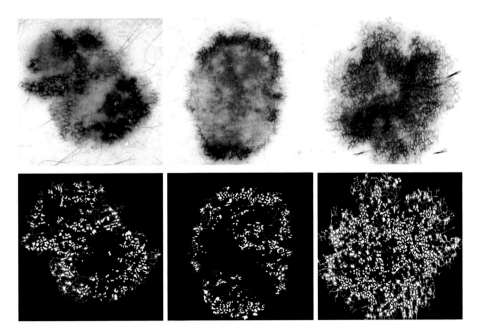

FIGURE 5.15 In the method proposed by Sadeghi et al.: work 2, three images: the top row shows the original ones of APN, APN, and TPN; the bottom row shows their corresponding pigment networks. (Reprinted with permission from Sadeghi, M. et al., *Lecture Notes in Computer Science*, vol. 6326, pp. 467–474, 2010.)

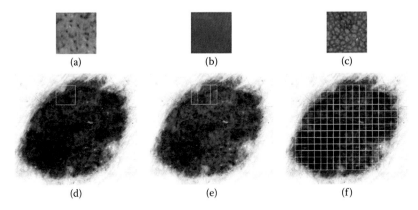

FIGURE 5.26 Examples of the two image sets used. (a–c) First set: Individual patches. 81×81 dermoscopic individual patches belonging to (a) globular pattern, (b) homogeneous pattern, and (c) reticular pattern. (d–f) Second image set: Complete lesions. (d) 81×81 sample extracted from the whole lesion. (e) Displacement equal to 27 rows or 27 columns is applied to obtain the following sample. (f) Overlapping samples to analyze the whole lesion. (Sáez, A. et al., *IEEE Transactions on Medical Imaging*, vol. 33, pp. 1137–1147. © 2014 IEEE.)

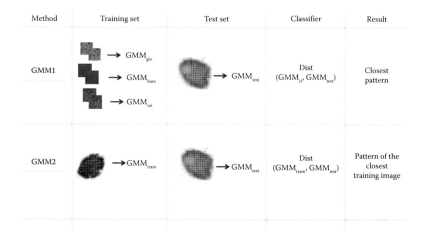

FIGURE 6.10 Classification methods based on Gaussian mixture model.

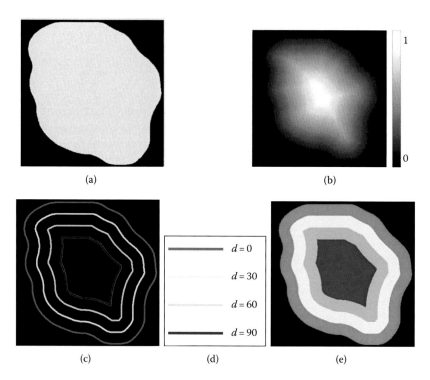

(a)

(b)

(c)

(d)

(e)

$d = 0$

$d = 30$

$d = 60$

$d = 90$

FIGURE 7.6 The isodistance contours and subbands of a lesion. (a) Lesion mask. (b) Distance transform of (a). (c) Isodistance contours C_d of the lesion, where d represents the distance between C_d and the lesion border in (a). (e) Bands of the lesion defined according to Equation 7.12 between the contours in (d).

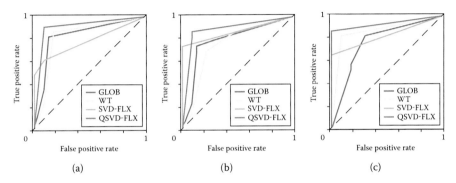

(a)   (b)   (c)

FIGURE 7.7 ROC curves of the pairwise classifiers resulting from using the different descriptors. Areas under the ROC curves are reported in Table 7.1. (a, b, c) represent binary classification results for ABS vs REG (a), ABS vs IRG (b), REG vs IRG (c).

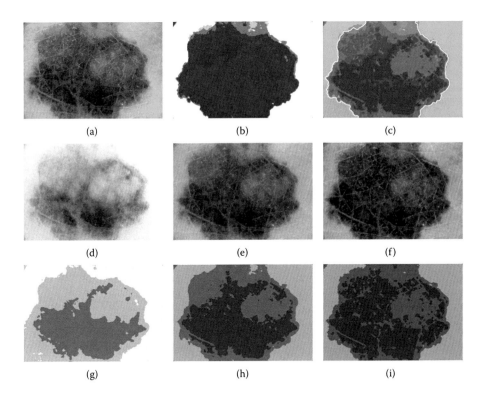

(a)   (b)   (c)

(d)   (e)   (f)

(g)   (h)   (i)

FIGURE 8.1 An example of the DMB system and lesion segmentation. (a) The original image. (b) The average color distance ratio image for determining the region of interest (ROI). (c) The result of automated segmentation for the pigmented lesion, where the lesion border is shown by the white line. (d–f) The red, green, blue channel images, respectively. (g–i) Three degrees of brightness images from d–f, respectively. (From Lee, G. et al., *Skin Research and Technology*, vol. 18, pp. 462–470, 2012.)

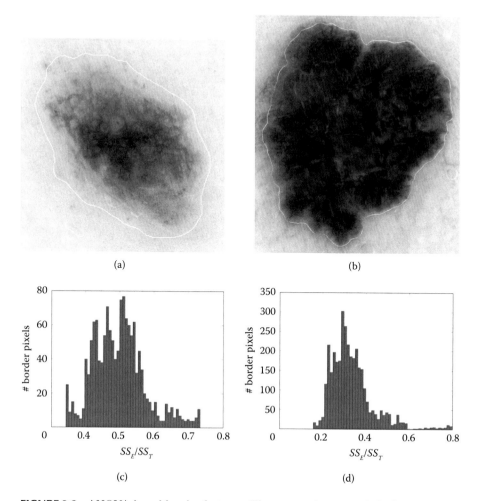

(a)

(b)

(c)

(d)

FIGURE 9.3 ANOVA-based border features. The gray region around the lesion border (white contour) in (a) and (b) indicates the samples used to derive the ANOVA-based border features in (c) and (d), respectively. While the color fading in the benign case is very smooth around the border, the malignant case has a much more abrupt color change across the border. This is summarized by the 25th, 50th, and 75th percentiles, corresponding to features f_7, f_8, and f_9, respectively. (Reprinted from *Artificial Intelligence in Medicine*, 60, M. Zortea et al., Performance of a dermoscopy-based computer vision system for the diagnosis of pigmented skin lesions compared with visual evaluation by experienced dermatologists, 13–26, Copyright 2014, with permission from Elsevier.)

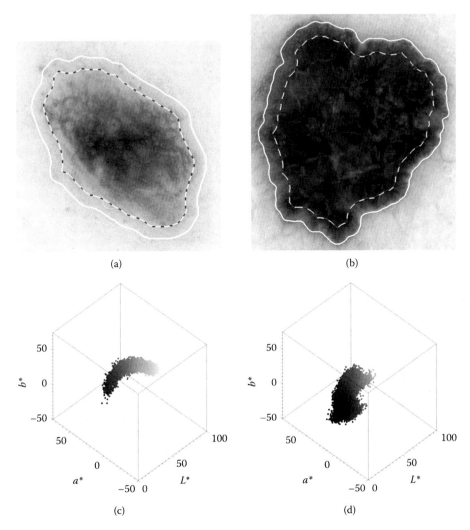

FIGURE 9.4 (a) Benign. (b) Malignant. (c, d) 3D histograms of $L^\star a^\star b^\star$ color space components of top row. (Reprinted from *Artificial Intelligence in Medicine*, 60, M. Zortea et al., Performance of a dermoscopy-based computer vision system for the diagnosis of pigmented skin lesions compared with visual evaluation by experienced dermatologists, 13–26, Copyright 2014, with permission from Elsevier.)

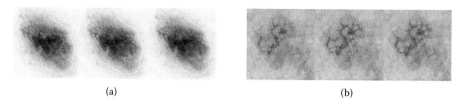

(a)   (b)

FIGURE 9.5 (a, b) Example of geometric features corresponding to the number of "lesion pieces" obtained by applying binary thresholds to the lesion area (delineated by the white contour) at different grayscale percentiles. From left to right: 25th, 50th, and 75th percentiles. (Reprinted from *Artificial Intelligence in Medicine*, 60, M. Zortea et al., Performance of a dermoscopy-based computer vision system for the diagnosis of pigmented skin lesions compared with visual evaluation by experienced dermatologists, 13–26, Copyright 2014, with permission from Elsevier.)

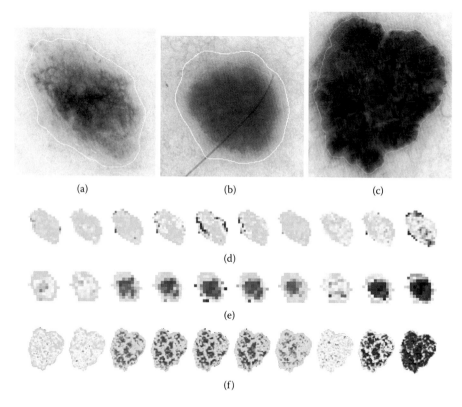

(a)   (b)   (c)

(d)

(e)

(f)

FIGURE 9.6 Example images (a) Benign *not cut*; (b) Benign *cut*; (c) Malignant. The following rows (d–f) of artificially colored images are texture images derived using the LBP algorithm and correspond to the three top images (rows [d–f] with top [a–c] images). Blue and red correspond to lower and higher values of texture, respectively. Maps 1–9 from left to right were linearly scaled in the range {0–0.18}, whereas 10 is in {0–0.36}. This is kept fixed for the three sets shown above, so the values are therefore directly comparable by visual inspection. (Reprinted from *Artificial Intelligence in Medicine*, 60, M. Zortea et al., Performance of a dermoscopy-based computer vision system for the diagnosis of pigmented skin lesions compared with visual evaluation by experienced dermatologists, 13–26, Copyright 2014, with permission from Elsevier.)

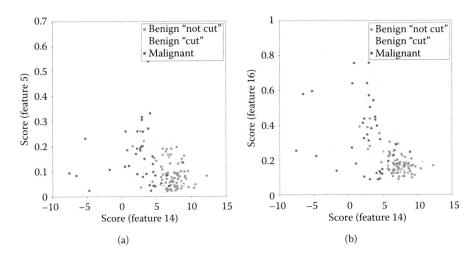

FIGURE 9.10 Examples of the first two features selected by LDA (a) and CART (b). All 206 samples are shown for visualization purposes (but not for feature selection). (Reprinted from *Artificial Intelligence in Medicine*, 60, M. Zortea et al., Performance of a dermoscopy-based computer vision system for the diagnosis of pigmented skin lesions compared with visual evaluation by experienced dermatologists, 13–26, Copyright 2014, with permission from Elsevier.)

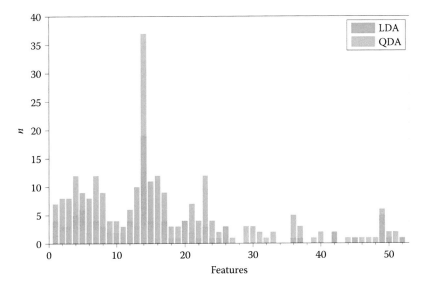

FIGURE 9.11 Number of times (n) each feature was included in the set of selected features in the 20 random data sets. The numbers for the two classifiers are stacked. (Reprinted from *Artificial Intelligence in Medicine*, 60, M. Zortea et al., Performance of a dermoscopy-based computer vision system for the diagnosis of pigmented skin lesions compared with visual evaluation by experienced dermatologists, 13–26, Copyright 2014, with permission from Elsevier.)

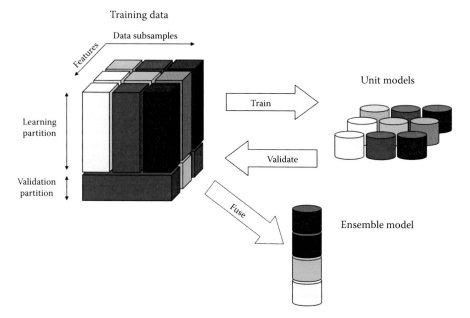

FIGURE 10.2 Ensemble learning approach. Training data are partitioned into learning and validation sets, which are further divided by features and data samples, referred to as bags. Unit models (SVMs) are trained for each bag, and an ensemble fusion approach fuses them.

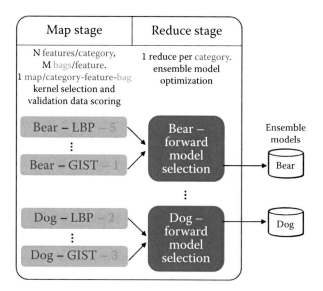

FIGURE 10.4 Large-scale ensemble modeling implementation in Hadoop MapReduce.

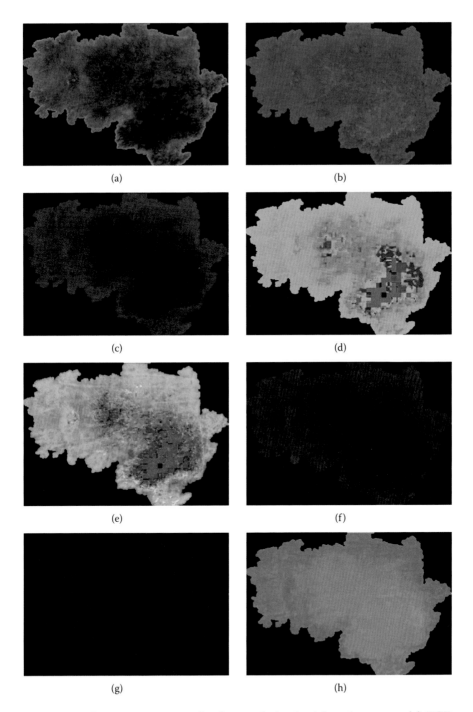

FIGURE 11.6 Dermoscopy image of melanoma lesion in eight color spaces. (a) RGB; (b) rgb; (c) $I_1/I_2/I_3$; (d) $L_1/L_2/L_3$; (d) hsv; (e) Luv; (f) Lab; (g) yCbCr.

TABLE 12.6
Color Reproduction

Reference Color	Samsung Galaxy S4		iPhone 5		
	DL1	DL3	DL1	DL3	Handyscope

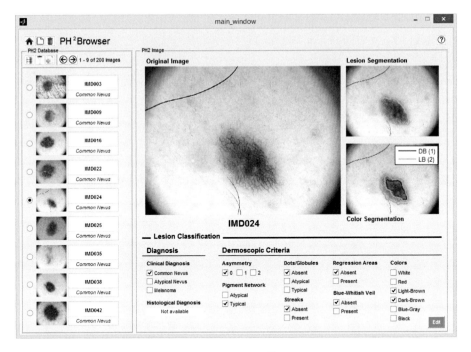

FIGURE 13.2 Graphical user interface of the PH² Browser.

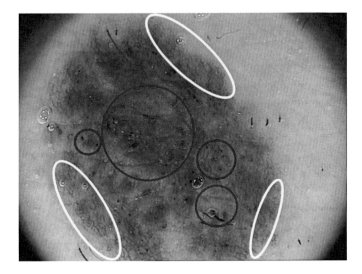

FIGURE 13.4 Dermoscopic feature identification: atypical pigment network (yellow ellipses), atypical dots/globules (red circles), and blue–white veil (blue circles).

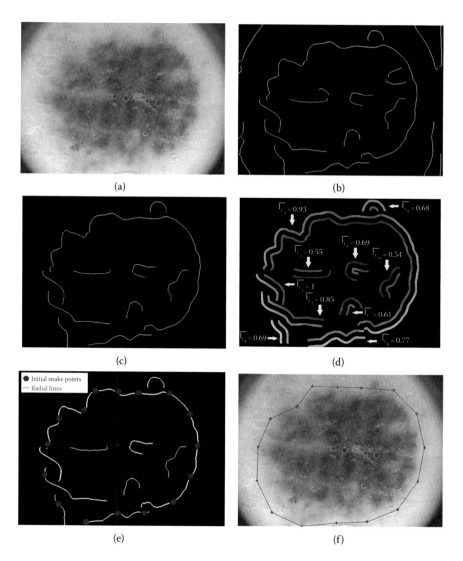

FIGURE 13.6 Automatic snake initialization method: (a) original RGB image, (b) edge map obtained through the Canny edge detector, (c) edge map after removing some false positive edge segments, (d) determination of the normalized mean intensity difference between the peripheral regions, (e) initial snake point finding process, and (f) initial snake curve.

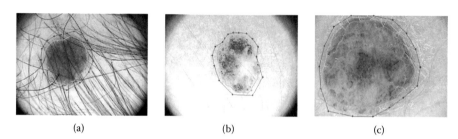

FIGURE 13.7 GVF snake segmentation in difficult dermoscopic images: (a) presence of hairs, (b) fragmented skin lesion, and (c) skin lesion with multiple colors. In these images the dotted red contour represents the initial snake curve, whereas the green contour corresponds to the final segmentation.

9 Improved Skin Lesion Diagnostics for General Practice by Computer-Aided Diagnostics

Kajsa Møllersen
University Hospital of North Norway
Tromsø, Norway

Maciel Zortea
University of Tromsø
Tromsø, Norway

Kristian Hindberg
University of Tromsø
Tromsø, Norway

Thomas R. Schopf
University Hospital of North Norway
Tromsø, Norway

Stein Olav Skrøvseth
University Hospital of North Norway
Tromsø, Norway

Fred Godtliebsen
University of Tromsø
Tromsø, Norway

CONTENTS

247

9.1   INTRODUCTION

9.1.1   SKIN CANCER AND MELANOMA

There are three main classes of skin cancer: basal cell carcinoma, squamous cell carcinoma, and melanoma [1, 2]. While the first two cancer types by far outnumber melanomas in incidence rate, the latter is the leading cause of death from skin cancer [1–3]. In fair-skinned populations, melanoma is responsible for more than 90% of all skin cancer deaths [1, 2]. Melanoma may arise at any age and is one of the most common cancer types for persons less than 50 years of age [1, 2].

Melanomas originate in the melanocytic cells (melanocytes), which produce melanin, the pigment of the skin [4]. Melanin is responsible for the various skin colors and it protects the body from solar UV radiation. Melanocytes are abundant in the upper layers of the skin. The cells can be scattered throughout the skin or nested in groups. When appearing in groups, they are often visible to the naked eye as common benign nevi [4].

In the majority of cases melanoma development starts in normal skin. However, approximately 25% of all melanomas originate in melanocytic cells within existing benign nevi [5, Chapter 27]. Single cells in the nevus change into cancer cells and behave abnormally.

Early-stage melanomas often resemble common nevi. If the patient already has many nevi, a new lesion may be hard to notice because it looks just like another mole. With time, the cancer lesion increases in size, and at some point most patients will notice a spot that looks different from other moles [5, Chapter 27]. If melanoma development begins within an existing mole, the patient may notice a change in its appearance, for example, a change in color or shape of the preexisting nevus.

There is usually horizontal growth in the early stages of the disease [4, 6]. The gross appearance is a mole increasing its diameter. Later, the lesion will grow vertically, gradually invading deeper layers of the skin. At this stage, melanoma cells may spread to other parts of the body, forming metastases. Some forms of melanoma may start the vertical growth very early, while it may take several years to occur in other types.

Melanoma may be cured if treated at an early stage. Mortality increases with increasing growth into deeper skin layers. More than 90% of melanoma patients are still alive after 5 years if treated early [7]. If distant spread of cancer cells has occurred, the proportion of patients alive after 5 years may be 20% or even lower [7].

The treatment of melanoma is surgery; that is, all cancer tissue is completely removed from the skin [8]. Removal of skin lesions suggestive of melanoma is fairly easy in the majority of cases. Many general practitioners (GPs) are able to perform this procedure themselves in primary health care practices. The main challenge is to decide which skin lesions to remove. A final diagnosis can only be made when a pathologist examines the removed tissue microscopically. When doctors decide to remove a skin lesion, it is based on clinical suspicion only, as there is no method to accurately diagnose skin cancer in advance by inspection.

Because overlooking a melanoma may have fatal consequences for the patient, the decision to remove a skin lesion is often based on a low grade of suspicion. Consequently, many surgically removed lesions turn out to be benign nevi when histopathologically examined.

9.1.2 DERMATOSCOPY

Dermatoscopy may be an aid to identify suspicious pigmented skin lesions suggestive of melanoma [8–10]. A dermatoscope is a magnifying lens with special illumination [11, Chapter 3, p. 7]. When inspecting a skin lesion through a dermatoscope, various anatomical structures in the upper layers of the skin become visible. Some of these structures are very small, for example, no more than 0.1 mm. Naturally, these structures are invisible to the naked eye. In addition to various anatomical structures, the dermatoscope also reveals a great variety of color shades [11, Chapter 4, p. 11]. These colors are generated mainly by hemoglobin and melanin in the skin. Hemoglobin is one of the main contents of blood and present throughout the skin. Melanin is the pigment produced in melanocytes. In melanoma and some other pigmented skin lesions, there may be an increased amount of melanin due to a change in the production rate of melanin. In addition to varying amounts of melanin, the localization of melanin within the skin influences the colors that can be seen through the dermatoscope. In order to reduce disturbing reflections from the skin surface, some dermatoscopes require the use of an immersion fluid (e.g., water, oil, alcohol) between the skin and the lens. Reduced reflections can also be achieved by the use of a polarized light source inside the dermatoscope.

Studies have shown that diagnostic accuracy may increase by using dermatoscopy [9, 10]. While using a dermatoscope is fairly easy, the interpretation of the findings may be challenging, as a great variety of features have been described. There is evidence that training and experience are required in order to improve diagnostic skills [12]. However, the amount of necessary training is uncertain. Since dermatoscopy requires training and regular use, it is mainly performed by dermatologists. Few reports exist on the use of dermatoscopy in general practice, with the exception of some reports from Australia [13, 14].

Several algorithms have been designed to help beginners of dermatoscopy. All these algorithms focus on a limited number of anatomical features. Typically, the examiner is asked to count specific features and the resulting numerical score may indicate if a lesion is suggestive of melanoma. There are also qualitative approaches where certain feature combinations are looked for.

Experienced dermatologists usually apply a method called *pattern analysis* for the dermatoscopic classification of pigmented skin lesions [15, 16]. The doctor systematically inspects a lesion for a large number of features and specific combinations of features. Certain anatomical regions have characteristic features, and common classes of lesions are often recognized instantly based on typical patterns. This concept requires a certain degree of previous experience and training, but dermatologists are familiar with this concept from the way they recognize other dermatologic diseases. In the remainder of this section we provide a brief overview of some dermatoscopic algorithms used by doctors.

The ABCD rule of dermatoscopy is a numerical scoring system based on the formula $A \cdot 1.3 + B \cdot 0.1 + C \cdot 0.5 + D \cdot 0.5$ [17]. The A, B, C, and D values are based on the dermatoscopic assessment of a melanocytic skin lesion.

A is connected to lesion asymmetry. If the lesion in question is completely symmetric, $A = 0$, whereas symmetry in one axis gives $A = 1$, and if there is no symmetry in two perpendicular axes, then $A = 2$. B assesses the border sharpness, and equals the number of segments (maximum eight) in which there is an abrupt peripheral cutoff in the pigmentation pattern. C is the color count (range 1–6: black, light brown, dark brown, red, white, blue–gray), and in D the number of dermatoscopic structures present in the lesion is counted (range 1–5: dots, globules, homogeneous areas, network, branched streaks). The resulting total dermatoscopy score will range from 1 to 8.9. A score larger than 5.45 indicates melanoma.

The Menzies' method applies a two-step approach [18]. First, symmetry and color are assessed. If the lesion is symmetrical and only one color is present, the appearance of the lesion is benign and no further assessment is necessary. If asymmetry or more than one color is observed, nine further features must be looked for: blue–white veil, pseudopods, scar-like depigmentation, multiple colors (five or six), broadened network, multiple brown dots, radial streaming, peripheral black dots/globules, and multiple blue–gray dots. If at least one of these features is present, the lesion is defined as suspicious.

The seven-point checklist defines major and minor criteria [19]. There are three major criteria; each is assigned a score of 2: atypical pigment network, blue–white veil, and atypical vascular pattern. The four minor criteria are each assigned a score of 1: irregular streaks, irregularly distributed dots/globules, irregularly distributed blotches, and regression structures. A total score of 3 or more indicates a suspicious lesion.

The three-point checklist is a simple algorithm including only three features: asymmetry, atypical pigment network, and blue–white structures [20]. The presence of two or more features indicates malignancy.

The chaos and clues algorithm applies a two-step approach [21]. First, symmetry and color are assessed dermatoscopically. Symmetrical lesions with one color do not require further assessment. If asymmetry or more than one color is observed, eight clues of malignancy are searched for: eccentric structureless areas, thick reticular/branched lines, blue/gray structures, peripheral black dots/clods, segmental radial lines/pseudopods, white lines, polymorphous vessels, and parallel lines/ridges at acral sites. The presence of one of these features indicates malignancy.

The acronym BLINCK refers to six steps, including both clinical and dermatoscopic findings [22]. In the first step (Benign), the doctor has to assess if the lesion immediately can be classified as a common benign pigmented skin lesion. In this case, no further assessment is needed. Otherwise, the examination continues with the next steps: If this is the only lesion with this particular pattern on that body region, the lonely score is 1. An irregular dermatoscopic appearance (asymmetrical pigmentation pattern and more than one color) scores 1 on irregularity. If the patient is anxious that the lesion may be skin cancer or if the lesion appears to change, the nervous and change score is 1 (even if both criteria are positive). In the known clues part, the presence of seven known clues are assessed: atypical pigment network, pseudopods/streaks, black dots/globules/clods, eccentric structureless zone, blue/gray color (irregularly distributed), atypical vessels, and acral pigmentation pattern (parallel ridge pattern, diffuse irregular brown/black pigmentation). The presence of any of the clues scores 1 (maximum score 1). A total score of 2 or more out of 4 indicates possible malignancy.

These algorithms have in common that they are easier to use than pattern analysis and therefore are suited for beginners or doctors not using dermatoscopy on a regular basis, but there are several drawbacks. The more complex algorithms (e.g., the ABCD algorithm) are time-consuming and it is questionable if doctors can use them regularly in a busy clinic. Some of the algorithms are not applicable to special anatomical sites (e.g., face, palms, and soles). Also, the usefulness for nonmelanocytic lesions is limited in most algorithms. A typical example is the identification of the common (benign) seborrheic keratoses, which often fails using these algorithms. In this setting, a certain knowledge of pattern analysis is required.

Due to time constraints, it may be impossible to dermatoscopically examine all pigmented skin lesions of a patient. Doctors have to select lesions after an initial brief assessment (without dermatoscopy), which is a challenging process [23]. A basic concept is the ugly duckling sign [24]. In most patients, a certain kind of benign-looking nevi can be identified in a body region. Any outlier that looks somewhat different (based on size, shape, structure) may represent malignancy and warrants a dermatoscopic examination. Another concept is the clinical ABCDE rule [25] (not to be confused with the ABCD rule of dermatoscopy). This clinical algorithm may help to identify suspicious pigmented skin lesions based on the inspection with the naked eye (without any additional tool). This method is commonly used as the only way of assessment by many GPs not familiar with dermatoscopy. ABCDE is an acronym for asymmetry, border, color, diameter, and evolution. An asymmetric appearance, an irregular or tagged border, variation in color, a diameter larger than 6 mm, or changing appearance over time may raise the level of suspicion. However, the clinical ABCDE rule has several drawbacks [26, 27]. It does not explain how to weight the different criteria. Many atypical (benign) nevi may fulfill these criteria with the consequence of being classified as malignant [28]. Also, all melanomas initially have a diameter of less than 5 mm [29]. Furthermore, early-stage melanomas may have a regular appearance and can easily be overlooked using this algorithm.

9.1.3 COMPUTER-AIDED DIAGNOSIS SYSTEMS

With the exception of Australia, dermatoscopy is not in regular use in most primary health care systems. Therefore, as many studies show, diagnostic accuracy of pigmented skin lesions and melanoma is lower in general practice than in specialist practice [30]. Computer-aided diagnosis (CAD) systems are designed to interpret medical information with the purpose of assisting a practitioner in the diagnostic process. CAD systems based on dermatoscopy may provide GPs with additional information to increase diagnostic accuracy. CAD systems available on the market so far are mainly intended for specialist doctors. To our knowledge, no system has been specifically designed for general practice.

To succeed in dermatoscopy, intensive training and long experience are needed. Dolianitis et al. [31] compared the diagnostic accuracy of four dermatoscopy algorithms in the hands of 61 medical practitioners in Australia. The study group was a mixture of primary care physicians, dermatologist trainees, and dermatologists. More than half used the dermatoscope on daily basis and 40% diagnosed more than five melanomas per year. Even if training is successful, the capacity for a GP to be trained for a range of different diseases is a limitation. Dolianitis et al. reported that the time necessary to complete the study was a significant factor for the low response rate (30% of those who initially showed interest).

The potential of a CAD system to increase diagnostic accuracy for inexperienced doctors is evident, as already discussed by the authors in a previous publication [32]. There have been many efforts to develop computer programs to diagnose melanoma based on lesion images. Roughly, these studies follow intuitive steps in a standard pattern recognition processing chain: (1) image segmentation to separate the lesion area from the background skin, (2) extraction of image features for classification purposes, and (3) final classification using statistical methods. A wide range of ideas have been used in these three steps; see Korotkov and Garcia [33] for an overview and categorizations. Reporting sensitivity and specificity, Rosado et al. [34] presented a thorough overview of state-of-the-art methods at the time. No statistically significant difference between human diagnosis and computer diagnosis under experimental conditions was found. In addition, no studies met all of the predetermined methodological requirements. Day and Barbour [35] attempted to reproduce algorithmically the perceptions of dermatologists as to whether a lesion should be excised or not; Arroyo and Zapirain [36] built a CAD system on the ABCD rule of dermoscopy; Fabbrocini et al. [37] built a CAD system on the seven-point checklist

Comparing performance of different systems is difficult because results are very sensitive to the data set used for validation, and a major problem is the lack of publicly available databases of dermatoscopic images. For a fair and representative comparison, a data set with a large number of examples of all types of lesions and all types of features expected to be encountered in clinical practice should be made available.

Following this, the research question stated in Zortea et al. [32, p. 14] was:

Assume identical information is made available to both computers and doctors for the same set of skin lesion images. Then, how does the accuracy of the computer system compare with the accuracy of the doctors?

An answer to the question above would make it easier to objectively assess the performance of new and existing methods, and would provide an indication of how difficult the lesion images in the data sets used in the experiments were to diagnose. In a data set with a clear distinction between classes, high accuracy is expected. Despite this being a conceptually rather simple experiment to conduct, the study could be demanding because it would require substantial effort by dermatologists to evaluate a large number of lesion images. Also, a more difficult question to answer is whether the data set is sufficiently representative. To be so, it needs to approximate the variability of cases found in a true clinical setting, including the prior information regarding the occurrence of each type of lesion.

Several studies have been reported where the diagnostic accuracy of a computer system is directly compared with human diagnosis. Most studies tend to compare the performance of their system exclusively with histopathological diagnosis, leaving it an open question how difficult the lesions are to diagnose by dermatologists. Korotkov and Garcia [33] recently listed 10 CAD systems for the diagnosis of melanoma based on dermatoscopy. As a rule, the systems use powerful and dedicated video cameras. Also, current limitations of state-of-the-art CAD systems motivate the development of new algorithms for analysis of skin lesions, and low-cost data acquisition tools (e.g., digital cameras and dermatoscopes) are becoming commonly available. A simple image acquisition setup with camera and dermatoscope has been previously discussed, for instance, in Gewirtzman and Braun [38], and has been used in the visual comparison system of Baldi et al. [39].

The clinical impact of CAD systems has been limited. Perrinaud et al. [40] reported on an independent clinical evaluation of some of these systems, and they found little evidence that such systems benefit dermatologists. The costs related to the acquisition material and proprietary technologies are likely substantial barriers to the systems gaining widespread popularity among physicians [41].

Day and Barbour [35] point out two main shortcomings: (1) a CAD system is expected to reproduce the decision of pathologists (malignant/benign) with only the input available to a dermatologist (image) and (2) histopathological data are not available for clearly benign lesions, resulting in a very skewed data set.

A CAD system aimed at dermatologists must be substantially better than the dermatologist. A CAD system whose diagnostic accuracy is not significantly different from that of a dermatologist can still be a valuable tool for GPs. GPs tend to excise more benign lesions per melanoma than dermatologists [42]. It is important to keep the image acquisition tool cost low, since a GP may not use it on a daily basis. Complementary and interpretable feedback beyond the posterior probability of the lesion being malignant can also be more valuable to a GP. If a lesion is flagged as suspicious, a dermatologist can take a closer look for evidence of malignancy. A GP will not have the necessary training to benefit from a closer look, unless being told what to look for. The algorithmic features should preferably relate to clinical features. Together with the suggested diagnosis from the CAD system, an indication of which features were the most significant for the diagnosis of this specific lesion will lead to better user–system interaction, and hopefully better diagnosis accuracy. A classifier with complex interaction between the features will appear as a "black box" to the user. Not only must the features themselves be interpretable, but also their contribution to the classification must be interpretable.

The CAD system presented here, called *Nevus Doctor*, is aimed at GPs by meeting the requirements of low-cost acquisition tool, clinical-like features, and interpretable classification feedback.

In a previous study [32], in addition to the histopathological results, we compared the results of the computer system with those of three dermatologists to provide an indication of how challenging our data set is to either type of analysis. The results suggest that *Nevus Doctor* performs as well as a dermatologist under the described circumstances. The study is done on a very limited data set. The results from a new study with a bigger data set from the same source are presented here. The focus is on giving the GP a recommendation, *not-cut* or *cut*, and an interpretation of the classification. The CAD system is therefore trained and tested on the two classes *not-cut* or *cut*. The *not-cut* class contains the non-suspicious looking nevi that were histopathologically confirmed to be benign. The *cut* class contains all melanomas confirmed by histopathology and, in addition, suspicious looking nevi that turned out to be benign. With this setup, where the CAD system is trained also with benign lesions in the *cut* class, the number of benign lesions being classified as *cut* will be high. In a classical benign/malignant setup, this would correspond to low specificity. But as long as we cannot guarantee close to 100% sensitivity, we believe that a melanoma-per-excised-lesion rate comparable to that of a dermatologist will improve lesion classification in the GP's office.

9.2   CAD SYSTEMS

A CAD system for skin lesions will necessarily be complex with several interacting pieces in the chain, from image acquisition, segmentation, and analysis to final response. Important steps in building a CAD system are feature selection and choice of classifier [43]. The quality of the images and limited computational resources are no longer the main obstacles. Correct classification depends on accurate feature values, which in turn depend on accurate segmentation. The success of both segmentation and feature value calculation depend on the data set. Evaluating the components of a CAD system can be tricky, since they are so dependent on each other. Multiple observers are needed for human evaluation, since the interobserver variation can be quite substantial.

9.2.1 IMAGE ACQUISITION AND PREPROCESSING

Image acquisition can be done in a number of ways: recording visible or invisible light, ultrasound, magnetic resonance, or electric impedance [44]. The cheapest way is to use a digital camera and a dermatoscope to record visible light. Both digital cameras and attachable dermatoscopes are off-the-shelf equipment. In addition to being cheap and available, the images are interpretable to any doctor. Normally, some preprocessing is done. This includes image filtering to remove noise and downsampling to cut computational costs for the feature calculation.

9.2.2 SEGMENTATION AND HAIR REMOVAL

Segmentation of a skin lesion image consists of detecting the borders of the skin lesion. This is a crucial first step in CAD systems. Most features for classification are computed from the segmented area and depend on correct segmentation, particularly shape- and border-related features.

Irregular shape, nonuniform color, and ambiguous structures make accurate segmentation challenging [45]. It can easily go wrong when the contrast between the lesion and the skin is low [46]. The presence of hairs and skin flakes is an additional undesirable feature that may interfere with segmentation. Hairs can be identified [47, 48] and given special treatment during the processing [49, 50 and references therein].

Supervised and unsupervised techniques have been developed for segmentation of dermatoscopic images. Supervised segmentation methods require input from the analyst, such as examples of skin and lesion pixels, a rough approximation of the lesion borders to be optimized, or a final refinement of a proposed solution [51, 52]. Generally, in such settings the user needs to provide a priori input for each particular image being analyzed. This task relies on the experience and knowledge of the user. Besides its accuracy, supervised approaches may be particularly time-consuming for health care professionals. For the sake of reproducibility, the fully manual segmentation may not be preferable in a computerized system. Indeed, reproducibility is an important feature of all segmentation procedures. Note that even under the best effort to counter this, different images of the same lesion will differ slightly in illumination, rotation, and shear, due to the flexibility of the skin.

Conversely, automatic segmentation methods (also called unsupervised methods) attempt to find the lesion borders without any input from the user. This reduces subjectivity and the burden on the analyst, at the expense of increased uncertainty in the accuracy of the final segmentation. Several approaches have been proposed in this direction. Most common automatic segmentation algorithms rely on techniques based on histogram thresholding [49, 52–55], where most commonly red, green, blue (RGB) information is mapped to a one- or two-dimensional color space through the choice of one of the channels, luminance, or principal component analysis. Other approaches include region-based techniques [52, 56–59], clustering [45, 60–62], contour-based approaches [52, 63, 64 and references therein], segmentation fusion techniques [65, 66], wavelets [67, 68], unsupervised iterative classification [46], and watershed transform [69].

Evaluation of the performance of segmentation techniques is difficult and suffers from the lack of a gold standard to refer to. Even trained dermatologists differ significantly when delineating the same lesion in separate incidents [70], so validation of any technique has to be treated with care. Strategies for evaluating the performance of border detection in dermatoscopic images can be divided into two main groups; qualitative and quantitative [46, 71]. In the qualitative evaluation approach, the dermatologist is asked to provide an overall score or grade to the segmentation result (e.g., good, acceptable, poor, and bad) based on visual assessment. In the quantitative evaluation the role of the dermatologist is reversed. Specifically, the dermatologist is asked to manually draw the border around the lesion, which is assumed to be the ground truth. Assessing the accuracy of the segmentation requires definition of a similarity score between the ground truth and a candidate border, and a strategy to deal with the different ground truths from different doctors.

From a practical perspective, it is important that a segmentation algorithm does not take too much time and that the users are not asked to perform a task that they are not trained for, for example, the GP having to draw the lesion border in dermatoscopic images.

9.2.3   IMAGE FEATURES

The term *feature* can refer to both a clinical/dermatoscopic feature, as those described in the ABCD rule, and an image feature, whose value is the input of a classifier. An image feature can be constructed to mimic some dermatoscopic feature, for example, asymmetry or detection of globules. Other image features are independent of dermatoscopic features, such as features on the pixel level [72]. The usefulness of image features is evaluated by stability to image acquisition, stability to segmentation, interpretability for the doctor, and improved performance of the CAD system. Dermatoscopic images of the same lesion taken with the same equipment at approximately the same time will to some extent still not be identical. How firmly the glass plate is pressed onto the skin will affect the blood flow. How the lesion is positioned can have an effect since light intensity often degrades toward to edges of the dermatoscope. This can in turn affect the segmentation. Therefore, it is desirable that slightly different segmentations influence the feature values as little as possible. A feature that is interpretable for the doctor can provide valuable feedback, especially since no CAD system has yet proved to be effective in a clinical setting. On the other hand, a feature that improves the performance of the CAD system significantly need not necessarily be interpretable.

Many features have been described in the literature. Korotkov and Garcia [33] give an overview and also categorize the features according to the clinical ABCDE rule, the dermatoscopic ABCD rule, pattern analysis, and others. As a rule, the features are not evaluated in any sense, except their contribution to the performance of the CAD system. Therefore, to go "feature shopping" among already described features is not straightforward. Evaluating features according to the aforementioned criteria can be difficult. For the stability criterion, the setup is relatively easy; it only requires the doctors to take multiple images of each lesion. Interpretability is a more tricky task, especially since the dermatoscopic features are somewhat subjective [31]. An image feature with high interpretability would necessarily have high correlation with the dermatoscopic feature. Because of the diversity of how doctors evaluate features in the same image, it would require the work of several doctors. A feature that improves the performance of the CAD system doesn't necessarily add anything to other CAD systems with a different classifier or another subset of features.

Some of the features presented here mimic dermatoscopic features, and others don't. They have not been evaluated yet, but we hope that this can be done soon. Future research in the field of pigmented skin lesion CAD systems could benefit from concentrating more on the features.

9.2.3.1 Color

Color is an important feature in all dermatoscopic lesion diagnosis algorithms. The lesions are evaluated according to color variegation, color asymmetry, number of colors, and presence of specific colors, such as red, blue, and white. A challenge when constructing a color feature is that the human color perception varies. Different physiology (e.g., red–green color deficiency) can play a part, but the psychology is probably more important. There are a number of effects (often referred to as optical illusions) that influence how a color is interpreted. A visual system is said to be color constant if the assigned color is determined by the spectral properties. The color constancy of the human vision fails dramatically under some circumstances and holds up under others. The factors that affect color constancy in human vision are not fully known, but numerosity, configural cues, and variability are known to have an effect [73].

A digital camera will record color unaffected by the factors that influence the human interpretation of color. But, factors such as light and camera white point will still affect the color.

A color space can be understood as a mathematical model and a reference, such that each color is represented by a set of numbers (typically three or four). The standard RGB color space (which is the default color space for most cameras and computer monitors) consists of the RGB model and a specific color reference and gamma correction. The Munsell color space was the first color space where hue, value, and chroma were separated into approximately perceptually uniform and independent dimensions, and is still in use today. A *perceptually uniform* color space is where the distance between two colors in the color space is proportional to the distance perceived by the human eye. Because human vision is not color constant, this is not a trivial task. In 1931 the CIE XYZ color space was introduced as a perceptually uniform color space, whereas the CIE $L^\star a^\star b^\star$ color space was defined in 1976 [74]. RGB color spaces are widely used, but they may not be the best ones for statistical calculations, since they are not perceptually uniform.

The number of color spaces in use today is huge and the best color space depends on the task at hand. We have chosen the CIE $L^\star a^\star b^\star$ because of its perceptual uniformity and wide use.

Strictly speaking, one can say that if two pixels don't have the exact same values, they don't represent the same color. In practice, when constructing features that can account for variegation, the number of colors, or the detection of specific colors, we look for groups of pixel values that represent the same color.

9.2.4 FEATURE SELECTION

Feature selection is an important step prior to classification [75]. The main goal of feature selection is to select a subset of p relevant features from the original feature set of dimension $d > p$. A feature is irrelevant if it is not correlated with or predictive of a classification class. Irrelevant features should be removed because their noisy behavior can lead to worse performance of the classifier. A feature is redundant if it is highly correlated with other features in the subset and therefore does not contribute to improved performance of the classifier. Redundant features should also be removed [76, p. 52], as they can actually worsen the performance of the classifier.

There can also be several reasons for restricting the number of features for classification. Classifier instability, interpretability, and computational burden are among the arguments most often used.

A high number of features, if compared to the number of observations, leads to an unstable classifier, in the sense that the replacement of one of the observations in the training set with another observation may change the classifier and features selected.

If the contribution of the different features to the classification result is meant to be interpreted by a human observer, it is crucial that the number of features is kept reasonably low. Classification trees [77] are a good example of this. When there are few features, a classification tree is maybe one of the most interpretable classifiers, but as the number of features grows, interpretation becomes very time-consuming. The more features, the longer time it takes to train a classifier, and the longer time it takes to compute the feature values for a new observation. Often the time spent on training the classifier is not of importance, since this is done before the clinical setting. Even if the classifier is updated for each new observation with verified class (a lesion with confirmed histopathology), the updating can be done offline, for instance, between patient visits. Conversely, the time spent on feature calculation is more crucial, as the doctor probably wants a result from the CAD system very fast. Many feature values can be calculated in a fraction of a second, while others need several tens of seconds. The inclusion of the different classifier features must be considered with respect to extra time consumption versus increased classifier performance.

Automatic feature selectors can be divided roughly into two categories: filters and wrappers. The filter method is independent of the classifier; it evaluates the general characteristics of the data and the classes. The wrapper method includes the classifier and chooses the subset that gives the best classification. The wrapper is generally more computationally intensive, since for each set of observations the classifier must be trained and tested (usually by cross-validation). If the data set is small or if the features are highly correlated, wrappers can act very unstable; a different cross-validation partition may lead to a different selection of feature subset. Filters are more stable, because no training and testing of a classifier are involved. Wrappers normally lead to better classification, but only if the data set is big enough for stable feature selection.

Correlation-based feature selection (CFS) [76] is an example of a filter. The acceptance of a feature into the final subset depends on its correlation to the classes, for areas in the observation space where the other features have low correlation to the classes. The feature subset evaluation function is

$$M_S = \frac{k\overline{r_{cf}}}{\sqrt{k + k(k-1)\overline{r_{ff}}}} \tag{9.1}$$

where M_S is the merit of a subset S containing k features, $\overline{r_{cf}}$ is the mean feature–class correlation, and $\overline{r_{ff}}$ is the mean feature–feature correlation.

Sequential feature selection (SFS) [78] is a simple search strategy that may be implemented with either the wrapper or the filter. The SFS algorithm comes in two versions: (1) forward, where it starts with an empty set of features and sequentially adds the feature that gives the best score and (2) backward, where it starts with all features and removes the feature that results in the best score for the remaining subset. An SFS wrapper is obtained when the error rate of the classifier is used to score the subset. An SFS filter is implemented when a proxy measure, such as an interclass distance, rather than the error rate, is used to score the subset. Examples of interclass distance measures that could be used in the filter case include the divergence, Chernoff, and Bhattacharyya distances [79].

Ultimately, the best feature selector depends on the task at hand. Automatic feature selection can be a good help for a first reduction of the number of features and to detect irrelevant and redundant features. Additional knowledge/preferences should be taken into account. Since feature selection can be done once and for all, it gives the opportunity to do a semiautomatic selection.

9.2.5 CLASSIFICATION

Correct classification (diagnosis) is the ultimate goal of the CAD system. If sensitivity and specificity near 100% are achieved, nothing else matters, assuming that the accuracy is measured on a separate and real-world representative test set. With lower sensitivity and specificity, other criteria must also be taken into account. Studies show that we cannot expect a CAD system to reach classification rates close to 100% [33, 34, 80]. Common statistical classifiers for skin lesion CAD systems are k-nearest neighbors (k-NNs), logistic regression, artificial neural networks (ANNs), decision trees (CART), support vector machines (SVMs), and discriminant analysis, among others [33]. The outcome of a classifier depends on both the set of lesions available for training and the image features chosen for classification. Therefore, it is difficult to compare classifier results from different studies [34].

When the data set used for training is small, additional care is needed to ensure that the classifier is stable in the sense that it is not overfitted [81]. Often, some parameters need to be tuned or chosen. The stability with regard to small changes in parameter value should also be considered. Another criterion is interpretability of the result. Interpretability is difficult when many low-level image features are designed for classification purposes, resulting in high-dimensional feature spaces and sparse representation due to the limited number of training instances. Since the doctor cannot blindly trust the classification, additional classifier feedback is desirable. The posterior probability indicates how certain the classification is. Benign 98% would feel different than benign 53%. But for this to have any meaning, often certain assumptions about the features and observations must be fulfilled (e.g., Gaussian distribution). If the classifier is simple and the number of features is kept low, the whole classification procedure can be interpreted by the user. Decision trees are an example where the whole tree can be displayed as a graph, and the decision flow can easily be understood if there are few features. With logistic regression, the feature weights tell something about how important each feature is in the classification, and together with the feature values (and their range), the grounds upon which the classification is done can be interpreted. For more advanced classifiers with complex interaction between the features, the interpretability is lost. The same goes for decision trees when the number of features is high. Note that a simple classifier might provide slightly lower classification rates, but it might be preferable if the result is interpretable.

A hybrid classifier combining parametric and nonparametric approaches can also be chosen. An example would be to use linear discriminant analysis (LDA) [82] for the subset of features that are approximately Gaussian distributed. The LDA outcome is then used as a feature of a classification tree together with the non-Gaussian features.

As the above-mentioned studies suggest, not much is gained by choosing the best classifier compared to a reasonably good one. Therefore, it might be wiser to allocate additional CAD development efforts elsewhere, like in the design of small sets of robust and easy-to-interpret features for classification.

9.3 FEATURE EXTRACTION

The features presented here are the 53 features described in Zortea et al. [32] and, in addition, six new features. All features are calculated in the CIE $L^\star a^\star b^\star$ color space, even if some of the features in Zortea et al. were calculated in sRGB. When grayscale is used, this corresponds to the $L^\star$ component. The features that did not end up in the final subset after feature selection are described in lesser detail, but a full description can be found in [32].

The image features try somehow to quantify dermatoscopic features and are named thereafter. There is seldom a one-to-one correspondence and we often use several image features to quantify the same dermatoscopic feature. Not all dermatoscopic features are covered by our image feature set, which is a drawback that can explain some of the missed melanomas in the final classification.

Most of the features described here are developed in-house, for instance, the analysis of variance for the lesion border, geometric features, and our choice of textures. The color and shape-related features are inspired by previous studies in the literature (e.g., [33, 83, 84], among others).

9.3.1 ASYMMETRY: DIFFERENCE IN GRAYSCALE (f_1, f_2)

Figure 9.1a is a schematic representation of the binary mask of a lesion with a coordinate system centered on the center of mass. Denote $I_{i,j}$ as the grayscale level of pixel (i, j), where the first index is along the horizontal dimension of Figure 9.1a. Set $I_{i,j} = 0$ if (i, j) is outside the binary mask of Figure 9.1a. We now compare the following regions:

1. $(A_1 \cup A_2)$ versus $(A_3 \cup A_4)$
2. $(A_1 \cup A_4)$ versus $(A_2 \cup A_3)$

For these two combinations, we evaluate

$$\Delta S_1 = \sum_i \sum_{j>0} |I_{i,j} - I_{i,-j}| \quad \text{and} \quad \Delta S_2 = \sum_{i>0} \sum_j |I_{i,j} - I_{-i,j}| \qquad (9.2)$$

We divide ΔS_1 and ΔS_2 by the area of the binary mask containing the lesion, so that the scores for lesions of different sizes are easily comparable. A large value of ΔS_1 or ΔS_2 indicates that there is a strong asymmetry of shape. The symmetry axes are rotated in steps of 10 degrees. We retain the rotation with the lowest average scores of ΔS_1 and ΔS_2. For the retained axes, we sort the scores of the two orthogonal axes, so that these will correspond to the asymmetry of shape features. Examples are shown in Figure 9.2a–c. Note that Equation 9.2 calculates the relative differences of grayscale values of

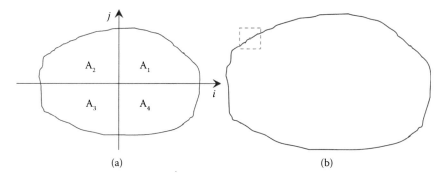

FIGURE 9.1 (a) Lesion with reference regions A_m, $m = 1,\ldots,4$. (b) Lesion border with a square region in red centered on a border pixel. (Reprinted from *Artificial Intelligence in Medicine*, 60, M. Zortea et al., Performance of a dermoscopy-based computer vision system for the diagnosis of pigmented skin lesions compared with visual evaluation by experienced dermatologists, 13–26, Copyright 2014, with permission from Elsevier.)

the lesion. Therefore, this is not strictly an asymmetry description feature, but serves as one.

9.3.2 ASYMMETRY: GRAYSCALE DISTRIBUTION (f_3, f_4)

The computation is similar to Equation 9.2. For the two combinations of regions, we evaluate

$$\Delta C_1 = \sum_{a=0}^{255} \left| \widehat{C}_{A_1 \cup A_2}(a) - \widehat{C}_{A_3 \cup A_4}(a) \right|$$

$$\Delta C_2 = \sum_{a=0}^{255} \left| \widehat{C}_{A_1 \cup A_4}(a) - \widehat{C}_{A_2 \cup A_3}(a) \right|$$

(9.3)

where, for instance, $\widehat{C}_{A_1 \cup A_2}$ is the estimated distribution of the 256 grayscales a using pixels belonging to either region A_1 or A_2, and is computed using Gaussian kernel density estimation [85]. Large values of ΔC_1 and ΔC_2 indicate that there is a strong asymmetry between the domains compared. The symmetry axes are rotated in steps of 10 degrees. We retain the rotation with the lowest average scores of ΔC_1 and ΔC_2. For the retained axes, we sort the scores for the two orthogonal axes that correspond to our proposed asymmetry features. Examples are shown in Figure 9.2d–f.

9.3.3 ASYMMETRY OF GRAYSCALE SHAPE (f_5, f_6)

A set of alternative binary masks, with mass centers (x_t, y_t), is generated by applying a threshold to the grayscale values inside the lesion border at

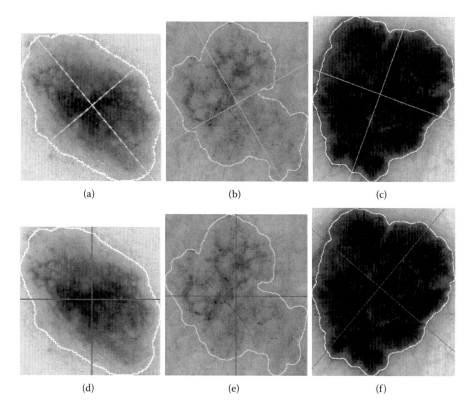

FIGURE 9.2 Upper row, from left to right: Asymmetry, difference in grayscale axes (light gray) of one benign and two malignant lesions. Lower row: Asymmetry, grayscale distribution axes (in dark gray) of the same lesions as in the upper row. (Reprinted from *Artificial Intelligence in Medicine*, 60, M. Zortea et al., Performance of a dermoscopy-based computer vision system for the diagnosis of pigmented skin lesions compared with visual evaluation by experienced dermatologists, 13–26, Copyright 2014, with permission from Elsevier.)

percentiles $t = [0.10, 0.20, \ldots, 0.90]$. We compute a vector v whose elements are the Euclidean distances between the original center of mass and the different (x_t, y_t). The features are the mean and standard deviation of v, respectively. These features were not included in the classifier.

9.3.4   BORDER: ANOVA-BASED ANALYSIS (f_7, f_8, f_9)

Suppose we have a segmented lesion such as the one in Figure 9.1b. For a particular region around the border pixel k, we have the pixels $X_{11}, X_{21}, \ldots, X_{n_1 1}$ inside the skin lesion and $X_{12}, X_{22}, \ldots, X_{n_2 2}$ outside the skin lesion, where

X_{ij} is the grayscale observation number i in tissue type $j = 1, 2$. The standard analysis of variance (ANOVA) then yields

$$SS_T(k) = SS_E(k) + SS_R(k) \quad \implies \quad R_k \equiv \frac{SS_E(k)}{SS_T(k)} \qquad (9.4)$$

where $SS_T(k)$ is the total sum of squares of the pixels within the border box, partitioned into two components related to the effects of the error $SS_E(k)$, and the pixel treatment $SS_R(k)$ (location inside/outside the lesion) in the model.

The above approach is implemented using a sliding window around the border, as illustrated in Figure 9.1b, using the grayscale version of the image. A square region of size 61×61 pixels is centered at each border pixel. This is an empiric choice, and corresponds to about 0.50 mm of the skin surface. The statistics are computed using the pixels inside and outside the lesion border that are contained within the sliding window. In general, for each pixel $k = 1, \ldots, K$ at the border of the lesion, we calculate R_k. Now, by observing the distribution of $\{R_k\}_{k=1}^{K}$, values close to 1 represent vague differences between the lesion area and the skin. For clear differences, values should be close to 0.

Our proposed features are the 25th, 50th, and 75th percentiles. Figure 9.3 shows two examples of the suggested features.

9.3.5 COLOR DISTRIBUTION (f_{10}, f_{11}, f_{12})

The three-dimensional (3D) histogram is computed using 10,000 randomly selected pixels. The bin size is set to 2. Only the nonempty bins are considered for the score computation. We use the average number of samples in each bin, the variance, and the percentage of nonempty bins in the color space. The $L^\star$ component values range from 0 to 100, while the $a^\star$ and $b^\star$ components vary between -127 to 127. Figure 9.4 shows the distribution of the three $L^\star a^\star b^\star$ components for two example images.

9.3.6 COLOR COUNTING AND BLUE–GRAY AREA (f_{19}, f_{20})

A palette approach, reported to efficiently estimate the number of colors of pigmented skin lesions in [83, 84], is used for feature extraction. The linear discriminant analysis classifier is trained on the colors white, red, light brown, dark brown, blue–gray, and black obtained from a training image. From these sample colors a statistical classifier is trained to recognize colors in unseen images. We classify the image into different regions and store the number of distinct colors as a feature. In addition, we retain the percentage of the lesion area classified as blue–gray as a feature. These features were not used in the final CAD system.

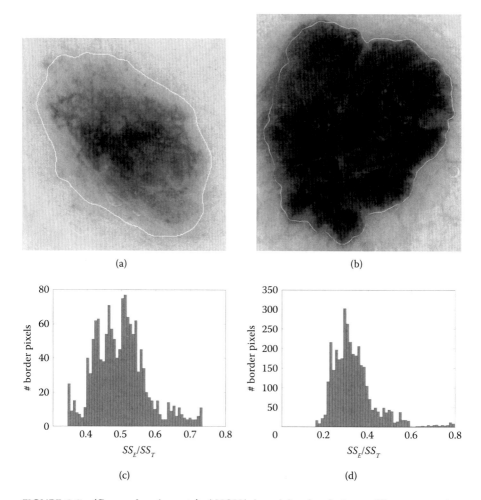

(a)   (b)

(c)   (d)

FIGURE 9.3 **(See color insert.)** ANOVA-based border features. The gray region around the lesion border (white contour) in (a) and (b) indicates the samples used to derive the ANOVA-based border features in (c) and (d), respectively. While the color fading in the benign case is very smooth around the border, the malignant case has a much more abrupt color change across the border. This is summarized by the 25th, 50th, and 75th percentiles, corresponding to features f_7, f_8, and f_9, respectively. (Reprinted from *Artificial Intelligence in Medicine*, 60, M. Zortea et al., Performance of a dermoscopy-based computer vision system for the diagnosis of pigmented skin lesions compared with visual evaluation by experienced dermatologists, 13–26, Copyright 2014, with permission from Elsevier.)

9.3.7 BORDERS: PERIPHERAL VERSUS CENTRAL (f_{13}, f_{14}, f_{15}, f_{16}, f_{17}, f_{18})

The lesion area is divided into the inner and the outer part separated by an internal border, indicated by the dashed lines in the two upper images of Figure 9.4. This border is found by iteratively shrinking the original border until the outer/inner regions contain 30%/70% of the original pixels,

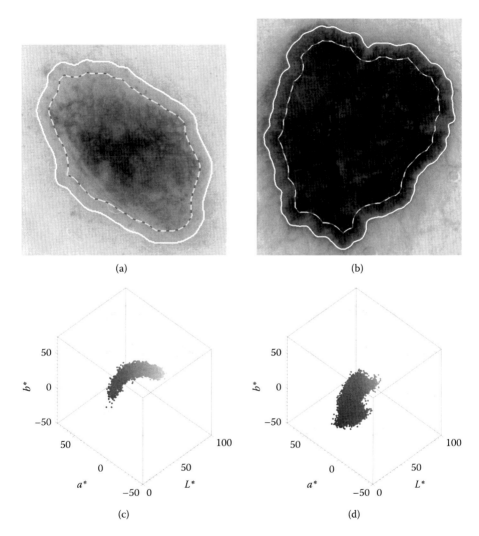

FIGURE 9.4 (See color insert.) (a) Benign. (b) Malignant. (c, d) 3D histograms of $L^{\star}a^{\star}b^{\star}$ color space components of top row. (Reprinted from *Artificial Intelligence in Medicine*, 60, M. Zortea et al., Performance of a dermoscopy-based computer vision system for the diagnosis of pigmented skin lesions compared with visual evaluation by experienced dermatologists, 13–26, Copyright 2014, with permission from Elsevier.)

respectively. We compute the mean value of the three $L^\star a^\star b^\star$ components in the inside and outside sets, and take the difference between them. These are the f_{13}, f_{14}, f_{15} features for the $L^\star a^\star b^\star$ channels. Similarly, we compute the probability density estimate of the samples of each $L^\star a^\star b^\star$ channel in the innermost and outermost parts of the regions. The density estimate is based on a Gaussian kernel function, using a window parameter (bandwidth) that is a function of the number of points in the regions [86]. For each channel, we compute the overlapping area of the densities. The resulting features for the $L^\star a^\star b^\star$ channels are referred to as f_{16}, f_{17}, f_{18}, respectively.

9.3.8   GEOMETRIC (f_{21}, f_{22}, f_{23})

We attempt to capture the lesion disorder by computing what we refer to as the number of lesion pieces resulting from applying binary thresholds to the grayscale version of the lesion. The thresholds are applied at the 25th, 50th, and 75th percentiles of the grayscale values of the skin lesion. To reduce noise, the number of pieces is computed after morphological opening using a disk element with a radius of five pixels that is applied to the binary masks obtained using each percentile. Figure 9.5 shows a benign and a malignant case, where the proposed scores are low and high, respectively.

9.3.9   TEXTURE OF THE LESION ($f_{24}, \ldots, f_{53}$)

Here we attempt to capture local spatial information in the skin lesions. We sample the segmented lesion using boxes of size 41×41 pixels that are displaced around the image in partially overlapping 20 pixels to reduce computational requirements. For each box, a feature vector containing spatial descriptors that consist of image textures is computed. We use textures in an attempt to discriminate between some of the anatomical structures that dermatologists consider (e.g., the D part of the ABCD rule corresponds

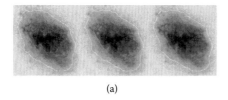 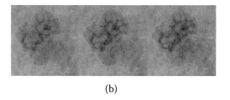

(a)   (b)

FIGURE 9.5   **(See color insert.)** (a, b) Example of geometric features corresponding to the number of "lesion pieces" obtained by applying binary thresholds to the lesion area (delineated by the white contour) at different grayscale percentiles. From left to right: 25th, 50th, and 75th percentiles. (Reprinted from *Artificial Intelligence in Medicine*, 60, M. Zortea et al., Performance of a dermoscopy-based computer vision system for the diagnosis of pigmented skin lesions compared with visual evaluation by experienced dermatologists, 13–26, Copyright 2014, with permission from Elsevier.)

to the presence of up to five structural features: network, structureless (or homogeneous) areas, branched streaks, dots, and globules). Texture should at a minimum be invariant to rotation and not very sensitive to acquisition issues. We focus on the use of uniform rotation-invariant local binary pattern (LBP) histograms proposed by Ojala et al. [72], computed from the grayscale version of the images. LBP is among the state-of-the-art methods for describing image textures, a powerful tool for rotation-invariant texture analysis and robust in terms of grayscale variations since the operator is, by definition, invariant against any monotonic transformation of the grayscale [72]. We compute LBP features using eight sampling points on a circle of radius 2 pixels (see [72] for additional details). This choice results in a 10-dimensional feature vector, corresponding to the occurrence histogram of unique uniform rotation-invariant binary patterns that can occur in the circularly symmetric neighbor set.

The retained feature scores for classification are the 25th, 50th, and 75th percentiles of each of the 10 texture images (an example is shown in Figure 9.6). Note that some of the maps appear to be spatially correlated, while others suggest good potential for discrimination. Despite the very similar colors of the two benign cases, some texture maps are very different. The presence of anatomical structures such as networks in the top and bottom cases are plausible reasons for the differences in the textures.

9.3.10 AREA AND DIAMETER (f_{54}, f_{55})

The area of the lesion is used as a feature. The same is the diameter, defined as the length of the major axis of the fitted ellipse. These two features are a bit questionable, since they might lead to misclassification of small melanomas.

9.3.11 COLOR VARIETY (f_{56})

Unsupervised cluster analysis tries to divide a data set into clusters (groups) without any previous knowledge about the characteristics of each cluster or the number of clusters. Estimating the number of clusters has shown to be a particularly difficult task [81]. Doing unsupervised cluster analysis in pixel values from a lesion would correspond to clustering the pixels according to color, without knowing which colors or even how many are present in the lesion. Mixture modeling combined with some estimator for the number of components [87] is a widely used method for unsupervised cluster analysis. We use the Gaussian mixture model (GMM), with parameters fitted by an expectation-maximization (EM) algorithm [88]. The Bayesian information criterion (BIC) [89] is used to estimate the correct number of components in the model. BIC consists of the negative log likelihood (a measure of how well the model fits the data) and a penalty term to avoid overfitting.

The number of components is the same as the number of clusters only if the clusters have Gaussian distribution, which cannot be assumed here. Even for a

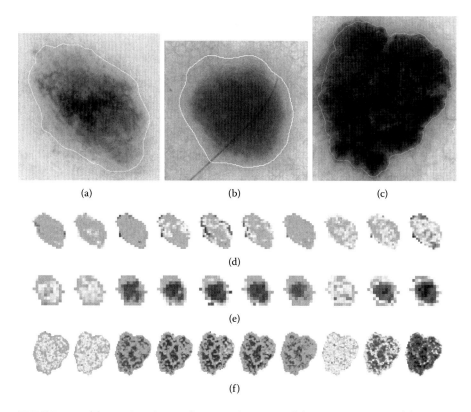

(a) (b) (c)

(d)

(e)

(f)

FIGURE 9.6 (See color insert.) Example images (a) Benign *not cut*; (b) Benign *cut*; (c) Malignant. The following rows (d–f) of artificially colored images are texture images derived using the LBP algorithm and correspond to the three top images (rows [d–f] with top [a–c] images). Blue and red correspond to lower and higher values of texture, respectively. Maps 1–9 from left to right were linearly scaled in the range {0–0.18}, whereas 10 is in {0–0.36}. This is kept fixed for the three sets shown above, so the values are therefore directly comparable by visual inspection. (Reprinted from *Artificial Intelligence in Medicine*, 60, M. Zortea et al., Performance of a dermoscopy-based computer vision system for the diagnosis of pigmented skin lesions compared with visual evaluation by experienced dermatologists, 13–26, Copyright 2014, with permission from Elsevier.)

lesion with few colors, as the one in Figure 9.6a, the BIC gives 7 components, while for the lesion in Figure 9.6c, BIC gives 15 components. The problem with using the number of components giving minimum BIC as a feature, even if it is related to the number of colors, is that fitting the GMM for several number of components takes a lot of time. For most lesions, the pixel values get a very bad fit (measured by BIC) for less than about five components. As seen in Figure 9.7, the BIC curve drops rapidly from $k = 1$ to $k = 5$, reaches the minimum, and slowly starts rising again.

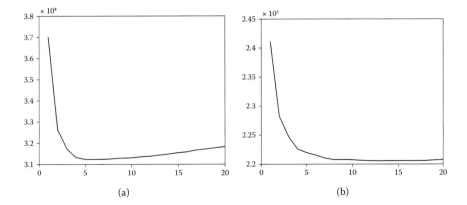

(a) (b)

FIGURE 9.7 The BIC value as a function of number of components in a fitted Gaussian mixture model, for (a) Figure 9.6a and (b) Figure 9.6c.

The BIC value in Figure 9.7a is much lower than that in Figure 9.7b. The feature of the presented algorithm is the BIC value for a 10-component GMM, fitted by an EM algorithm. If the lesion has few colors, then a 10-component GMM will result in a very good fit, but if the lesion has a great variety of colors, then the fit for a 10-component GMM is worse. By fixing the number of components, much time is saved when calculating the feature value. For additional time saving, the image is downsampled using coordinate-wise median binning with 7×7 pixel squares.

9.3.12 SPECIFIC COLOR DETECTION (f_{57}, f_{58}, f_{59})

Some colors are more frequent in melanomas than in benign lesions. This is particularly the blue–white veil [90], but also the red color should alarm the doctor. The CIE $L^\star a^\star b^\star$ color space can be transformed into its cylindrical counterpart $(L^\star, hue, chroma)$, where $hue = \arctan(a^\star, b^\star)$. Different angles represent different colors. The blue color lies in the lower quadrants, the whitish veil is found at very low positive angles with a magenta hue, while red is found approximately in the middle of the first positive quadrant. Red is a tricky color in this setting because it fades into orange, and brown and orange have the same hue, only different lightness. While blue and whitish can be distinguished only by hue, to differentiate red from brown, the lightness must be taken into consideration. The image is downsampled by 7×7 pixel coordinate-wise medians, and then a k-means clustering [81] with 20 clusters is performed. The 20 cluster centers then represent the 20 colors of that lesion. If the lesion is all brown, then the 20 colors will be 20 different brown hues.

Blue is defined as hue value of <0.10. Whitish is defined as hue values between 0.10 and 0.40. Red is defined as hue values between 0.40 and 0.60 in combination with $L^\star > hue \cdot 50 - 15$, where the $hue \cdot 50 - 15$ line was found empirically from the training data set. If $C_1, \ldots, C_K$ are the cluster centers with a specific color, and the upper hue value for that color is t_{hue}, then the amount of that color is calculated as $\sum_{k=1}^{K}(t_{hue} + 0.10) - C_k$. The value of a specific color feature is a function of how many cluster centers have that color and how distinct the hue is. The area covered by that color is not evaluated. The 0.10 is to ensure that even if a cluster center is very close to the hue threshold, the feature value is still significantly different from zero.

9.4 EARLY EXPERIMENT

We here briefly describe an early experiment in building and testing a CAD system based on the first 53 features described in Section 9.3. All details are found in [32]. The experiences from this experiment form the basis for further developments of a CAD system for lesion diagnoses.

9.4.1 IMAGE ACQUISITION AND DATA

Dermatoscopic images of 206 pigmented skin lesions were acquired using a portable dermatoscope (DermLite FOTO, 3Gen LLC, San Juan Capistrano, California) attached to a consumer-grade digital camera (Canon G10, Canon, Inc., Tokyo, Japan). Images were acquired at two locations: 113 images were obtained consecutively from all patients requiring biopsy or excision of a pigmented skin lesion because of diagnostic uncertainty. In addition, we added 93 images (60 images represented benign common lesions not requiring biopsy or excision and 33 images of melanomas). A total number of 206 lesion images was decided on because this number appeared realistic regarding the workloads of the three dermatologists participating in the evaluation of this study.

Printed images were given to three dermatologists familiar with dermatoscopy and who were not otherwise involved in the data collection. They were asked to provide, for each case, an indication regarding whether they would recommend excision of the skin lesion. In Table 9.1 the characteristics of the lesions used in the study are summarized. Notably, the Breslow depth is less than 1 mm in all cases except three, where a Breslow depth of <1 mm indicates early-stage melanoma. Pigmented Bowen's disease and basal cell carcinoma are examples of malignant nonmelanoma skin cancers.

The benign lesion class was split into two subclasses by a dermatologist (author T.R.S.), who was not involved in the accuracy assessment performed by the other three dermatologists. Based on the dermatoscopic images, out of the 169 benign lesions, 89 were labeled *not-cut* (i.e., representing a complete benign appearance) and 80 *cut* (i.e., displaying an equivocal appearance, where *cut* simply means recommending the lesion to be excised because malignancy cannot be ruled out). The low sensitivity scores achieved by two of the three dermatologists (shown in Section 9.4.3) suggest that the malignant class was very challenging.

TABLE 9.1

Histopathologic Findings for Lesions Used in the Study with Breslow Tumor Depths for Nodular and Superficial Spreading Melanomas

Benign/other[‡] lesions		**169**
	Melanocytic nevi	154
	Seborrheic keratoses	10
	Pigmented Bowen's disease[‡]	3
	Sarcoidal granuloma	1
	Basal cell carcinoma[‡]	1
Malignant melanoma		**37**
	Superficial spreading melanoma	13
	In situ melanoma	10
	Lentigo maligna	6
	Nodular melanoma	2
	Melanoma metastasis	2
	Undetermined	4
Breslow tumor depth	Median (mm)	0.61
	Interquartile range (mm)	0.33–0.825

Source: Reprinted from *Artificial Intelligence in Medicine*, 60, M. Zortea et al., Performance of a dermoscopy-based computer vision system for the diagnosis of pigmented skin lesions compared with visual evaluation by experienced dermatologists, 13–26, Copyright 2014, with permission from Elsevier.

[‡] Pigmented Bowen's disease and Basal cell carcinoma.

Figure 9.8a and b show examples of skin lesions where all three doctors agree and provide the correct excision recommendation according to the histopathological diagnosis. Figure 9.8c shows a case with agreement between the doctors, but with the incorrect diagnosis. The skin lesion is malignant, but all doctors diagnose it as benign and do not recommend excision. Two doctors label the benign lesion in Figure 9.8d as suspicious and recommend excision. One doctor concludes it is benign and that it should not be excised.

9.4.2 SETUP

Automatic segmentation was performed [46] on all images. Given the unfavorable ratio between the reduced number of training samples available, especially for the malignant class, and the dimensionality of the input feature vector, feature reduction was considered before training a statistical classifier. In particular, we focused on feature selection. For feature selection, a sequential forward selection algorithm was used [81]. The search depth (maximum number of features selected) was empirically set to 10 features in our application.

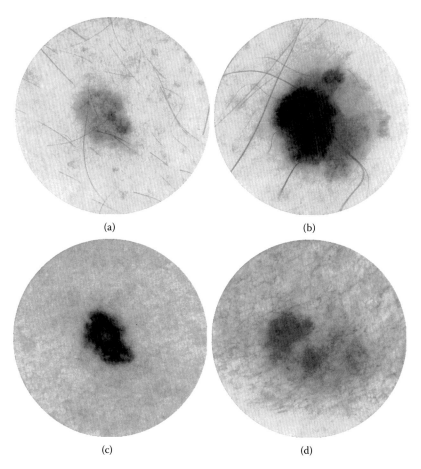

(a)   (b)

(c)   (d)

FIGURE 9.8 Examples of feedback from dermatologists, showing cases where all, none, and some of the three doctors give the correct recommendation. (a) Benign. All agree; *not cut*. (b) Malignant. All agree; *cut*. (c) Malignant. Mistake by all; *not cut*. (d) Benign. One *not cut*, two *cut*. (Reprinted from *Artificial Intelligence in Medicine*, 60, M. Zortea et al., Performance of a dermoscopy-based computer vision system for the diagnosis of pigmented skin lesions compared with visual evaluation by experienced dermatologists, 13–26, Copyright 2014, with permission from Elsevier.)

The optimization score for feature selection is the accuracy (average of sensitivity and specificity), as it balances both detected and missing lesions. The optimization score is computed on the training set using five fold cross-validation (CV). CV is used to reduce the risk of overfitting our simple models during the feature selection stage. After training, we choose the subset of features corresponding to the peak of CV accuracy as the best subset for statistical classification.

For statistical classification, two classical parametric approaches, the LDA and quadratic discriminant analysis (QDA) [82], are considered. The classification and regression tree algorithm (CART) [77] was also included in the analysis as an example of a nonparametric decision tree learning technique.

9.4.3 RESULTS

First, we consider the classification task of separating clearly benign *not cut* and malignant lesions. Out of the 37 malignant lesions available, 27 were randomly selected for training, and the remaining 10 were used for testing. The same number of 37 benign lesions (27 plus 10) was used for training and testing, respectively. Here, all the benign lesions were randomly sampled from the clearly benign subclass containing 89 lesions. Table 9.2 shows the classification scores, where each score is computed as the average result based on 20 realizations. Notice that the sensitivity and specificity outcomes of the doctors are divergent.

Secondly, we add atypical benign lesions that resemble melanomas to the test set, those lesions in the set labeled *cut*. Table 9.3 shows the classification scores after adding the benign *cut* lesions.

The reason for training the classifier using only clearly benign *not-cut* and malignant is illustrated in Figure 9.9. In short, given our proposed set of explanatory features, the statistical distributions of the subclass benign *cut* often seems to be closer to the malignant class than to the benign *not-cut*.

TABLE 9.2

Average Scores for a Test Set Including Clearly Benign (*not cut*) and Malignant Lesions in 20 Realizations

	SE	SP	AC	# Excisions
Doctor 1	85.0	57.5	71.3	12.8
Doctor 2	58.5	83.0	70.8	7.6
Doctor 3	44.5	95.0	69.8	5.0
LDA	80.5	83.5	82.0	9.7
QDA	86.0	73.0	79.5	11.3
CART	79.0	85.0	82.0	9.4

Source: Reprinted from *Artificial Intelligence in Medicine*, 60, M. Zortea et al., Performance of a dermoscopy-based computer vision system for the diagnosis of pigmented skin lesions compared with visual evaluation by experienced dermatologists, 13–26, Copyright 2014, with permission from Elsevier.

Note: Sensitivity (SE), specificity (SP), and accuracy (AC) scores are in percent. The average number of excisions is also included (ideally it should be 10 in this case). LDA, linear discriminant analysis; QDA, quadratic discriminant analysis; CART, decision tree.

TABLE 9.3

Average Scores for a Test Set Including Clearly Benign (*not cut*), Suspicious Benign (*cut*), and Malignant Lesions for 20 Realizations

	SE	SP	AC	# Excisions
Doctor 1	85.0	47.8	60.2	19.0
Doctor 2	58.5	72.5	67.8	11.4
Doctor 3	44.5	87.8	73.3	6.9
LDA	80.5	62.3	68.3	15.6
QDA	86.0	52.0	63.3	18.2
CART	79.0	63.0	68.3	15.3

Source: Reprinted from *Artificial Intelligence in Medicine*, 60, M. Zortea et al., Performance of a dermoscopy-based computer vision system for the diagnosis of pigmented skin lesions compared with visual evaluation by experienced dermatologists, 13–26, Copyright 2014, with permission from Elsevier.

Note: Sensitivity (SE), specificity (SP), and accuracy (AC) scores are in percent. The average number of excisions is also included (ideally it should be 10 in this case). LDA, linear discriminant analysis; QDA, quadratic discriminant analysis; CART, decision tree.

This is the main reason for our experimental choice, where the important subclass of difficult benign was not considered during the training phase, but only in the testing of the classifier.

Tables 9.2 and 9.3 also show the number of excisions for the test set containing 10 malignant cases in each random realization. Ideally, the 10 malignant lesions should be excised. Note that the addition of the difficult benign cases in the second experiment significantly increased the average number of excisions recommended by doctor 1 (from 12.8 to 19.0). The increment was slightly lower for the computer methods (from 11.3 to 18.2).

9.4.4 DISCUSSION

Figure 9.10 shows examples of scatter plots of features selected during the experiments. The plots suggest that in terms of feature values, the melanoma class is very hard to distinguish from the benign (both *not cut* and *cut*) class. By distinguishing instead between the *cut* (melanoma and benign *cut*) and the *not-cut*, well-separated classes become more feasible.

Different subsets of training lesions often lead to the selection of different combinations of features. Figure 9.11 shows how many times each feature was selected in the 20 realizations by LDA and QDA. Apart from feature 14, it is not easy to pick the most relevant features.

The goal of this study was to investigate feature extraction and classification in pigmented skin lesions. The data set contained all common types of nevi, including the most prevalent subclasses of melanoma. The findings

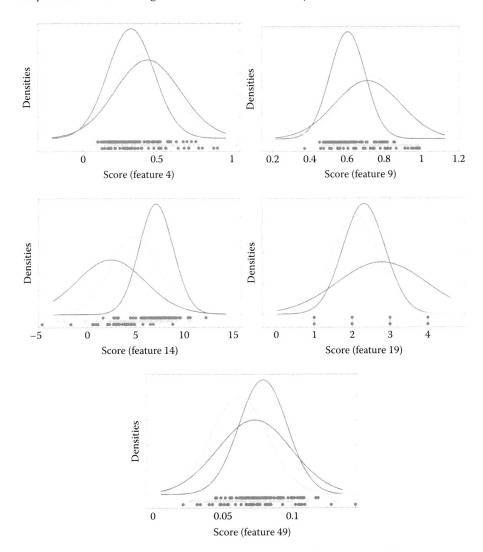

FIGURE 9.9 Examples of different feature scores. The colored dots mark feature scores connected to cases of benign *not cut* (dark gray, upper row), benign *cut* (light gray, middle row), and malignant (dark gray, lower row). The solid lines (dark gray, small variance; light gray; dark gray, large variance) are fitted Gaussian density estimates of the respective class of cases. (Reprinted from *Artificial Intelligence in Medicine*, 60, M. Zortea et al., Performance of a dermoscopy-based computer vision system for the diagnosis of pigmented skin lesions compared with visual evaluation by experienced dermatologists, 13–26, Copyright 2014, with permission from Elsevier.)

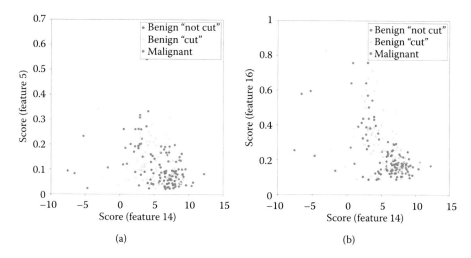

FIGURE 9.10 (**See color insert.**) Examples of the first two features selected by LDA (a) and CART (b). All 206 samples are shown for visualization purposes (but not for feature selection). (Reprinted from *Artificial Intelligence in Medicine*, 60, M. Zortea et al., Performance of a dermoscopy-based computer vision system for the diagnosis of pigmented skin lesions compared with visual evaluation by experienced dermatologists, 13–26, Copyright 2014, with permission from Elsevier.)

were evaluated on the basis of histopathology reports as the gold standard. In addition, we compared the results of the classifiers with the performance of three physicians practicing dermatology. The dermatologists made their assessments on the basis of dermatoscopic images only; that is, no clinical data were provided. This was done in order to evaluate how the doctors would assess the dermatoscopic features. In order to develop useful features and classifiers, we believe that the classifiers should be compared to doctors' assessment of dermatoscopic features in both simulated and real clinical environments. The proposed system performs as well as or better than dermatologists on both sensitivity and specificity when the only information available is the dermatoscopic image.

9.5 CAD SYSTEM FOR THE GP

Based on our experiences from the early study, a new version of the CAD system was developed and tested. One of the drawbacks of the first study was the limited number of images. Although we have a considerable database (about 3000 dermatoscopic images of excised lesions with histopathology), we only have 104 melanomas. The literature suggests that CAD systems are not significantly better than dermatologists. A CAD system mimicking a dermatologist is clearly not very valuable for a dermatologist, but could it be valuable for the GP?

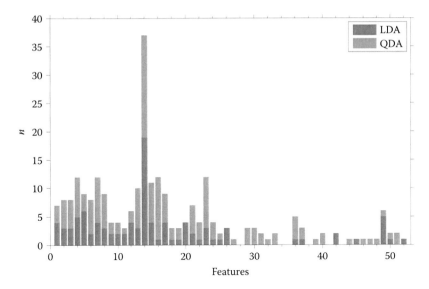

FIGURE 9.11 **(See color insert.)** Number of times (n) each feature was included in the set of selected features in the 20 random data sets. The numbers for the two classifiers are stacked. (Reprinted from *Artificial Intelligence in Medicine*, 60, M. Zortea et al., Performance of a dermoscopy-based computer vision system for the diagnosis of pigmented skin lesions compared with visual evaluation by experienced dermatologists, 13–26, Copyright 2014, with permission from Elsevier.)

Lindelof and Annehedblad [42] have investigated the ratio between melanoma and benign nevi for samples investigated by six different pathological laboratories in Stockholm, Sweden, in 2000 and 2005. The overall ratio is about 90 benign nevi per melanoma in 2000 and 58 in 2005. The ratio varies much between laboratories, where laboratories that receive samples from primary care have a higher ratio than those receiving samples from dermatology departments at the hospital. Even though the cost for excising a skin lesion at the dermatology department is higher (about two times higher), the cost per excised melanoma/dysplastic nevus is lower. With higher competence of primary care physicians, the excision rate of obviously benign lesions will decrease.

In Norway, 1718 new cases of melanoma were registered in 2011 [1]. There are 4289 GPs in Norway (serving a population of five million). On average, a GP will see a melanoma every $2\frac{1}{2}$ years, if we assume that all patients see their GP first. Even if the GPs can achieve higher competence, maintaining that competence will also require substantial effort. Lindelof and Annehedblad [42] point out that the extra burden that should be put on primary care physicians is limited.

With this in mind, we aim to construct a CAD system that can be a decision support for the GP, not for the dermatologist. The aim is not to outperform the dermatologist, but to give a second opinion as good as a dermatologist would give. This means that the focus is not on benign/malignant, but on *not cut/cut*. In addition, the interpretability of the outcome is valued.

9.5.1   IMAGE ACQUISITION, DATA, AND SEGMENTATION

The image acquisition equipment and the data source are the same as described in Section 9.4. We have included all 104 melanomas in the database. In addition, we have 941 unique benign lesions. The benign lesions are labeled *not-cut* or *cut* by the same dermatologist as in Section 9.4, with no additional information available. We then got 488 benign lesions in the *not-cut* class and 453 lesions in the *cut* class. As opposed to the first experiment, the *not cut* lesions were not handpicked. From the three subsets, 80% of the images are used for training and 20% are used for testing. The test set is the latest gathered images for each subset, to avoid that images used in the first study ended up in the test set in the follow-up study. The test images are kept totally independent from all steps in the development of the CAD system. Automatic segmentation was performed [46] on all images.

9.5.2   FEATURE SELECTION AND CHOICE OF CLASSIFIER

The high number of features (59) should be reduced for the sake of both interpretability and performance. To evaluate the stability of the feature selection methods, we chose to do a cross-validation study on the training sample. For 20 repetitions, the training sample was randomly partitioned into a training class and a test class, where the training class consisted of 80% of the images in each of the three subsets (*not-cut*, *cut*, melanoma). In the first study, described in Section 9.4.2, we used a sequential forward feature selector. With only 54 lesions in the training set, and 53 features, a backward selector could not be used (since the 54 lesions must be divided into a training set and a test set for feature selection). Here, we chose to use the backward selector.

As shown in Tables 9.2 and 9.3, the LDA classifier is not inferior to QDA and CART. Since LDA is simpler, and possibly more interpretable, we chose the LDA. An important parameter in the LDA classifier is the cost parameter α, as it weights the two types of misclassifications differently in the training phase (typically a *cut* lesion classified as *not cut* should have greater cost than a *not-cut* lesion classified as *cut*). The cost parameter directly controls the sensitivity–specificity balance. Based on previous experience [32], we set $\alpha = 2$, chosen to balance the sensitivity and specificity scores.

As seen in Figure 9.12, the wrapper is not as stable as we would hope for, considering the high number of images. The instability is probably caused by high correlation between the features. Several features are constructed as 25th, 50th, and 75th percentiles, and correlation is expected. All features are chosen at least once. Blindly eliminating those features that are chosen the fewest times is risky. The border features f_7, f_8, f_9 are all chosen in less than

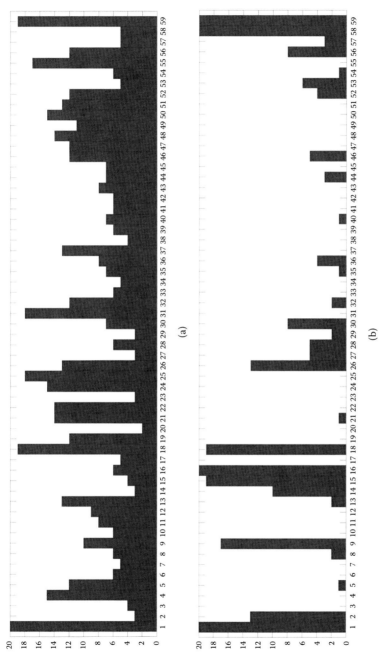

FIGURE 9.12 Feature selection for 20 cross-validations. (a) Sequential backward feature selection with LDA correct classification rate. (b) CFS filter.

half of the repetitions, but studying each repetition reveals that at least one of them is chosen every time.

The correlation-based feature selector (CFS) shows more stability, but leads to lower performance of the classifier. Notice how the two selectors totally disagree for many of the features.

Another aspect is how well the features meet the assumptions of an LDA classifier. Feature f_{58} (whitish veil) is chosen every time by CFS, but quite seldomly by SFS. For almost all lesions in the *not-cut* class, and most of the lesions in the *cut* class, the value of f_{58} is 0. It clearly does not resemble a Gaussian distribution, which is the distribution assumed by the LDA classifier. By identifying the features that have a similar behavior as f_{58} (small value for almost all lesions, but where high value appears only in the *cut* class), we can make a hybrid classifier as follows:

1. Identify the *cut*-specific features and set a threshold for each.
2. From the remaining features, select a subset for the LDA classifier.
3. A new lesion is classified as *cut* if either
   a. The LDA classifies it as *cut*.
   b. The LDA classifies it as *not-cut* with posterior probability below some predefined threshold and at least one of the *cut*-specific feature values exceeds its threshold.

Apart from improving the performance of the original LDA classifier, this hybrid model has the advantage that it provides easily interpretable feedback to the user. While the features in the LDA classifier interact with each other, the *cut*-specific features are evaluated one by one.

To find the *cut*-specific features, cross-validation was used on the training set. For the lesions in the *not-cut* class in the CV training set, the 2.5th upper percentile of the feature values was used as the threshold. If there were at least five times as many lesions from the *cut* class as from the *not-cut* class exceeding this threshold, the feature was considered a *cut*-specific feature. The chosen features were f_1 (asymmetry), f_8 (border), f_{13} (border), f_{16} (border), f_{23} (geometry), f_{54} (area), f_{56} (color variation), f_{57} (blue), f_{58} (whitish), and f_{59} (red). The f_{20} feature was also chosen, but removed since f_{57} classifies the same lesions as *cut*, in addition to some other *cut* lesions. The texture features f_{24}–f_{53} were not considered because of their lack of interpretability.

With the *cut*-specific features removed from the feature pool, a new attempt for automatic feature selection was made, using the correct rate of the hybrid classifier as criterion for the wrapper. By subjectively combining the results from the wrapper and the filter, we ended up with the features f_2, f_4, f_9, f_{11}, f_{14}, f_{18}, f_{21}, f_{22}, f_{24}, f_{25}, f_{30}, f_{31}, f_{32}, f_{37}, f_{39}, f_{46}, f_{48}, f_{53}, and f_{55}.

With the feature selection done, the whole training set was used to calculate the thresholds for the *cut*-specific features, and train the LDA classifier. The limit for the posterior probability was heuristically set to 90%. This means that if there is at least a 10% posterior probability of this lesion coming from the *cut* class, then it will be classified as *cut* if at least one *cut*-specific feature exceeds its threshold.

9.5.3 RESULTS

The test set consisted of 98 benign nonsuspicious lesions, 91 benign suspicious lesions, and 21 melanomas. Among the melanomas, the dermatologist classified 5 as nonsuspicious and 15 as suspicious, while 1 lesion was undecidable because the image was out of focus. All 21 melanomas were included in the test set.

For the sensitivity and specificity score, the *not-cut* class consists of the 98 nonsuspicious lesions, while the *cut* class consists of the 91 benign suspicious lesions and the 21 melanomas. The red curve in Figure 9.13 shows the receiver operating characteristic (ROC) curve with varying cost parameter α. The best correct rate with sensitivity higher than specificity is 81% (sensitivity 83% and specificity 80%).

The blue curve in Figure 9.13 shows the number of excised melanomas as a function of excised lesions, varying with α. The black square marks the position of the dermatologist, assuming that he would excise the undecidable lesion (cutting 107 lesions, among them 16 melanomas). If the CAD system cuts only 16 melanomas (as the dermatologist did), then the total number of excised lesions is 91. If the CAD system excises a total number of 107 lesions

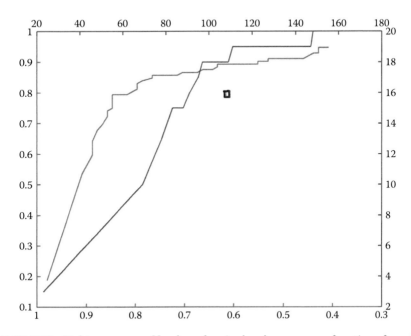

FIGURE 9.13 Light gray curve: Number of excised melanomas as a function of number of excised lesions. Dark gray curve: Sensitivity and specificity.

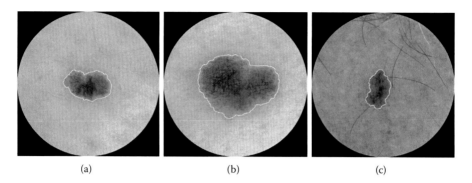

(a)   (b)   (c)

FIGURE 9.14   (a–c) Melanomas falsely classified as *not-cut*.

(as the dermatologist did), then the number of excised melanomas is 18. In that sense, the·CAD system has a better rate for excised lesions per melanoma than the dermatologist.

Figure 9.14 shows the three melanomas that would not be excised, if the maximum number of excisions would be 107. They are all in situ melanoma and (c) is a lentigo maligna. By the decision of the dermatologist, only melanoma (b) would have been excised.

9.5.4   DISCUSSION

When comparing the ratio of excised lesions per melanoma, the CAD system performs better than the dermatologist. Cross-validation studies on the training set gave a standard deviation of 1.4 for the number of excised melanomas and a standard deviation of 6.1 for the number of excised lesions. For the dermatologist, the standard deviation was 2.3 for the number of excised melanomas. (Standard deviation for the number of excised lesions could not be evaluated for the dermatologist, as this was used as the ground truth.) Even if the CAD system performs better than the dermatologist on this specific test set, we cannot conclude that it is better in general. For a better understanding of how the CAD system works compared to dermatologists, the opinion of more than one dermatologist would have been needed. The heavy workload of giving an opinion on more than 1000 images prevented us from including more dermatologists in the study.

The sensitivity and specificity scores presented in Section 9.5.3 are based on the opinion of one dermatologist and the histopathology reports as the gold standard. Another dermatologist's opinion would have led to a different gold standard, so the scores must be read with great care. The reason for including them is that we want the CAD system to be comparable to a dermatologist's opinion also for the benign lesions that are excised.

The only exclusion criterion used on the images in the data set is duplicates of lesions. Among the images we have nonmelanocytic lesions, lesions occluded

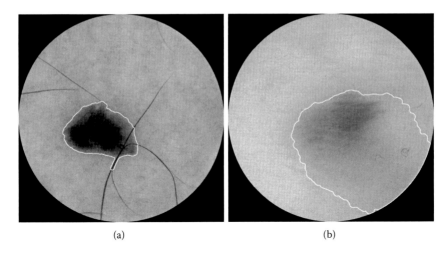

(a)   (b)

FIGURE 9.15 Inadequate segmentation. (a) Lesion occluded by hair. (b) Lesion situated in palm.

by hair, and lesions where the segmentation fails. Figure 9.15a shows a benign lesion in the *not-cut* class from the test set. It is classified as *not-cut* by the LDA classifier, with a posterior probability of 89%. Because of the bad segmentation, caused by the hair in the lower part, it gets a high score on the *cut*-specific asymmetry feature, and the class is changed to *cut*. Figure 9.15b shows another benign lesion in the *not-cut* class from the test set, where the segmentation seems to be inadequate.

9.6   CONCLUSIONS

In a study with an independent test set and no exclusion criteria except for duplicates, we have shown that the presented CAD system is able to perform comparably to the dermatologist in the sense of excised lesions per melanoma ratio. The data set suffers from consisting of only excised lesions. In a clinical setting, the decision of excising a lesion is based on more than just the dermatoscopic image. Indeed, all the lesions in our data set have been excised, even though roughly half of them were considered nonsuspicious by the dermatologist based solely on the dermatoscopic image. The extra information leading to excision can be relevant for diagnosis, such as knowing that the lesion has changed recently, but it can also be based on the patient's concerns or even aesthetic. A complete CAD system should include this kind of information, but this information has not been available for the study.

The presented CAD system does not differ from CAD systems presented earlier in the literature when it comes to the performance being comparable to an expert opinion. The novelty lies in the attempt to make a CAD system for the GPs, with a focus on interpretable features and the classification process, without having inferior performance. This seems like a reasonable turn to take in the CAD-system-for-skin-lesions field, as long as near-to-100% sensitivity (combined with reasonable specificity) is out of reach. By showing that interpretability of the CAD system can be combined with high performance, it gives justification to spend more effort on developing stable and interpretable features, even if they do not lead to improved performance. For the features used in the present CAD system, there is room for improvement. The texture features do not have a very obvious interpretation that can be linked directly to patterns in the lesion. Stability of the feature values should be verified by the use of duplicate images. Interpretability must ultimately be verified by the user of the CAD system.

Although there is room for improvements, we believe that the CAD system as presented here can be a valuable decision support tool for the GP, but a clinical trial is needed.

9.6.1 CLINICAL TRIAL

The CAD system described here has been named *Nevus Doctor* and is part of a planned pilot study for a clinical trial. In addition to the dermatoscopic image, the user will also be asked some questions regarding the patient. The pilot study will investigate if *Nevus Doctor* is suited as decision support tool in Norwegian GP offices, and how it can be adjusted and improved based on feedback from users.

ACKNOWLEDGMENT

We are indebted to Dr. Herbert Kirchesch, who generously helped us to collect dermatoscopic images for this study.

REFERENCES

1. I. Larsen, T. Grimsrud, T. Johannesen, A. Johansen, H. Langseth, S. Larnningen, J. Martinsen et al., Cancer in Norway 2010: Cancer incidence, mortality, survival and prevalence in Norway, tech. rep., Cancer Registry of Norway, Oslo, Norway, 2012.
2. C. Holterhues, E. de Vries, M. W. Louwman, S. Koljenović, and T. Nijsten, Incidence and trends of cutaneous malignancies in the Netherlands, 1989–2005, *Journal of Investigative Dermatology*, vol. 130, no. 7, pp. 1807–1812, 2010.
3. C. Garbe and U. Leiter, Melanoma epidemiology and trends, *Clinics in Dermatology*, vol. 27, no. 1, pp. 3–9, 2009.
4. G. Massi and P. E. LeBoit, *Histological Diagnosis of Nevi and Melanoma*, Springer, Berlin, 2004.
5. D. S. Rigel, J. K. Robinson, M. I. Ross, R. Friedman, C. J. Cockerell, H. Lim, and E. Stockfleth, *Cancer of the Skin*, 2nd ed., Saunders, Philadelphia, PA, 2011.
6. B. A. Solky, M. C. Mihm, H. Tsao, and A. J. Sober, 15 factors influencing survival in melanoma patients, *Cancer of the Skin*, vol. 1, p. 189, 2005.

7. C. M. Balch, J. E. Gershenwald, S.-J. Soong, J. F. Thompson, M. B. Atkins, D. R. Byrd, A. C. Buzaid et al., Final version of 2009 AJCC melanoma staging and classification, *Journal of Clinical Oncology*, vol. 27, no. 36, pp. 6199–6206, 2009.

8. Australian Cancer Network Melanoma Guidelines Revision Working Party. Clinical practice guidelines for the management of melanoma in Australia and New Zealand. The Cancer Council Australia and Australian Cancer Network, Sydney and New Zealand Guidelines Group, Wellington, New Zealand, 2008.

9. H. Kittler, H. Pehamberger, K. Wolff, and M. Binder, Diagnostic accuracy of dermoscopy, *Lancet Oncology*, vol. 3, no. 3, pp. 159–165, 2002.

10. M. Vestergaard, P. Macaskill, P. Holt, and S. Menzies, Dermoscopy compared with naked eye examination for the diagnosis of primary melanoma: a meta-analysis of studies performed in a clinical setting, *British Journal of Dermatology*, vol. 159, no. 3, pp. 669–676, 2008.

11. W. Stolz, O. Braun-Falco, P. Bilek, M. Landthaler, W. H. C. Burgdorf, and A. B. Cognetta, *Color Atlas of Dermatoscopy*, 2nd ed., Blackwell Publishing, Berlin, Germany, 2002.

12. M. Binder, M. Schwarz, A. Winkler, A. Steiner, A. Kaider, K. Wolff, and H. Pehamberger, Epiluminescence microscopy: a useful tool for the diagnosis of pigmented skin lesions for formally trained dermatologists, *Archives of Dermatology*, vol. 131, no. 3, p. 286, 1995.

13. C. Rosendahl, G. Williams, D. Eley, T. Wilson, G. Canning, J. Keir, I. McColl, and D. Wilkinson, The impact of subspecialization and dermatoscopy use on accuracy of melanoma diagnosis among primary care doctors in Australia, *Journal of the American Academy of Dermatology*, vol. 67, no. 5, pp. 846–852, 2012.

14. D. Wilkinson, D. A. Askew, and A. Dixon, Skin cancer clinics in Australia: workload profile and performance indicators from an analysis of billing data, *Medical Journal of Australia*, vol. 184, no. 4, p. 162, 2006.

15. G. Argenziano, H. P. Soyer, S. Chimenti, R. Talamini, R. Corona, F. Sera, M. Binder et al., Dermoscopy of pigmented skin lesions: results of a consensus meeting via the Internet, *Journal of the American Academy of Dermatology*, vol. 48, no. 5, pp. 679–693, 2003.

16. H. Pehamberger, A. Steiner, and K. Wolff, In vivo epiluminescence microscopy of pigmented skin lesions. I. Pattern analysis of pigmented skin lesions, *Journal of the American Academy of Dermatology*, vol. 17, no. 4, pp. 571–583, 1987.

17. F. Nachbar, W. Stolz, T. Merkle, A. B. Cognetta, T. Vogt, M. Landthaler, P. Bilek, O. Braun-Falco, and G. Plewig, The ABCD rule of dermatoscopy: high prospective value in the diagnosis of doubtful melanocytic skin lesions, *Journal of the American Academy of Dermatology*, vol. 30, no. 4, pp. 551–559, 1994.

18. S. Menzies, C. Ingvar, and W. McCarthy, A sensitivity and specificity analysis of the surface microscopy features of invasive melanoma, *Melanoma Research*, vol. 6, no. 1, pp. 55–62, 1996.

19. G. Argenziano, G. Fabbrocini, P. Carli, V. De Giorgi, E. Sammarco, and M. Delfino, Epiluminescence microscopy for the diagnosis of doubtful melanocytic skin lesions: comparison of the ABCD rule of dermatoscopy and a new 7-point checklist based on pattern analysis, *Archives of Dermatology*, vol. 134, no. 12, pp. 1563–1570, 1998.

20. H. P. Soyer, G. Argenziano, I. Zalaudek, R. Corona, F. Sera, R. Talamini, F. Barbato et al., Three-point checklist of dermoscopy, *Dermatology*, vol. 208, no. 1, pp. 27–31, 2004.

21. C. Rosendahl, A. Cameron, I. McColl, and D. Wilkinson, Dermatoscopy in routine practice: "chaos and clues," *Australian Family Physician*, vol. 41, no. 7, p. 482, 2012.

22. P. Bourne, C. Rosendahl, J. Keir, and A. Cameron, BLINCK: a diagnostic algorithm for skin cancer diagnosis combining clinical features with dermatoscopy findings, *Dermatology Practical and Conceptual*, vol. 2, no. 2, 2012.

23. M. van Rijsingen, S. Hanssen, J. Groenewoud, G. van der Wilt, and M. Gerritsen, Referrals by general practitioners for suspicious skin lesions: the urgency of training, *Acta Dermato-Venereologica*, 2013.

24. A. Scope, S. W. Dusza, A. C. Halpern, H. Rabinovitz, R. P. Braun, I. Zalaudek, G. Argenziano, and A. A. Marghoob, The ugly duckling sign: agreement between observers, *Archives of Dermatology*, vol. 144, no. 1, pp. 58–64, 2008.

25. R. J. Friedman, D. S. Rigel, and A. W. Kopf, Early detection of malignant melanoma: the role of physician examination and self-examination of the skin, *CA: A Cancer Journal for Clinicians*, vol. 35, no. 3, pp. 130–151, 1985.

26. F. Brehmer, M. Ulrich, and H. A. Haenssle, Strategies for early recognition of cutaneous melanoma: present and future, *Dermatology Practical and Conceptual*, vol. 2, no. 3, 2012.

27. N. R. Abbasi, M. Yancovitz, D. Gutkowicz-Krusin, K. S. Panageas, M. C. Mihm, P. Googe, R. King et al., Utility of lesion diameter in the clinical diagnosis of cutaneous melanoma, *Archives of Dermatology*, vol. 144, no. 4, pp. 469–474, 2008.

28. P. Cyr, Atypical moles, *American Family Physician*, vol. 78, no. 6, p. 735, 2008.

29. M. Inskip, J. Magee, D. Weedon, and C. Rosendahl, When algorithms falter: a case report of a very small melanoma excised due to the dermatoscopic "ugly duckling" sign, *Dermatology Practical and Conceptual*, vol. 3, no. 2, p. 59, 2013.

30. M. D. Corbo and J. Wismer, Agreement between dermatologists and primary care practitioners in the diagnosis of malignant melanoma: review of the literature, *Journal of Cutaneous Medicine and Surgery*, vol. 16, no. 5, pp. 306–310, 2011.

31. C. Dolianitis, J. Kelly, R. Wolfe, and P. Simpson, Comparative performance of 4 dermoscopic algorithms by nonexperts for the diagnosis of melanocytic lesions, *Archives of Dermatology*, vol. 141, no. 8, pp. 1008–1014, 2005.

32. M. Zortea, T. R. Schopf, K. Thon, M. Geilhufe, K. Hindberg, H. Kirchesch, K. Møllersen, J. Schulz, S. O. Skrøvseth, and F. Godtliebsen, Performance of a dermoscopy-based computer vision system for the diagnosis of pigmented skin lesions compared with visual evaluation by experienced dermatologists, *Artificial Intelligence in Medicine*, vol. 60, no. 1, pp. 13–26, 2014.

33. K. Korotkov and R. Garcia, Computerized analysis of pigmented skin lesions: a review, *Artificial Intelligence in Medicine*, vol. 56, no. 2, pp. 69–90, 2012.

34. B. Rosado, S. Menzies, A. Harbauer, H. Pehamberger, K. Wolff, M. Binder, and H. Kittler, Accuracy of computer diagnosis of melanoma: a quantitative meta-analysis, *Archives of Dermatology*, vol. 139, no. 3, pp. 361–367, 2003.

35. G. Day and R. Barbour, Automated skin lesion screening: a new approach, *Melanoma Research*, vol. 11, no. 1, pp. 31–35, 2001.

36. J. L. G. Arroyo and B. G. Zapirain, Automated detection of melanoma in dermoscopic images, in *Computer Vision Techniques for the Diagnosis of Skin Cancer* (J. Scharcanski and M. E. Celebi, eds.), pp. 139–192, Springer, Berlin, 2013.

37. G. Fabbrocini, V. D. Vita, S. Cacciapuoti, G. D. Leo, C. Liguori, A. Paolillo, A. Pietrosanto, and P. Sommella, Automatic diagnosis of melanoma based on the 7-point checklist, in *Computer Vision Techniques for the Diagnosis of Skin Cancer* (J. Scharcanski and M. E. Celebi, eds.), pp. 71–107, Springer, Berlin, Germany, 2013.

38. A. Gewirtzman and R. Braun, Computerized digital dermoscopy, *Journal of Cosmetic Dermatology*, vol. 2, no. 1, pp. 14–20, 2003.

39. A. Baldi, R. Murace, E. Dragonetti, M. Manganaro, O. Guerra, S. Bizzi, and L. Galli, Definition of an automated content-based image retrieval (CBIR) system for the comparison of dermoscopic images of pigmented skin lesions, *Biomedical Engineering Online*, vol. 8, pp. 1–10, 2009.

40. A. Perrinaud, O. Gaide, L. French, J. Saurat, A. Marghoob, and R. Braun, Can automated dermoscopy image analysis instruments provide added benefit for the dermatologist? A study comparing the results of three systems, *British Journal of Dermatology*, vol. 157, no. 5, pp. 926–933, 2007.

41. A. Tenenhaus, A. Nkengne, J. Horn, C. Serruys, A. Giron, and B. Fertil, Detection of melanoma from dermoscopic images of naevi acquired under uncontrolled conditions, *Skin Research and Technology*, vol. 16, no. 1, pp. 85–97, 2010.

42. B. Lindelof and M. Annehedblad, Ratt kompetens vid diagnostik ger lagre kostnader, *Lakartidningen*, vol. 105, no. 39, pp. 2666–2669, 2008.

43. M. E. Celebi, H. A. Kingravi, B. Uddin, H. Iyatomi, Y. A. Aslandogan, W. V. Stoecker, and R. H. Moss, A methodological approach to the classification of dermoscopy images, *Computerized Medical Imaging and Graphics*, vol. 31, no. 6, pp. 362–373, 2007.

44. M. E. Vestergaard and S. W. Menzies, Automated diagnostic instruments for cutaneous melanoma, in *Seminars in Cutaneous Medicine and Surgery*, vol. 27, pp. 32–36, Elsevier, 2008.

45. R. Melli, C. Grana, and R. Cucchiara, Comparison of color clustering algorithms for segmentation of dermatological images, in *SPIE Medical Imaging: Image Processing*, vol. 6144, San Diego, CA, 2006.

46. M. Zortea, S. O. Skrøvseth, T. R. Schopf, H. M. Kirchesch, and F. Godtliebsen, Automatic segmentation of dermoscopic images by iterative classification, *Journal of Biomedical Imaging*, vol. 2011, pp. 1–19, 2011.

47. T. Lee, V. Ng, R. Gallagher, A. Coldman, and D. McLean, Dullrazor®: a software approach to hair removal from images, *Computers in Biology and Medicine*, vol. 27, no. 6, pp. 533–543, 1997.

48. K. Thon, H. Rue, S. O. Skrøvseth, and F. Godtliebsen, Bayesian multiscale analysis of images modeled as Gaussian Markov random fields, *Computational Statistics and Data Analysis*, vol. 56, no. 1, pp. 49–61, 2012.

49. K. Møllersen, H. M. Kirchesch, T. G. Schopf, and F. Godtliebsen, Unsupervised segmentation for digital dermoscopic images, *Skin Research and Technology*, vol. 16, no. 4, pp. 401–407, 2010.

50. Q. Abbas, I. F. Garcia, M. E. Celebi, and W. Ahmad, A feature-preserving hair removal algorithm for dermoscopy images, *Skin Research and Technology*, vol. 19, pp. e27–e36, 2013.

51. M. E. Celebi, H. Iyatomi, G. Schaefer, and W. Stoecker, Lesion border detection in dermoscopy images, *Computerized Medical Imaging and Graphics*, vol. 33, no. 2, pp. 148–153, 2009.

52. M. Silveira, J. Nascimento, J. Marques, A. Marcal, T. Mendonca, S. Yamauchi, J. Maeda, and J. Rozeira, Comparison of segmentation methods for melanoma diagnosis in dermoscopy images, *IEEE Journal of Selected Topics in Signal Processing*, vol. 3, no. 1, pp. 35–45, 2009.

53. C. Grana, G. Pellacani, R. Cucchiara, and S. Seidenari, A new algorithm for border description of polarized light surface microscopic images of pigmented skin lesions, *IEEE Transactions on Medical Imaging*, vol. 22, no. 8, pp. 959–964, 2003.

54. D. Gomez, C. Butakoff, B. Ersboll, and W. Stoecker, Independent histogram pursuit for segmentation of skin lesions, *IEEE Transactions on Biomedical Engineering*, vol. 55, no. 1, pp. 157–161, 2008.

55. R. Garnavi, M. Aldeen, M. E. Celebi, G. Varigos, and S. Finch, Border detection in dermoscopy images using hybrid thresholding on optimized color channels, *Computerized Medical Imaging and Graphics*, vol. 35, no. 2, pp. 105–115, 2011.

56. H. Iyatomi, H. Oka, M. Saito, A. Miyake, M. Kimoto, J. Yamagami, S. Kobayashi et al., Quantitative assessment of tumour extraction from dermoscopy images and evaluation of computer-based extraction methods for an automatic melanoma diagnostic system, *Melanoma Research*, vol. 16, no. 2, p. 183, 2006.

57. M. E. Celebi, H. Kingravi, H. Iyatomi, Y. Aslandogan, W. Stoecker, R. Moss, J. Malters et al., Border detection in dermoscopy images using statistical region merging, *Skin Research and Technology*, vol. 14, no. 3, pp. 347–353, 2008.

58. M. E. Celebi, Y. Alp Aslandogan, W. V. Stoecker, H. Iyatomi, H. Oka, and X. Chen, Unsupervised border detection in dermoscopy images, *Skin Research and Technology*, vol. 13, no. 4, pp. 454–462, 2007.

59. H. Iyatomi, H. Oka, M. E. Celebi, M. Hashimoto, M. Hagiwara, M. Tanaka, and K. Ogawa, An improved Internet-based melanoma screening system with dermatologist-like tumor area extraction algorithm, *Computerized Medical Imaging and Graphics*, vol. 32, no. 7, pp. 566–579, 2008.

60. P. Schmid, Segmentation of digitized dermatoscopic images by two-dimensional color clustering, *IEEE Transactions on Medical Imaging*, vol. 18, no. 2, pp. 164–171, 1999.

61. T. Lee, M. Atkins, M. King, S. Lau, and D. McLean, Counting moles automatically from back images, *IEEE Transactions on Biomedical Engineering*, vol. 52, no. 11, pp. 1966–1969, 2005.

62. H. Zhou, G. Schaefer, A. H. Sadka, and M. E. Celebi, Anisotropic mean shift based fuzzy c-means segmentation of dermoscopy images, *IEEE Journal of Selected Topics in Signal Processing*, vol. 3, no. 1, pp. 26–34, 2009.

63. B. Erkol, R. Moss, R. Joe Stanley, W. Stoecker, and E. Hvatum, Automatic lesion boundary detection in dermoscopy images using gradient vector flow snakes, *Skin Research and Technology*, vol. 11, no. 1, pp. 17–26, 2005.

64. H. Zhou, X. Li, G. Schaefer, M. E. Celebi, and P. Miller, Mean shift based gradient vector flow for image segmentation, *Computer Vision and Image Understanding*, vol. 117, no. 9, pp. 1004–1016, 2013.

65. H. Ganster, A. Pinz, R. Rohrer, E. Wildling, M. Binder, and H. Kittler, Automated melanoma recognition, *IEEE Transactions on Medical Imaging*, vol. 20, no. 3, pp. 233–239, 2001.

66. M. E. Celebi, Q. Wen, S. Hwang, H. Iyatomi, and G. Schaefer, Lesion border detection in dermoscopy images using ensembles of thresholding methods, *Skin Research Technology*, vol. 19, no. 1, pp. e252–e258, 2013.

67. H. Castillejos, V. Ponomaryov, L. Nino-de Rivera, and V. Golikov, Wavelet transform fuzzy algorithms for dermoscopic image segmentation, *Computational and Mathematical Methods in Medicine*, vol. 2012, 2012.

68. A. R. Sadri, M. Zekri, S. Sadri, N. Gheissari, M. Mokhtari, and F. Kolahdouzan, Segmentation of dermoscopy images using wavelet networks, *IEEE Transactions on Biomedical Engineering*, vol. 60, no. 4, pp. 1134–1141, 2013.

69. H. Wang, R. H. Moss, X. Chen, R. J. Stanley, W. V. Stoecker, M. E. Celebi, J. M. Malters et al., Modified watershed technique and post-processing for segmentation of skin lesions in dermoscopy images, *Computerized Medical Imaging and Graphics*, vol. 35, no. 2, pp. 116–120, 2011.

70. P. Wighton, M. Sadeghi, T. K. Lee, and M. S. Atkins, A fully automatic random walker segmentation for skin lesions in a supervised setting, in *Medical Image Computing and Computer-Assisted Intervention: MICCAI 2009* (G.-Z. Yang, D. Hawkes, D. Rueckert, A. Noble, and C. Taylor, eds.), vol. 5762 of *Lecture Notes in Computer Science*, pp. 1108–1115, Springer, Berlin, 2009.

71. R. Garnavi, M. Aldeen, and M. E. Celebi, Weighted performance index for objective evaluation of border detection methods in dermoscopy images, *Skin Research and Technology*, vol. 17, no. 1, pp. 35–44, 2011.

72. T. Ojala, M. Pietikäinen, and T. Mäenpää, Multiresolution gray-scale and rotation invariant texture classification with local binary patterns, *IEEE Transactions on Pattern Analysis and Machine Intelligence*, vol. 24, no. 7, pp. 971–987, 2002.

73. L. T. Maloney and J. A. Schirillo, Color constancy, lightness constancy, and the articulation hypothesis, *Perception*, vol. 31, pp. 135–139, 2002.

74. E. Carter, Y. Ohno, M. Pointer, A. Robertson, R. Seve, J. Schanda, and K. Witt, Colorimetry: publication 15, tech. rep., CIE Central Bureau, Vienna, Austria, 2004.

75. Y. Chang, R. J. Stanley, R. H. Moss, and W. Van Stoecker, A systematic heuristic approach for feature selection for melanoma discrimination using clinical images, *Skin Research and Technology*, vol. 11, no. 3, pp. 165–178, 2005.

76. M. A. Hall, Correlation-based feature selection for machine learning, PhD thesis, University of Waikato, 1999.

77. L. Breiman, J. Friedman, C. Stone, and R. Olshen, *Classification and Regression Trees*, Chapman & Hall/CRC, Boca Raton, FL, 1984.

78. J. Kittler, Feature search algorithms, *Pattern Recognition and Signal Processing*, pp. 41–60, 1978.

79. K. Fukunaga, *Introduction to Statistical Pattern Recognition*, Academic Press, San Diego, CA, 1990.

80. J. Frühauf, B. Leinweber, R. Fink-Puches, V. Ahlgrimm-Siess, E. Richtig, I. Wolf, A. Niederkorn, F. Quehenberger, and R. Hofmann-Wellenhof, Patient acceptance and diagnostic utility of automated digital image analysis of pigmented skin lesions, *Journal of the European Academy of Dermatology and Venereology*, vol. 26, no. 3, pp. 368–372, 2012.

81. T. Hastie, R. Tibshirani, and J. Friedman, *The Elements of Statistical Learning: Data Mining, Inference, and Prediction*, 2nd ed., Springer, New York, 2009.

82. R. Johnson and D. Wichern, *Applied Multivariate Statistical Analysis*, vol. 4, Prentice Hall, Englewood Cliffs, NJ, 1992.

83. S. Seidenari, G. Pellacani, and C. Grana, Computer description of colours in dermoscopic melanocytic lesion images reproducing clinical assessment, *British Journal of Dermatology*, vol. 149, no. 3, pp. 523–529, 2003.

84. G. Pellacani, C. Grana, and S. Seidenari, Automated description of colours in polarized-light surface microscopy images of melanocytic lesions, *Melanoma Research*, vol. 14, no. 2, pp. 125–130, 2004.

85. M. Wand and M. Jones, *Kernel Smoothing*, Chapman & Hall/CRC, Boca Raton, FL, 1995.

86. A. Bowman and A. Azzalini, *Applied Smoothing Techniques for Data Analysis: The Kernel Approach with S-Plus Illustrations*, Oxford University Press, New York, 1997.

87. G. McLachlan and D. Peel, *Finite Mixture Models*, Wiley Series in Probability and Statistics, John Wiley and Sons, New York, 2000.

88. A. P. Dempster, N. M. Laird, and D. B. Rubin, Maximum likelihood from incomplete data via the EM algorithm, *Journal of the Royal Statistical Society: Series B (Methodological)*, vol. 39, no. 1, pp. 1–38, 1977.

89. G. Schwarz, Estimating the dimension of a model, *Annals of Statistics*, vol. 6, no. 2, pp. 461–464, 1978.

90. M. E. Celebi, H. Iyatomi, W. V. Stoecker, R. H. Moss, H. S. Rabinovitz, G. Argenziano, and H. P. Soyer, Automatic detection of blue-white veil and related structures in dermoscopy images, *Computerized Medical Imaging and Graphics*, vol. 32, no. 8, pp. 670–677, 2008.

10 Accurate and Scalable System for Automatic Detection of Malignant Melanoma

Mani Abedini
IBM Research Australia
Melbourne, Australia

Qiang Chen
IBM Research Australia
Melbourne, Australia

Noel C. F. Codella
IBM T. J. Watson Research Center
Yorktown Heights, New York

Rahil Garnavi
IBM Research Australia
Melbourne, Australia

Xingzhi Sun
IBM Research Australia
Melbourne, Australia

CONTENTS

10.1 INTRODUCTION

Malignant melanoma is the deadliest form of skin cancer; it makes up only 2.3% of all skin cancers, yet is responsible for 75% of skin cancer deaths. The American Cancer Society reported 76,100 new cases of melanoma in the United States in 2013, with 9710 melanoma deaths, maintaining an increasing trend over the last decades [1]. In Australia, melanoma is the most common cancer in people aged 15–44 years. It represents 10% of all cancers and its per-capita incidence is four times higher than in Canada, the UK, and the United States, with more than 10,000 cases diagnosed and around 1250 deaths annually [2]. The worldwide steady increase in incidence of melanoma in recent years [3], its high mortality rate, and the massive respective medical cost have made its early diagnosis a continuing priority of public health.

Early diagnosis of melanoma is particularly important for two reasons [4–6]: First, the prognosis of melanoma patients depends highly on tumor thickness. If melanoma is detected at an early stage, when the tumor thickness is less than 1 mm, it is highly curable, with a 10-year survival rate between 90% and 97%. However, thickened melanoma is lethal, and diagnosis at a more advanced stage decreases the 5-year survival rate to 10%–15%. Second, melanoma is a skin cancer that in a majority of cases is localized to the skin and is therefore detectable by simple examination. However, it is more likely to metastasize and spread to other organs than other skin tumors. It has been shown [3] that an early detection campaign may lead to mortality reduction more quickly than sun protection efforts. Nevertheless, the early diagnosing of melanoma is not always trivial even for experienced dermatologists and more particularly for primary care physicians and less experienced dermatologists [7–9].

Much effort has been made in the last two decades to improve the clinical diagnosis of melanoma. These include alternative imaging technologies such as dermoscopy [7] and several diagnostic algorithms such as pattern analysis [10], the ABCD rule of dermoscopy [11], Menzies method [12], the 7-point checklist [13], the CASH algorithm [14], CHAOS and clues [15], and the BLINCK algorithm [16].

Meta-analysis of studies conducted before 2001 showed that using the mentioned diagnostic algorithms along with dermoscopy improves the diagnosis of melanoma compared to simple naked-eye examination or traditional clinical examinations by 5%–30%, depending on the type of skin lesion and the experience of the dermatologist [3, 7]. However, it has been demonstrated that dermoscopy can reduce the diagnostic accuracy in the hands of inexperienced dermatologists [17] or sometimes make no improvements compared with clinical examinations [3]. Furthermore, clinical diagnosis of melanoma is inherently subjective, highly reliant on clinical experience and visual perception of individuals, and its accuracy has been an issue of concern, especially with equivocal pigmented lesions [7]. Even with the use of technologies such as dermoscopy and applying the above-mentioned algorithms, clinical diagnosis is still challenging, and its accuracy is considered to be limited, especially with equivocal pigmented lesions [7]. Despite the use of dermoscopy, the accuracy of expert dermatologists in diagnosing melanoma is estimated to be about 75%–84% [18]. Moreover, clinical diagnosis of melanoma is inherently subjective and suffers from inter- and intraobserver variabilities. This issue highlights the demand for receiving an *in vivo* second opinion, which increases the accuracy of diagnosis, thus saving more lives, and decreases the number of false excision of benign lesions, hence reducing the medical and emotional costs imposed on individuals by unnecessary surgeries. Image processing and computer vision techniques have been applied in an attempt to solve this problem since 1985. A computer-aided diagnosis of melanoma provides quantitative and objective evaluation of the skin lesion, versus the subjective clinical assessment. It allows for reproducible diagnosis by diminishing the interobserver and intraobserver variabilities that could be found in dermatologists' examinations. It also automates the analysis, and thereby reduces the amount of repetitive and tedious tasks to be done by clinicians. For further reading, please see [19–21].

Due to enhancements in skin imaging technology and image processing techniques in recent years, and owing to the repetitive patterns in skin lesions, which make skin lesion pattern recognition an intriguing problem to work on, there has been a significant increase in interest in development of computer-based diagnostic systems for melanoma. Various groups around the world have been trying to develop effective systems and devices to assist in the evaluation of pigmented skin lesions, some of which include the following.

SolarScan [22], developed by Polartechnics Ltd., Sydney, Australia, analyzes dermoscopy images of the pigmented skin lesion according to 103 variables based on color, pattern, and geometry of the lesion. The system was tested [23] on an image set of 2430 lesions, among which 382 were melanomas with median Breslow thickness of 0.36 mm. Seven specialist referral centers and two general practice skin cancer clinics from three continents were engaged in the study, and the SolarScan diagnosis results were compared with those of 13 clinicians, including 3 dermoscopy experts, 4 dermatologists, 3 trainee dermatologists, and 3 general practitioners. Applying statistical analysis and calculating the area under the ROC* curve (AUC), the system obtained a sensitivity of 86%–96% and specificity of 64%–72%.

DermoGenius Ultra [24], wherein the ABC features were calculated to approximate the A, B, and C parameters of the ABCD clinical algorithm, was developed by LINOS Photonics, Inc. Instead of the D parameter in the ABCD rule of dermoscopy, which identifies the dermoscopic structures, in this system D was to approximate the degree of heterogeneity in the lesion. The system was tested on 187 patients at risk for melanoma, resulted in identifying 52 lesions to be removed, which were labeled as unsuspicious in the clinical examination by physicians. Biopsy of these lesions showed that nine of them were potentially dangerous and the removal was required.

The DBDermo MIPS system [25], developed at the University of Siena, Italy, analyzed 147 pigmented skin lesions (selected from an archive of more than 10,350 images collected between 1991 and 2000, with 3220 of them being excised). The clinical criteria for inclusion of lesions in the study were asymmetrical, pigmented, impalpable lesions with variegated color, with diameter of 0.4 ± 1 cm. Using an artificial neural networks (ANN) classifier, the obtained diagnostic accuracy was about 93%.

The DANAOS expert system [26] also applied ANN, and the system was tested during a multicenter study in 13 dermatology centers in nine European countries in 1997. The resulting performance of the system on 2218 skin lesions was shown to be similar to that of dermatologists as published in the literature, which was dependent on the size and quality of the images.

While the above-mentioned systems used dermoscopy images, MelaFind [27–29] (developed by Electro-Optical Sciences, Inc., Irvington, New York) and SIAscope[†] [30] (developed by Astron Clinica, Cambridge, UK) have applied a different technology to capture skin images, using multispectral narrow bands ranging from 400 to 1000 nm. Because of the multilayered structure

---

* Receiver operator characteristic.
† Spectrophotometric intracutaneous analysis.

of skin, light of different wave-lengths penetrates the skin to different depths. MelaFind takes 10 images of each lesion using 10 different narrow spectral bands from 430 to 950 nm. Eight of these ten images were used for each lesion, and wavelet analysis along with a linear classifier was applied. The classification accuracy on a difficult image set, including dysplastic and congenital nevi, was reported to be 89% [27].

SIAscope produced eight narrow-band spectrally filtered images of the skin with radiation ranging from 400 to 1000 nm. The purpose of the analysis was to identify the amount, distribution, and depth of certain critical features, including collagen, melanin, and hemoglobin, within the epidermis and papillary dermis layers of skin. Over an image set of 348 pigmented lesions with lesions greater than 6 mm, the system obtained sensitivity and specificity of about 83% and 80%, respectively [30].

Some other computerized image analysis systems available in the market or under development include [31] MoleMax II developed by Derma Instruments L.P., MicroDerm by VisioMED, NevusScan by Romedix, FotoFinder by Derma Edge Systems Corp., and VideoCap100 by DS Medica. It is acknowledged that [32] the cost efficiency of the existing digital imaging systems (computer-aided diagnosis systems of melanoma) is still an issue of concern. Some of these devices are undergoing clinical trials before final approval and are not for sale.

In this chapter, in Section 10.2, we provide a comprehensive literature review on existing methods and techniques for implementing different components of a computer diagnostic system of melanoma. In Section 10.3, we propose a novel and highly scalable melanoma detection system and discuss the experimental result in Section 10.4. This chapter concludes with Section 10.5.

10.2 BACKGROUND

A computer-aided diagnosis of melanoma generally comprises five main components: image acquisition, image segmentation (or border detection), feature extraction, feature selection, and classification. A summary of the methods applied to implement each of these components in some of the studies is provided in the following.

10.2.1 IMAGE ACQUISITION

The first step in a computer-based diagnostic system of melanoma is the acquisition of the digital image of the lesion. The main techniques used for this purpose in the literature include [8] digitized color slides, which were used in early melanoma analysis studies [33]; acquisition of clinical images using still or video cameras; Epiluminescent Microscopy (ELM) or dermoscopy, which captures detailed information about the surface of the lesion and has been widely utilized in the literature [8, 26, 34–37]; and transmission electron microscopy (TEM) [38], which is useful for studying growth and inhibition of melanoma. Nevoscope [39–41], introduced by Dhawan in 1985, is a noninvasive transillumination-based imaging modality for analysis and diagnosis of melanoma. It involves three modes of illumination: (1) surface illumination, which is achieved by directing light perpendicular to the skin surface through fiber optic cables; (2) transillumination performed by directing light into the skin at a 45° angle through a ring light source; and (3) epi-illumination obtained from the combination of surface illumination and transillumination. The main advantage of transillumination is its sensitivity to imaging increased blood flow and vascularization, and also to viewing the subsurface pigmentation in a nevus.

Confocal scanning laser microscopy (CSLM) [31, 42] is a noninvasive imaging technology used for the *in vivo* examination of skin. It uses laser light to focus on a specific spot within the tissue and captures high-resolution images of cellular structures of skin lesions, which are comparable to detailed histologic images. The imaging depth is limited by the condition of the stratum corneum and the wavelength of the laser. Currently, the maximum depth of imaging is 200–300 μm at the level of the papillary dermis. Confocal images obtained from melanomas are clearly different from those of melanocytic nevi [42]. In addition to exhibiting the morphologic differences between melanoma and melanocytic nevi, CSLM technology has been applied to determining the border of melanoma lesions [43]. Currently, application of the CSLM to the diagnosis of melanoma is in the research stage [31, 44].

Ultrasound is also applied to clinical dermatology, more in Europe than in the United States [31]. The technology works based on the acoustic properties of skin tissue. There are three modes of ultrasound scan [31]: (1) A-mode is one-dimensional and shows the amplitude of the intensity at different levels in the skin tissue; (2) B-mode, commonly used in clinical settings, creates two-dimensional images from the brightness level of multiple A-mode scans; and (3) C-mode, which is still at an experimental stage, creates a three-dimensional (3D) display using computer assistance. The image resolution and tissue penetration are largely dependent on the frequency of the scanner; that is, an ultrasound scanner with a high frequency has a short wavelength and has less tissue penetration but higher image resolution. Even though ultrasound alone cannot provide a reliable means of differentiating between melanomas and common melanocytic nevi [45], it is shown to be potentially useful for differentiating melanoma from seborrheic keratosis [46]. Moreover, an important application of the ultrasound technology is the *in vivo* assessment of melanoma thickness [45, 47]. Other imaging modalities used for dermoscopy image analysis include computed tomography (CT) [48], positron emission tomography (PET) employing fluorodeoxyglucose [49], which has shown high sensitivity and specificity in diagnosing the staging of melanoma, MRI [50], multifrequency electrical impedance [51], and Raman spectra [52].

10.2.2   SEGMENTATION

Image segmentation is the process of dividing an image into disjoint and homogeneous partitions with respect to some characteristics, such as color, texture, and so forth [53]. Alternatively, it is the process of locating the boundaries between the regions, called border detection [54]. Segmentation is a prerequisite in the development of any computer vision system. Similarly, it is the first step toward the automated analysis and evaluation of medical images in a computer-aided diagnostic system. The accuracy of the segmentation result is of high importance due to the bias it can impose on the subsequent steps of the diagnostic system, that is, in the feature extraction and the ultimate classification result. In computer-aided diagnosis of melanoma, the purpose of segmentation is to detect the border of the lesion, in order to separate the lesion, the region of interest (ROI), from the background skin. The accuracy of the detected border is crucial, as exclusion of any part of the lesion my lead to loss of dermoscopic patterns, color, and texture-based information that can be extracted from the interior of the lesion. Moreover, the geometric shape of the lesion and structural properties of the border have diagnostic importance, all of which depend on the detected border (the segmentation results). Low contrast between the lesion and the background skin, irregularity and blurriness of the lesion border, image artifacts such as black frames, skin lines, blood vessels, hairs, and air bubbles, and scars, as well as the presence of various colors within the lesion, make border detection a challenging task [55].

Different image features, such as shape, color, texture, and brightness, can be employed to perform skin lesion segmentation. Accordingly, numerous methods have been developed for automated border detection in dermoscopy images in recent decades. As suggested by Celebi et al. [55], segmentation methods can be categorized into the following class of techniques: (1) histogram thresholding, which involves the determination of one or more threshold values that separate the ROI from the background, used in [56–60]; (2) color clustering methods, which partition the color space into homogeneous regions using unsupervised clustering algorithms, applied by [61–68]; (3) edge-based methods, which apply edge operators to determine the edges between the background and foreground regions applied by [69–71]; (4) region-based methods, which use region-merging and region-splitting algorithms to group the pixels into homogeneous regions [72–75]; (5) morphological methods, which start from predetermined seeds and apply the watershed transform in order to detect the contours of the object [76–78]; (6) model-based methods, which model the image as random fields and apply optimization to determine the parameters of the model [73]; (7) active contour methods, such as snakes, which use curve evolution techniques to determine the contours of the shape, as applied in [70, 79–83]; and (8) soft computing methods, which classify pixels using soft computing techniques such as neural networks, fuzzy logic, and evolutionary computation [84, 85].

Some previous studies have combined the results of different border detection methods to come up with the final ROI. For example, Pagadala [86] developed a skin segmentation method combining the segmentation results of three thresholding-based methods independently applied on red, green, and blue color channels of the dermoscopy image. Al-abayechi [87] proposed using a smooth filter (bilateral filtering with spline) to select the optimal color channel. Ganster et al. [35] also used a fusion process (logical OR operation on resultant binary segmented images) and combined three basic segmentation algorithms, to detect the border of lesions in dermoscopy images. The three basic segmentation methods involved global thresholding, dynamic thresholding, and a method based on a 3D color clustering concept adopted from [88]. The experimental results demonstrated that [35] thresholding with the blue channels of the red, green, blue (RGB) and CIE L*a*b* color spaces along with 3D color clustering on the X, Y, and Z channels of the CIE XYZ color channel produced the best segmentation results. Using an image set of 40 skin lesions, the thresholding algorithms achieved a good segmentation result in about 80% of the images. The 3D clustering approach, although it had poor performance in general (about 8%), performed reasonably well in cases where the other two methods were not successful [35].

Another similar approach to combine different segmentation methods is *thresholding fusion mechanism*. In this approach an ensemble of thresholding methods is proposed to incorporate multiple thresholding techniques to overcome the inefficiencies of each individual method. Although there are many generally good enough thresholding methods in the literature, there is no generic best method that appears robust enough on a variety of images. In other words, the effectiveness of a method normally depends on the statistical characteristics of images. Thus, different techniques have been used to combine the results obtained from multiple segmentations, such as majority voting, Markov random field (MRF) on a single channel (blue color) [89], or MRF on multichannels [90]. MRF allows us to combine multiple independent segmentation methods and take the advantage of each one in order to build a robust and accurate method.

Garnavi et al. proposed a hybrid border detection method [56] that encompasses two stages; the first stage applies global thresholding to detect an initial boundary of the lesion, and the second stage applies adaptive histogram thresholding on optimized color channels of X (from the CIE XYZ color space) to refine the border.

Based on the accepted assumption of color uniformity in the skin, unsupervised color clustering techniques have been frequently used in applications of skin lesion segmentation. Color clustering is used to reduce the number of colors such that they are quantized to the most representative colors. Melli et al. [66] combined an unsupervised clustering component with a supervised classification module to automatically extract the boundary of the skin lesion. In the clustering phase, they employed and compared four major clustering algorithms: median cut, k-means, fuzzy c-means, and mean shift (each will be explained in the following paragraph). The clusters obtained by these clustering processes were then merged and classified into two classes of *skin* and *lesion*. It was assumed that the lesion would occupy the central part of the skin image and the image's corners would belong to the *skin* class. The corner pixels were used as the *skin* training set to train the classifier, and the clusters obtained from the clustering module were merged and classified as *skin* class if they contained a particular number of pixels whose colors have been trained as *skin* color. After completion of classification and merging procedures, the major object within the image was identified as the *lesion* and the lesion boundary was detected. Over a set of 117 dermoscopy images, the resultant lesion boundaries were compared with the results obtained from dermatologists' manually drawn borders. The comparison, which was performed in terms of sensitivity, specificity, and the average of these two parameters, revealed that the best results were obtained from the mean-shift algorithm. Furthermore, they proposed a web-based test platform wherein all four segmentation algorithms were applied to a set of 5616 skin lesions. Dermatologists voted for the best segmentation results in each four-image set, and the overall verification test indicated that the mean-shift algorithm was the best. However, for those images that are corrupted and have no identifiable corners (which is sometimes the case in practice), this technique may not be applicable.

Hance et al. [61] compared the accuracy of six different color segmentation techniques and investigated their effectiveness in skin border extraction: adaptive thresholding, fuzzy c-means, spherical-coordinate transform/center split, principal component transform/median cut, split and merge, and multiresolution. For the spherical transform segmentation method, by algorithmic definition, the number of colors for segmentation was set to four, while for other algorithms it was kept constant at three. They showed that the principal component transform/median cut and adaptive thresholding algorithms provide the lowest average error. They also proposed a combined method of these six methods, which resulted in further improvement in the number of correctly identified tumor borders. Zhou [91] proposed a mean-shift-based fuzzy c-mean technique to reduce the computational costs and improve the segmentation performance. Schmid [62] also proposed a color-based segmentation algorithm in L*u*v* color space. They applied a modified version of fuzzy c-means, wherein the number of clusters depends on the number of maxima in the histogram information of the three color components.

In the dermatologist-like tumor extraction (DTEA) method [57, 92], the histogram thresholding technique based on Otsu's method [93] was applied to the blue color channel. This was followed by labeling the components, and merging the regions smaller than a predefined size. The region that met some heuristic criteria based on size, intensity, and distance to the margin of the image (defined in [57]) was taken as the initial lesion area. Lastly, the detected border was expanded by an iterative region-growing method to obtain the final border detection result. Ruiz et al. [94] also used Otsu's method for pixel segmentation and border detection by incorporating adaptive thresholding for each image.

Other recent methods include the following: The KPP* method [68] uses spatial constraints in the pigmented lesions and applies a two-stage clustering, based on the k-mean++ algorithm, to merge the homogeneous regions. The JSEG method [74], which is an unsupervised approach to border detection, is a modified version of an earlier JSEG algorithm [95]. In this method a color class map of the image is first formed during a color quantization step. Then, in a spatial segmentation step, similar regions are merged based on similarity in the CIE L*u*v* color space. The method was tested on a set of 100 dermoscopy images, using manually determined borders from a dermatologist as the ground truth. The results were compared with three other automated methods (discussed above) proposed by Pagadala [86], the DTEA method [57], and the KPP segmentation method [68], and were shown to be highly comparable with those. The authors acknowledge that the JSEG method may not, in certain circumstances, perform well on lesions with a lot of hair, and have suggested the use of a hair removal method such as DullRazor [96] might improve the results for such cases. Moreover, as acknowledged by the author, using a single dermatologist as the ground truth might not be reliable enough to validate the segmentation results. Amelio and Pizzuti [97] proposed a genetic algorithm–based segmentation method to build a graph of similar pixels and identify color clusters. In a similar approach, Wen [98] proposed a postprocess mechanism on the extracted pigmented regions by using Superpixel [99]. In their approach the superpixels are merged to form bigger superpixels considering texture, intensity, and color uniformity inside a superpixel. Sarrafzade et al. [100] applied wavelet transformation on a single channel (gray level) to enhance image by applying the inverse wavelet transform on the original images. Then morphology operators allow extracting of the borders and segments. Color mathematical morphology operators have been used in [101] to enhance the lesion contrast and color without modifying the characteristics of dermoscopy images.

Celebi et al. [55] outlined several issues to be considered when choosing a segmentation method: (1) scalar versus vector processing—the former is preferred to avoid excessive computational time requirements and the difficulty of choosing an appropriate color space, (2) automatic versus semiautomatic—the latter (e.g., active contour models) requires human interaction, and the former is preferred if we aim to develop a fully automated computer-based diagnosis system, and (3) number of parameters—the more the number of parameters, the harder the model selection. Parametric methods involve a process of determination of the optimal parameter values.

---

* K Plus Plus (k-mean++).

10.2.3 FEATURE EXTRACTION

Feature extraction is the process of extracting certain characteristic attributes and generating a set of meaningful descriptors from an image. The purpose of the feature extraction component in a computer-aided diagnosis system of melanoma is to extract various features from a given skin image that best characterize a given lesion as benign or malignant. The feature extraction methodology of many computerized melanoma detection systems has been generally based on the conventional clinical ABCD rule of dermoscopy due to its effectiveness and simplicity of implementation. Its effectiveness stems from the fact that it incorporates the main features of a melanoma lesion, such as asymmetry, border irregularity, color, and diameter (or differential structures), that are measurable and computable by computer. This section addresses some of the features employed by previous computer-based melanoma recognition studies.

10.2.3.1 Asymmetry

According to the ABCD rule of dermatoscopy, symmetry is given the highest weight among the four features [11]. In the Consensus Net Meeting on Dermoscopy [18], asymmetry, along with a few other criteria, was highlighted as a feature strongly associated with melanoma. In the ABCD rule of dermatoscopy [102], to quantify the asymmetry, the lesion is bilaterally segmented by two perpendicular axes positioned such that the resultant asymmetry score is minimized. The asymmetry score is calculated according to the contour (shape), color distribution, and internal structure of the lesion on either side of each axis.

Numerous approaches have been proposed to quantify the asymmetry in skin lesions. Some of the methods try to imitate the ABCD rule of dermatoscopy and investigate lesion asymmetry with respect to a symmetry axis passing through the lesion. In these approaches, the symmetry axis is determined in a variety of ways, such as principal axis [103–105], major axis of the best-fit ellipse [106, 107], Fourier transform [108], longest or shortest diameter [109], and so forth. Then, the difference between the area on both sides of the axis is calculated. In another technique, symmetry determination is based on geometrical measurements on the whole lesion, such as circularity [109–111]. Some others quantify the homogeneity of the lesion, wherein for certain patches the overall internal structure or coloration of the lesion is evaluated [105, 106, 112–114]. According to Stolz et al. [102], due to the fact that some equivocal lesions have symmetrical shapes, incorporating color and structural asymmetry is very crucial to scoring the symmetry of the lesion. In the following we provide a summary of existing methods in evaluating the symmetry measure in dermoscopy images, categorized as (1) shape asymmetry and (2) color and pattern asymmetry.

10.2.3.1.1 Shape Asymmetry

In numerous studies, a *circularity index* (also known as compactness, thinness, or roundness index) has been applied and claimed to be a proper indication of symmetry in skin lesions [109–111, 115]. This index is calculated as

$$Circularity = \frac{4A\pi}{P^2} \tag{10.1}$$

In this equation, A and P refer to the area and perimeter of the shape, respectively. This metric is scale independent, which makes it a handy tool for measuring the symmetry. However, it does not show enough efficacy in lesions with fuzzy and irregular borders. In such cases, the segmented region generally has a thick border, but a small internal area. Thus, the circularity index value attains a very small value, which does not reflect the actual circularity of the lesion. Therefore, the significance of this method tightly depends on the segmentation precision.

The *symmetry distance* (SD) measure is another concept applied to skin images in order to quantify the symmetry of the lesion. In 1995 Zabrodsky et al. proposed [116] SD as "quantifier of the minimum effort required to transform a given shape into a symmetric shape."

Ng et al. [109, 111] later applied the SD measure to investigate the symmetry property in skin lesions. They collected data of three types of melanocytic lesions: benign nevi, dysplastic nevi, and malignant melanoma. The purpose was to improve the performance of their system over their previous work, wherein the circularity index was applied. They selected boundary points at equal angles on the contour and established an *adaptive symmetry distance* (ASD) measure. Since the number of required representative points varies against the border's fuzziness and irregularity, it was not possible to have a predefined number of points as it is in SD. ASD calculates successive SDs by using an incremental number of boundary points, until the difference between two successive SDs hits a predefined threshold. However, due to inefficiency found in ASD when dealing with irregular and fuzzy borders, the *adaptive fuzzy symmetry distance* (AFSD) was proposed. AFSD involves a fuzzy factor f that represents the segmentation accuracy and implies that for any boundary point P_i, its actual location can be any point within a circle with P_i as center and $\|P_i - C\| \times f$ as radius. In order to test the efficacy of the proposed symmetry measurements in [111], that is, SD, ASD, AFSD, and circularity (CIRC), these measures were applied on 84 skin images of nonhairy melanocytic lesions. Each lesion was also labeled as either symmetrical or asymmetrical by a dermatologist. They compared the mean values obtained from each of the symmetry measures. Among all the methods, CIRC had a reasonably good performance, the SD method had the worst differential ability, and AFSD has the best performance among all.

The *bulkiness* concept was applied by Claridge et al. [117] in order to investigate the asymmetry of the lesion in terms of closeness to the equivalent ellipse, which has the same center of gravity and a moment of inertia similar to that of the lesion.

Stoecker et al. [103] proposed an objective definition for asymmetry. The authors dismissed the existing algorithms for their complexity and low performance, and thus suggested a new algorithm based on principal axis theory. Taking for granted that for a symmetric shape, at least one principal axis accords with the symmetry axis, they assumed that for an almost symmetrical contour, the principal axis can be considered a good approximation of the axis of symmetry. They proposed the method to determine the axis of symmetry, based on which the asymmetry index can be computed. Lastly, Clawson et al. [108] proposed a method based on Fourier descriptors to determine the optimal principal axes to quantify lesion symmetry.

10.2.3.1.2   Color and Pattern Asymmetry

This section provides a summary of some of the existing methods that measure the texture and color asymmetry of the skin lesion. Chang et al. [106] proposed a symmetry feature, called *solid pigment asymmetry index*. The pigment network beneath the epidermis is dominant in some parts of the lesion, producing a dark color term a solid pigment. An asymmetric solid pigment is considered an indication for the presence of melanoma. The authors applied the histogram-based thresholding technique on the luminance image to detect solid pigment areas inside the lesion and quantified the asymmetry of the position of solid pigmented areas within the lesion via a pigment asymmetry index.

Clawson et al. [112] proposed a technique to detect color asymmetry. The method analyzed the pigment distribution along radial paths connecting the center of the lesion to each of the boundary points. The proposed method started with converting the color lesion image to a grayscale image. Then for each radial path the mean grayscale value was estimated. Next, for each lesion a metric was defined to indicate the grayscale distribution over the whole lesion. Finally, for each boundary point a normalized color distance (NCD) was defined, in order to draw a new boundary for the lesion. Specifically, each NCD value showed the radial path length between the centroid and the corresponding boundary point. The authors stressed that hyperpigmentation areas lead to larger NCD, while regression areas result in small NCD values. In order to quantify the color asymmetry, they defined a mismatch metric by which the generated contour was compared with the circle, which is the symbol of perfect symmetry of pigment distribution.

Seidenari et al. [118] proposed a method to objectively evaluate pigment distribution in three types of skin lesions: early melanoma (MM), atypical nevi (AN), and benign nevi (BN). The aim was to investigate the efficacy of measured pigment distribution parameters in differentiating malignant lesions from normal ones. The authors noted that a big difference among the values of the distribution parameters indicates nonhomogeneity within the lesion.

In a similar study, Seidenari et al. [105] performed a numerical assessment of asymmetry based on comparison of CIE L*a*b* color components within the lesion color blocks. After finding the boundary, centroid, and principal axes of the lesion, the lesion was rotated along the principal axes, so that the major axis was aligned with the horizontal axis and the minor axis with the vertical one. Then, the image was subdivided with a grid of selected block size. They provide four block sizes corresponding to resizing of the image to 1%, 2%, 5%, and 8%. They presumed that colors were distributed as a multivariate distribution in each color block, so that they can be described via mean CIE L*a*b* vector and its corresponding covariance matrix. In the last step, they investigated the color asymmetry by finding the distance between each block and its symmetric pair with respect to the major and minor axes.

Manousaki et al. [113] suggested the fractal dimension of lesion surface (FDMB) to calculate the pigment distribution irregularity on the surface of the lesion. They applied the Minkowski–Boulingand algorithm, also known as box counting, to estimate FDMB. They also proposed a color texture feature of heterogeneity, which refers to uncompleted space filling within the lesion. The parameter, called grayscale lacunarity of lesion (Lac gray), shows the number and size of color voids inside the lesion. Holmstrom [114] stated that certain hue[†] values indicate malignancy. The areas containing these specific hue values were identified and their centroids calculated. The distance between these centroids and the center of gravity of the whole lesion was also estimated. Comparison between the acquired distance values was performed to reveal the color symmetry/asymmetry property of the lesion.

10.2.3.2 Border

Holmstrom [114] breaks down the border–feature problem into two separated problems of (1) border blurriness and (2) border irregularity. In the following we summarize some of the existing methods in quantifying each.

10.2.3.2.1 Border Blurriness

Day [119] investigated the blurriness of the lesion boundary by measuring the lightness gradient of the lesion along its border. Similarly to the clinical ABCD technique for measuring the B feature, the lesion was divided into eight segments, and in each segment five equally distant boundary points were chosen. The author defined the sharp pigment cutoff at each segment as a major difference between lightness values of skin and lesion in

---

[*] CIE L*a*b* is the most complete color space specified by the International Commission on Illumination. It describes all the colors visible to the human eye and was created to serve as a device-independent model to be used as a reference.

[†] Hue is the dominant wavelength of a color and is considered one of the main properties of a color described with names such as red or blue. Hue is also one of the three dimensions in some color spaces, such as HSV or HSL, along with saturation and value/lightness.

that segment. The L value from CIE L*a*b* color space was used as the lightness measure. To evaluate the lightness rate at each boundary point P_i, the lightness values of 30 pixels inside the border and 30 pixels outside the border were measured. These points were located along the line connecting P_i to the centroid of the lesion. Thus, for each of the five boundary points at each of the eight segments, 60 lightness values are recorded. Then, at each boundary point P_i, the slope of the lightness values is measured by using the method of least squares. For every segment, five lightness rates are obtained, the maximum of which was selected as the B score for that segment. These scores were compared with a given threshold to decide whether each segment has a sharp border ($Bscore = 1$) or a blurry one ($Bscore = 0$). The results were correlated with dermatologists' ratings, upon which a threshold value could be tuned to acquire a better scoring. The author acknowledged the shortcoming of the proposed method: when the scores obtained from the algorithm and those found by the dermatologists were compared, only the total B score was applied, meaning that the algorithm and dermatologists might have marked different segments as sharp cutoff. Manousaki et al. [113] measured the sharpness of the border by calculating the standard deviation (std) of gray intensity on the border of lesion. Moreover, they computed the coefficient of variation of std of gray intensity. The authors noted that these values indicate the degree of distinction of the lesion from the surrounding normal skin and that higher values correspond to sharper borders.

10.2.3.2.2   Border Irregularity

Different techniques have been introduced to measure the border irregularity of the skin lesions, some of which are discussed as follows. Claridge et al. [117] identified two types of irregularities on the border of the lesion and called them *textural* irregularity and *structural* irregularity. The former refers to small variations along the border of the lesion, which are sensitive to segmentation noise. The latter denotes the global indentations and protrusions on the whole shape, which show high correlations with malignancy of the lesion. Lee et al. [120–122] introduced a new shape descriptor that measures and locates structural irregularities (i.e., indentations and protrusions) along the border of the skin lesion.

In [104, 107, 123, 124], circularity or the *compactness index* (CI) has been also used to investigate the border irregularity of lesions. Holmstrom [114] recognizes two disadvantages of using such method: First, this index is too sensitive to noise and any error in calculating the perimeter of the shape will be squared. Second, while the method effectively responds to textural irregularities, it fails to recognize structural irregularities, which have higher correlation with melanoma [114, 121]. Lee [125] also noticed that the same compactness index can be obtained from lesions with different boundary shapes. Maglogiannis [126] calls this index the *thinness ratio*.

There are other types of measures proposed to evaluate the border irregularity of the skin lesion, including *smoothness* by Bono et al. [115], *fractal dimension* (FD) by Ng and Lee [127], *best-fit ellipse* by Chang et al. [106], and *conditional entropy* by Aribisala et al. [128].

10.2.3.3 Color

Color is another indicative feature in the classification of skin lesions, which is carefully considered in clinical practices such as the ABCD rule of dermatoscopy [11], Menzies method [12], and the CASH algorithm [14]. We observed three different trends in assessing the color feature in computer-aided diagnosis systems of melanoma: (1) developing a color palette that comprises certain defined color groups and associating different areas within each skin image with these color groups, (2) evaluating the relative color histogram to define melanoma colors, and (3) extracting statistical parameters from different color channels. We present a more detailed review of each of these approaches in the following.

10.2.3.3.1 *Color Palette*

Seidenari et al. [129] established an approach to imitate the human perception of colors in skin lesions. In an interactive process incorporating dermatologists' opinions, they created a color palette constituting six color groups (i.e., black, dark brown, light brown, red, white, and blue–gray). The palette involved different numbers of color patches for each color group; for example, the light brown group comprises 28 different light brown patches, all being perceived as light brown by human observers. To test the method and detect the color regions within the lesions, each pixel of the lesion was attributed to its corresponding color patch. This correspondence was obtained by finding the color patch with a minimum Euclidean distance of the RGB value to the pixel. After assigning all the pixels to the most relevant color patch, those pertaining to the same group were connected to form the unified segment of that particular color. Thus, for each lesion, the number and type of the colors were investigated and the results compared with clinical data by using statistical analysis. They also applied discriminant analysis to investigate the accuracy of the proposed method in diagnosis of melanoma. The results revealed a high correlation between computer results and dermatologists' opinions; that is, both methods found that the black, white, and blue–gray colors occurred more frequently in melanoma cases.

10.2.3.3.2 *Relative Color Histogram Analysis*

Faziloglu et al. [130] presented a three-dimensional relative color histogram analysis method to specify the color characteristics pertaining to melanoma, termed *melanoma colors*. Using relative colors in melanoma image analysis was first suggested by Umbaugh et al. [131] and has been widely used since [106, 124, 130, 132–135]. The relative color, in which the surrounding skin color is subtracted from the lesion color, aims to handle the color distortion in the image acquisition. Color distortion occurs for several reasons: variations in film type, camera settings and lighting condition, different color skin and pigmentations, and the Tyndall effect* for different patients.

10.2.3.3.3   Statistical Parameters

In order to quantify the color features of the skin lesion, various statistical parameters of different color spaces have been used. Celebi et al. [37] measured mean and standard deviation statistical parameters over the three channels of six different color spaces: RGB, rgb (normalized RGB), HSV, I1/I2/I3 (Ohta space), L1/2/3, and *CIE L*u*v*. The *mean* parameter represents the average color and the *standard deviation* shows the color variegation over each channel. A total number of 108 color features were calculated: (6 color spaces) × (3 channels in each color space) × (2 parameters: mean and std) × (3 regions: lesion, inner periphery, outer periphery). Furthermore, the differences and ratios of the two parameters (mean and std) over the three defined regions (lesion, inner periphery, outer periphery) were computed: (outer/inner), (outer/lesion), (inner/lesion), (outer/inner), (outer/lesion), and (inner/lesion). These relative parameters revealed significant information; for example, a big difference between inner and outer periphery might indicate malignancy of the lesion.

Sboner et al. [60] analyzed the color features of the image in RGB and HSV color space and calculated the *mean* and *standard deviation* of hue and saturation components. They also computed the fractal dimension of blue, green, hue, and saturation channels. Moreover, they measured the distances between the centroids of red, green, blue, hue, saturation, and value channels and the lesion centroid, average distance from the centroid of the RGB and HSV channels to the lesion centroid, and the difference, mean, and standard deviation of hue and saturation channels over the lesion border.

In another study [136] the *average* and *variance* of pixels in three color spaces, RGB, HIS (hue, intensity, saturation), and spherical coordinates CIE L*a*b*, were measured. She et al. [107] defined the color variegation as the normalized standard deviation of red, green, and blue color channels. The authors put great emphasis on the normalization process due to fact that in skins with higher pigmentation of surrounding normal skin, the lesion also exhibits higher pigmentation values. Furthermore, several color parameters were suggested by Manousaki et al. [113]: minimum, maximum, mean, and standard deviation values of gray, red, green, and blue intensities. They also measured the skewness from the Gaussian curve over each color channel, that is, the deviation of the histograms of the gray, red, green, and blue color channels from the normal (Gaussian) distribution curve.

---

* The Tyndall effect is the visible scattering of light along the path of a beam of light as it passes through a system containing discontinuities.

10.2.3.4 Differential Structures

In this section we briefly review the existing methods on analyzing differential structures in dermoscopy images.

Grana et al. [137] proposed a method based on Gaussian derivative kernels and Fisher linear discriminant analysis to detect and localize network patterns. Fischer et al. [138] proposed a multistep approach consisting of transforming RGB color space by the Karhunen–Loeve transform [139] and applying color segmentation on the new color components, with histogram equalization and grayscale morphology to enhance and filter pigment network patterns. Another algorithm was suggested by Fleming et al. [140], which aimed to analyze pigment networks and also measure the network line width and network hole size. Murali et al. [141] developed a texture-based algorithm to detect blotchy areas. They also aimed to determine the degree of importance of this feature in differentiating between malignant and benign lesions. Stoecker et al. [142] analyzed areas of granularity (or multiple blue–gray dots defined as accumulation of tiny, blue–gray granules in dermoscopy images) to discriminate granularity in melanoma from visually similar areas in nonmelanoma skin lesions. The granular areas in dermoscopy images of 88 malignant (including 14 melanomas *in situ* and 74 invasive melanoma) were manually selected. For 200 nonmelanoma dermoscopy images, those areas that most closely matched granularity, in terms of size, color, and texture, were similarly selected. The texture measures, including the average and range of energy, inertia, correlation, inverse difference, and entropy (based on co-occurrence matrix), and color measures, including absolute and relative RGB averages, absolute and relative RGB chromaticity averages, absolute and relative G/B averages, CIE X, Y, Z, X/Y, X/Z, and Y/Z averages, R variance, and luminance, were measured for each granular area of the melanomas and similar areas in the nonmelanoma images. ROC analysis revealed that the best classification result is obtained by using a combination of six texture and five relative color measures, resulting in an accuracy of 96.4%.

Sadeghi et al. [143] proposed a graph-based algorithm to detect and visualize pigment network structures. In this work, first an edge detection algorithm is performed on dermoscopy images. Then the binary edge images are converted to graphs. Their assumption is that pigmented network structures can be identified by analyzing cyclic subgraphs. Sadeghi et al. [144] extended that work to identify streak lines in skin lesions by modeling the lesion texture using joint probability distribution. Three different features are proposed to model geometric pattern and the distribution and coverage of the pigment network structures. For the classification model, they used a simple logistic classifier and achieved 85% AUC for identifying regular versus irregular streak lines on a collection of 945 dermoscopy images. In a similar approach, Barata et al. [145] detected a pigmented network by looking at the geometry and spatial organization of the lines. The assumption is that in a pigment network structure there are connected/circular lines. Also, another measure is to look for intensity transition between dark lines and surrounding brighter holes.

Lately, G. Arroyo et al. built a statistical rule-based classifier using low-level features (such as color, spectral, and statistical features) to generate candidate masks of pixels. These submasks are part of the general pigment network mask [146]. Abbas et al. [147] extracted color features and texture features to build an adaptive boosting multilabel learning algorithm that can identify seven global patterns (reticular, globular, cobblestone, homogeneous, parallel ridge, starburst, and multicomponent) in pigment networks. Saez et al. [148] used Markov random field (MRF) for texture analysis for identifying global patterns. Then three different models (Gaussian model, Gaussian mixture model, and bag-of-features histogram model) were carried out to capture the distribution of the texture features for each pigment network.

10.2.3.5   High-Level Intuitive Features

Another branch of feature extraction work [149–152], done by R. Amelard et al., focused on high-level intuitive features (HLIFs). In [152], HLIF was defined as "a mathematical model that has been carefully designed to describe some human-observable characteristic, and whose score can be intuited in a natural way." The authors argued that although usually requiring more up-front design time, HLIFs can provide image characteristics that are general and intuitive to a human observer. Compared with classic low-level features, HLIFs can decrease dimensionality of the feature space, which relieve the issues caused by high dimensionality, such as curse of dimensionality, high computational complexity, data sparsity, and so forth. Furthermore, the classification results based on HLIFs may have less overfitting problems (caused by sparsity) and are more easily interpreted by human observers. Specifically in [152], the authors defined 10 HLIFs for describing a lesion skin in terms of the asymmetry [149, 151], border irregularity [150, 151], and color complexity. The classification was performed based on three feature settings: state-of-the-art low-level features (LFs), HLIFs, and a combination of LFs and HLIFs. The results showed that HLIFs increased the classification accuracy of LFs, and HLIFs could convey diagnostic rationale to the user.

10.2.4   FEATURE SELECTION

Feature selection is an important component in data preprocessing/analysis in various applications, such as computer vision, data mining, image mining, and so forth. It reduces the number of features by removing irrelevant, redundant, or noisy data, and has an immediate effect on application by accelerating the classification, clustering, or data mining algorithm, as well as improving performance [153]. A typical feature selection process consists of four basic steps [154] (shown in Figure 10.1): subset generation, subset evaluation, stopping criterion, and result validation. Subset generation is a search

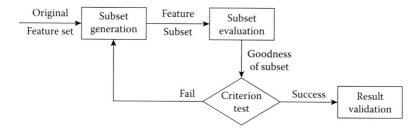

FIGURE 10.1 Basic steps of a typical feature selection process. (From Liu, H. and Yu, L., *IEEE Transactions on Knowledge and Data Engineering*, vol. 17, pp. 491–502. © 2005 IEEE.)

procedure that produces candidate feature subsets based on a certain search strategy [155, 156]. Each candidate subset is then evaluated and, based on a certain evaluation criterion, compared with the previous best subset. If the new subset defeats the previous one, the old subset is replaced by the new one. The process of producing and evaluating the subsets is repeated until a given stopping criterion is satisfied. Ultimately, the selected best subset will be validated and testified by prior knowledge or different tests using simulated or real-world data [153].

Feature selection algorithms can be categorized in three classes [153]: (1) the filter model [157], which uses the general characteristics of the data to evaluate the features and select the optimal feature subset(s) with no classification or learning algorithm, such as methods based on correlation [158, 159], entropy, mutual information, and so forth; (2) the wrapper model [160], which uses a learning algorithm and searches for features that improve the learning performance, such as methods based on greedy or genetic algorithms [161–163]; and (3) the hybrid model, which combines the two approaches [164–166]. Filter model feature selectors are less computationally expensive than wrapper-based approaches.

Some existing computer-based melanoma diagnosis systems have applied feature selection in their study; for example, principal component analysis was used by Walvick et al. [167] to obtain an optimal set of four features from an initial set of 11 features. Roß et al. [168] performed feature selection by applying the sequential forward selection (SFS) method, reducing the feature set from 87 to 5 features. Nimunkar et al. [169] applied a statistical feature selection approach (unpaired t-test for normally distributed features and Wilcoxon rank-sum test for nonnormally distributed features), to cut down the feature vector from 34 to 5 optimal features.

Celebi et al. [170] proposed a hybrid approach by using conventional feature selection methods (ReliefF, mutual information-based feature selection, and correlation-based feature selection) to rank the features and then applied an optimization approach to select optimal feature subsets. The AUC measure obtained from trained SVM were taken into account to evaluate each feature subset. They reported a specificity of 92.34% and a sensitivity of 93.33% over a diverse collection of dermoscopy images (564 images). In [59] a neural network was applied and node pruning was used to reduce the set size from 21 features to 6. Ganster et al. [35] started with 122 features and used three statistical approaches of sequential floating forward selection (SFFS), sequential floating backward selection (SFBS), and leave one out (LOO) to reduce the number of the selected features to 21. Iyatomi et al. [171] developed an automated method to detect the dermoscopic criteria for diagnosing melanomas, based on two diagnostic algorithms of the ABCD rule and the 7-point checklist. A total of 356 features were extracted from a set of 105 dermoscopy images, and their dermoscopic findings determined by four dermatologists were used as the gold standard. They applied correlation-based feature selection to reduce the feature space to 163 features and built multiple regression models for the 15 clinical findings defined by the two diagnostic algorithms. The model reportedly provides results comparable to those of dermatologists in recognizing almost all of the dermoscopic criteria. Garnavi et al. [172] used gain ratio to identify optimal features to be used in the classification of melanoma lesions, and achieved a significant reduction in dimension of feature space—the number of features was reduced from 35,455 to 23—while increasing the accuracy by 12% and decreasing the computational time by a factor of 50.

10.2.5 CLASSIFICATION

Classification is the process of distributing items into classes or categories of similar type. In a computer vision system, similarity is defined in terms of the features that have been extracted in the feature extraction module. This section provides a brief review of the most popular classification methods that have been applied to computer-based melanoma diagnostic systems.

10.2.5.1 Discriminant Analysis

Discriminant analysis has been employed to classify pigmented skin lesions in [60, 104, 126, 169, 173–175]. The main aim of discriminant analysis [176] is to classify a set of observations into predefined classes, based on the values of certain measurements, known as predictors. The discriminant analysis discovers the combination of these predictor variables that best characterizes the interclass differences. The coefficients are calculated and the obtained discriminant functions can be used to predict the class of a new observation with unknown class. For a k-class problem, k discriminant functions are constructed. Given a new observation, all k discriminant functions are evaluated and the observation is assigned to class i if the ith ($i = 1, 2, \ldots, k$) discriminant function has the highest value. Another application of this technique is to find out the most discriminating predictor, which is done either by successively eliminating those predictor variables that do not contribute significantly to the discrimination between classes or by successively identifying the predictor variables that have a major contribution. The likelihood function and Fisher's linear discriminant function are two common discriminant rules that are employed in this technique.

10.2.5.2   Artificial Neural Network

The artificial neural network (ANN) approach has been applied to classify skin lesion images in [36, 104, 126, 167, 168, 177]. Neural networks are nonlinear statistical data modeling tools that can be used to model complex relationships between inputs and outputs or to find patterns in data. The methodology of neural networks involves mapping a large number of inputs into a small number of outputs; therefore, it is frequently applied to classification problems [178]. The artificial neural network or neural network (NN) [179] is a mathematical or computational model that calculates posterior class membership probabilities by minimizing a cross-entropy error function. Based on biological neural networks, ANNs consist of highly interconnected processing units called artificial neurons. Information is propagated between neurons positioned in different layers and stored as connection weights between neurons. A minimization process is implemented as a rule that updates the weights in the network. An ANN is generally an adaptive system that changes its structure based on external or internal information (feedback) that flows through the network during the learning phase.

10.2.5.3   *k*-Nearest-Neighborhood

The k-nearest-neighborhood (k-NN) algorithm has been used to classify pigmented skin lesions in [35, 36, 60, 168, 175, 180]. The k-NN algorithm [181] is a popular density estimation algorithm for numerical data. It classifies objects based on closest training examples in the feature space. This algorithm uses the elements of the training set to estimate the density distribution of the data by applying a distance measure such as Euclidean distance. For a given distance measure, the only parameter of the algorithm is k, the number of neighbors, which determines the smoothness of the density estimation; larger values consider more neighbors, and therefore smooth over local characteristics. Smaller values consider only limited neighborhoods.

10.2.5.4   Support Vector Machine

The support vector machine has been applied to skin lesion classification in [8, 36, 37, 41, 104, 136, 180, 182, 183]. The support vector machine (SVM) [184] is a popular classification algorithm based on statistical learning theory. Considering input data as two sets of vectors (support vectors) in an n-dimensional space, SVM calculates a separating hyperplane in that space, which maximizes the distance (margin) between the two datasets. Celebi et al. [37] recognized several advantages of SVM over other classification algorithms such as neural networks. The advantage arises from the logic that since the training phase of

SVM involves optimization of a convex cost function, there is no risk of local minima to complicate the learning process, as in the case of backpropagation neural networks.

10.2.5.5   Decision Trees

Decision trees have been used to classify skin lesion images in [8, 36, 60, 135, 185, 186]. The decision tree, as described in [187, 188], provides a classification schema by dividing the dataset into smaller and more uniform groups, based on a measure of disparity (usually entropy). To achieve this separation, a variable and a corresponding threshold in the domain of this variable are identified, which can be used to divide the dataset into two groups. The best choice of variable and threshold is that which minimizes the disparity measures in the resulting groups. In these tree structures, leaves represent class labels and branches represent conjunctions of features that lead to those classifications.

10.2.5.6   Ensemble Classifiers

Ensemble methods have been used in prior literature to improve threshold-dependent performance under conditions of data imbalance, perform feature selection, and improve both efficiency and scalability of learning and subsequent recognition tasks [189–198].

With ensemble methods, a multitude of smaller unit models are trained (such as SVM or k-NN classifiers) from subsets of features and data. Each data subset typically controls imbalance, whereby all minority instances are utilized, and majority instances are randomly undersampled to balance each model's learning problem. The number of SVMs trained are usually chosen to ensure complete data coverage of the majority class and depend on the sampling strategy used. Two primary sampling strategies are seen in practice: replacement, whereby data exemplars can occur in multiple unit models, or nonreplacement, whereby each exemplar is assigned to at most one model in the ensemble.

Several algorithms exist for learning the ensemble fusion of smaller unit models. A common approach is to simply average the output of all trained models [189]. More complex techniques exist that attempt to optimize performance through optimized model selection, efficiency, or both [195–197]. In some cases, the same algorithms used to train models, such as SVMs, are also trained at this second layer, where the outputs of the smaller models are concatenated into a midlevel feature [198].

Garnavi et al. applied [172] random forest to classify melanoma from benign lesions on a dataset comprising 289 dermoscopy images and achieved an accuracy of 91.26%. The random forest classifier demonstrated higher accuracy in the classification of melanoma lesions than SVM, logistic model tree, and hidden naive Bayes.

10.2.5.7   Comparison of Different Machine Learning Methods

Dreiseitl et al. [36] utilized five machine learning (classification) techniques: k-nearest-neighborhood, logistic regression, artificial neural network, decision tree, and support vector machine, to classifying pigmented skin lesions as common nevi, dysplastic nevi, or melanoma. Regarding the experimental results, the authors recognized that the decision tree paradigm was not a good option to apply on skin lesion classification, since most of the variables (features) basically have continuous values in such applications. However, k-NN performed well, and logistic regression, ANN, and SVM claimed to exhibit very good performance over the given image set. Another comparison between different classification methods was performed by Burroni et al. [175], where the performance of two statistical classifiers, linear discriminant analysis and k-nearest-neighborhood, was evaluated. The experiments were conducted on an image set containing 391 melanoma and 449 melanocytic nevi images. Using independent test sets of lesions, the results achieved by the linear classifier and the k-nearest-neighborhood classifier revealed a mean sensitivity of 95% and 98% and a mean specificity of 78% and of 79%, respectively.

Sboner et al. [60] used a voting scheme integrating the outputs of three different classifiers of discriminant analysis, k-nearest neighbor, and decision tree, applied to a set of 152 skin images. The authors claimed that the voting scheme increases the diagnostic sensitivity and specificity over applying each individual classifier.

Maglogiannis and Doukas [8] presented a survey on existing computer vision systems for characterization of skin lesions in 2007 (published in 2009). They also utilized a fairly large set of 3707 images, extracted 31 features of color, border, and texture from those, and applied three feature selection methods based on correlation, principal component analysis, and generalized sequential feature selection (GSFS), aiming to (1) detect melanoma from nevus, (2) classify dysplastic (nevus) versus nondysplastic skin lesions, and (3) classify the three classes of melanoma, dysplastic, and nondysplastic. A group of classifiers were applied, for example, Bayes networks, SVM, classification and regression trees (CART), multinomial logistic regression (MLR), locally weighted learning (LWL), and neural network (multilayer perceptron). The result showed that regarding the first aim, MLR had the best performance, followed by SVM, LWL, and CART. For the second aim, all classifiers achieve lower accuracy, indicating the difficulty of differentiation between dysplastic and nondysplastic nevi. Among all three classifiers of multilayer perceptron, SVM and Bayes networks had the best performance. In the last experiment the majority of the examined classifiers performed satisfactorily, with accuracy ranges from 68.70% (Bayes networks) to 77.06% (SVM). The authors emphasized the overall superior performance of SVM, followed by regression and Bayes networks.

Table 10.1 shows the classification results of some of the existing computer-based melanoma diagnosis systems. Obviously, the results obtained from those studies with a reasonable number of images (e.g., at least 100), with balanced

TABLE 10.1

Classifier Performance Results from Existing Systems

Classifier	Performance Results	No. of Images	Reference
Discriminant analysis	TP 93%, FP 0%–21%	28	[169]
	SNS 65%, SPC 83%	152	[60]
	SNS 93%, SPC 100%	34	[104]
	ACC 71%	70	[173]
	SNS 100%, SPC 86%	29	[174]
	SNS 95%, SPC 78%	821	[175]
Artificial neural network	TP 100%, FP 23.5%	60	[167]
	SNS 91%, SPC 94%	1619	[36]
	SNS 93%, SPC 100%	34	[104]
	ACC 87%	—	[168]
	ACC 85%–89%	250	[177]
k-nearest-neighborhood	SNS 87%, SPC 92%	5393	[35]
	SNS 85%, SPC 90%	1619	[36]
	SNS 35%–68%, SPC 90%–97%	152	[60]
	ACC 93%	—	[168]
	SNS 98%, SPC 79%	821	[175]
Support vector machine	SNS 92%, SPC 95%	1619	[36]
	SNS 93%, SPC 92%	564	[37]
	SNS 86%, SPC 100%	34	[104]
	ACC 82.5%	4277	[182]
	SNS 100%, SPC 63.5%	977	[183]
	SNS 92%, SPC 93%	60	[41]
Decision trees	SNS 80%, SPC 90%	1619	[36]
	SNS 64%, SPC 84%	152	[60]
	ACC 70%	251	[185]
Random forest	ACC 91.26%, AUC 0.937	289	[172]

Note: The performance results has been reported based on True Positive (TP), False Positive (FP), Sensitivity (SNS), Specificity (SPC), Accuracy (ACC), and Area Under the ROC Curve (AUC).

distribution between classes of benign and malignant, and with separated image sets for training and testing the classifier, provide more validity and reliability.

10.3   METHODOLOGY: VISUAL RECOGNITION APPROACH

In this section we introduce a novel and highly scalable melanoma detection system. The system has multiple components, including feature extraction, feature selection, building classification models, and combining the trained classifiers into an ensemble model. The learning core of the system has a two-stage learning mechanism. In the first stage, models are trained over random subsets of low-level features and data. These are referred to as unit models. In the second stage, the unit models are input to an ensemble modeling algorithm that optimizes a combination of unit models that yield the best visual recognition results. The system is implemented in the Hadoop MapReduce environment for arbitrary scalability, in terms of both data and number of entities to be recognized.

Each component of this system is described in the following subsections. Low-level features used in experiments are described in Section 10.3.1. The ensemble modeling algorithm in its entirety is described in Section 10.3.2. Finally, the large-scale implementation is reviewed in Section 10.3.3.

10.3.1 LOW-LEVEL VISUAL FEATURES

All our experiments were based on a set of low-level visual features extracted at different spatial granularities. These have been used in prior reports related to medical image modality classification [199]. We selected a subset of the most useful features with the use of an 80%–20% train–validation split of the whole training set. The spatial granularities adopted were as follows:

- **Global**: Feature extracted from entire image.
- **Grid(7)**: 5×5 (7×7) image grid, with feature vector extracted from each grid block and concatenated. Increases dimensionality by factor of 25 (49).
- **Layout**: Five image regions including the center and the four quarters.
- **Pyramid(3)**: Spatial pyramid with global as first level and 2×2 (3×3) image grid as second level.

The pool of visual features we employed is a combination of global and local descriptors:

- **Color histogram**: Global color distribution represented as a 166-dimensional histogram in HSV color space.
- **Color correlogram**: Global color and structure represented as a 166-dimensional single-banded auto-correlogram in HSV space using eight radii depths.
- **Color moments**: Localized color extracted from a 5×5 grid and represented by the first three moments for each grid region in Lab color space as a normalized 225-dimensional vector.
- **Wavelet texture**: Localized texture extracted from a 3×3 grid and represented by the normalized 108-dimensional vector of the normalized variances in 12 Haar wavelet subbands for each grid region.
- **Edge histogram**: Global edge histograms with eight edge direction bins and eight edge magnitude bins, based on a Sobel filter (64-dimensional).

- **GIST**: Describes the dominant spatial structure of a scene in a low-dimensional representation, estimated using spectral and coarsely localized information. We extract a 512-dimensional representation by dividing the image into a 4×4 grid. We also extract histograms of the outputs of steerable filter banks on eight orientations and four scales.

- **Local binary pattern (LBP)** [200]: Extracted from the grayscale image as a histogram of 8-bit local binary patterns, each of which is generated by comparing the grayscale value of a pixel with those of its eight neighbors in circular order, and setting the corresponding bit to 0 or 1 accordingly. A pattern is called uniform if it contains at most two bitwise transitions from 0 to 1. The final histogram for each region in our granularity contains 59 bins, 58 for uniform patterns and 1 for all the nonuniform ones.

- **Multiscale LBP** [201]: Multiscale color LBP is an extension of the common grayscale LBP, whereby LBP descriptors are extracted across four color channels (red, green, blue, and hue), with one histogram per color channel. In our implementation, for each color channel, LBP descriptors are extracted across multiple scales $(1/1, 1/2, 1/4,$ and $1/8$ image size) and aggregated into the same histogram, weighted by the inverse of the scale. For a 59-bin LBP histogram, this results in $59*4 = 236$ total bins, including all scales.

- **Image type**: A set of global image statistics: mean saturation, hue entropy, variance, quantized color entropy, and switches (proportion of instances where a pixel has a different value than its right neighbor).

- **Image stats**: A series of statistics on the image: aspect ratio, isWhite, isBlack, isAllBW, isColor, entropy, variance, minimum value, maximum value, mean, median, standard deviation, central moments, average energy of the first-level 2D wavelet decomposition subbands, skin color, number of unique colors in quantized color space.

- **Fourier polar pyramid**: Computes the magnitude of a spatial pyramid in Fourier space, under the polar coordinate system, across all three color channels, red, green, and blue, in addition to a grayscale color channel. Pyramid levels in the radial dimension consist of 1, 2, 4, and 8 partitions. For each of these partitions, we construct a pyramid in the angular dimension, of partitions 1, 2, 4, 8, 16, and 32 segments. Due to the property of image symmetry in Fourier space, only the top half of the polar Fourier circle is sampled for the feature vector.

- **Maxi thumbnail vector**: The concatenated RGB pixel values of the image after downsampling to 24×24 dimensions.

10.3.2 ENSEMBLE MODELING APPROACH

Visual modeling is carried out by an ensemble learning approach, which is a common method for training classifiers under conditions of data imbalance [196, 197, 202–205]. Instead of training large single models by concatenating all features in early fusion, and training models from all available data, our system trains smaller unit models. For each concept, unit models are trained on a single feature, a single image granularity (such as a whole image, which results in a descriptor matching the dimensionality of the feature, or a 5×5 grid resulting in a descriptor 25 times the dimensionality of the original feature), and a random subsample of data, referred to as a bag (Figure 10.2). For each unit model, the system trains an SVM using linear approximation kernels with explicit kernel mapping [206] and logistically normalizes that SVM output via two fold cross-validation [207].

The most discriminative unit models for each concept are selected to be fused into an ensemble classifier based on their performance on a held-out validation set (Figure 10.3). In the first step, the unit model U_i that maximizes the average precision of the ensemble $AP(E_1)$ (which is initialized with no models) on the validation dataset is selected. A weight w_i may be applied, which is defined as the average precision of the unit model on the validation data, $AP(U_i)$. The second step is a loop, whereby additional unit models are

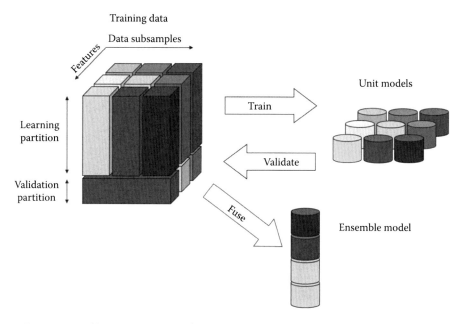

FIGURE 10.2 (See color insert.) Ensemble learning approach. Training data are partitioned into learning and validation sets, which are further divided by features and data samples, referred to as bags. Unit models (SVMs) are trained for each bag, and an ensemble fusion approach fuses them.

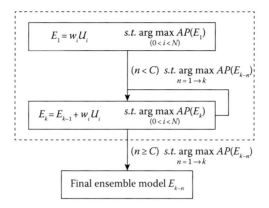

FIGURE 10.3 Ensemble fusion strategy using forward model selection. First, the best-performing unit model is selected for inclusion into the ensemble model. Subsequently, unit models that boost performance the most at each iteration of the loop are combined into the ensemble until performance ceases to improve.

added to the ensemble E_{k-1} that maximize the performance of E_k in each iteration. Once up to C unit models have been added with no improvement in performance ($C = 1$ for our experiments), the loop terminates.

Building models in this manner yields several desirable properties:

1. Data imbalance is markedly reduced. When a unit model is subsampled, a maximum data imbalance threshold is enforced. The whole of the majority class is covered by the generation of many unit models, each with a different sampling of examples.
2. The learning problem is much more efficient when training many smaller models, instead of one large model, since the computational complexity of training a model is polynomial in nature. For number of bags k, number of examples n, and some constant ($c = 2$), when calculating kernel matrices, we have

$$O\left(k \cdot \left(\frac{n}{k}\right)^c\right) << O\left(n^c\right) \tag{10.2}$$

especially for large k.
3. Since each unit model is an independent training task, we can easily parallelize to an arbitrary scale.
4. Our forward model selection algorithm will combine the most complementary unit models and features into the final ensemble classifier, rather than simply selecting the best unit models and features, which may be redundant with one another. This helps to boost performance as much as possible, while discarding unit models and features that do not yield any improvement or negatively impact performance.

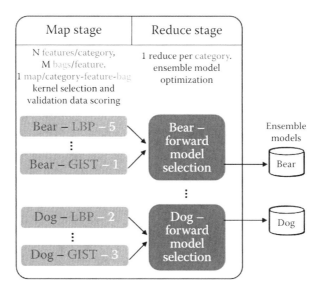

FIGURE 10.4 (**See color insert.**) Large-scale ensemble modeling implementation in Hadoop MapReduce.

10.3.3 LARGE-SCALE TRAINING

Due to the parallelizable nature of our ensemble algorithm, we used a Hadoop MapReduce implementation for large-scale ensemble classifier learning similar to that used in prior literature [196, 197, 204, 208]. In this method, unit models are learned in the Hadoop Map stage, where each task is independent, and ensembles are optimized in the Hadoop Reduce stage, where independent tasks are aggregated (Figure 10.4). We used a physical cluster of approximately 800 CPU cores, 3.1 TB of total system memory, and 70 TB of hard disk storage.

10.4 EXPERIMENTAL RESULTS

In the following sections, we describe the application of the ensemble modeling strategy to the task of diagnosing melanoma based on dermoscopic imaging. First, two datasets utilized for experiments are described. Subsequently, experimental results are reviewed. Two series of experiments have been conducted: (1) We conduct pattern classification. These patterns are dermoscopic criteria labeled by expert dermatologist on Pedro Hispano Hospital (PH2). (2) Then we try to solve the disease classification problem, that is, melanoma classification, using the low-level features and the pattern classifiers (i.e., midlevel or semantic features).

10.4.1 DATASETS

In the following experiments, we first use the Pedro Hispano Hospital [209] dermoscopic image dataset. The PH2 dataset includes the manual segmentation, the clinical diagnosis, and the identification of several dermoscopic structures, performed by expert dermatologists. The PH2 dataset has been made freely available for research and benchmarking purposes and contains a total number of 200 melanocytic lesions, including 80 common nevi, 80 atypical nevi, and 40 melanomas. Every image was evaluated by an expert dermatologist with regard to the following parameters: (1) manual segmentation of the skin lesion, (2) clinical and histological (when available) diagnosis, and (3) dermoscopic criteria (asymmetry, colors, pigment network, dots/globules, streaks, regression areas, blue–white veil).

We also utilize a dataset obtained through collaboration with the International Skin Imaging Collaboration (ISIC) [210]. This dataset includes 391 dermoscopy images of melanoma and 2314 dermoscopy images of benign lesions, a subset of which (225) are considered near-miss atypical lesions (visually similar to melanoma, as judged by medical professionals). The images of this dataset come without lesion segmentations. Therefore, for recognition of disease state, we simply analyzed regions defined by manually delineated bounding boxes around the areas of the skin lesions, in order to eliminate erroneous areas of the image that may influence recognition results.

10.4.2 PATTERN CLASSIFICATION

In this study, the objective is to validate the usefulness of the proposed ensemble modeling approach in building classification models to predict dermoscopy patterns (e.g., asymmetry, number of colors, etc.). In doing so, for each pattern, images for the PH2 database are partitioned per each label (pattern). For each label, a binary classifier is trained, and the final prediction is obtained by voting mechanism for multilabel classes (e.g., asymmetry pattern that can take the value of full symmetric, half symmetric, and full asymmetric) or based on threshold for binary classes (e.g., presence of the blue–white pattern). These experiments have used the original dermoscopy images (without segmentation). The reason is to be more consistent with ISIC data we will be using in our next experiments.

We have used leave-one-out cross-validation due to a limited number of samples; that is, one sample has been used for test (handheld), and the rest for training. From the training data, 80% for training the unit models and 20% for validating the SVM kernels.

The results are shown in Table 10.2, which indicates most of the patterns can be classified with more than 85% accuracy. Those patterns are guidelines for expert dermatologists to diagnose the melanoma disease. Thus, we would apply the pattern classifiers learned here, which are basically semantic

TABLE 10.2
Pattern Classification Results on PH2

Classifier Label	Accuracy	AUC	Average Precision
Asymmetry_0	66%	0.65	69%
Asymmetry_1	83%	0.49	14%
Asymmetry_2	79%	0.71	47%
BlueWhitishVeil_A	90%	0.96	99%
ColorBlack_A	83%	0.90	97%
ColorBlueGray_A	86%	0.89	97%
ColorDarkBrown_A	78%	0.72	41%
ColorLightBrown_A	74%	0.82	64%
ColorRed_A	95%	0.48	96%
ColorWhite_A	91%	0.74	97%
Dots_Globules_A	47%	0.53	47%
Dots_Globules_AT	61%	0.51	29%
Dots_Globules_T	70%	0.55	39%
NumColors_H	92%	0.30	91%
PigmentNetwork_T	74%	0.82	79%
RegressionAreas_A	89%	0.86	98%
Streaks_A	85%	0.79	95%

Note: Asymmetry_0, full symmetry; asymmetry_1, half asymmetry; asymmetry_2, full asymmetry; A, absent; AT, atypical; T, typical; NumColors_H, more than three colors.

or midlevel features, to the disease classification problem in the following subsection.

10.4.3 DISEASE CLASSIFICATION

The aim of the following experiments is to validate the proposed ensemble model for disease classification on the PH2 and ISIC datasets. The low-level and midlevel or semantic features (pattern classifiers) are applied on images, and the ensemble modeling approach is used for the final classification to ascertain whether a given lesion is benign or malignant.

10.4.3.1 Using Low-Level Feature Only on PH2

The goal is to evaluate the ensemble modeling approach performance on the PH2 dataset and compare the performance of our model with that in prior reports on PH2. The inputs are image data and output is the disease label (melanoma, nevus). Because of the extreme scarcity of exemplars in the PH2 dataset, we used a variant of IMARS that trains a single unit model with early fusions of features. Twofold cross-validation is still used for logistic score fitting in order to address data imbalance. Evaluations are carried out in accordance with prior literature, utilizing a leave-one-out strategy: one example is left out of training, while models are trained on the remaining data and used to make a judgment of the sample left out. This is repeated until all samples have been left out.

Our experimental approach was to start with a simple feature to describe color and iteratively add features that better describe texture or interactions between color and texture. We expected to see an improvement in performance as additional image statistics were involved in the training process, until the feature combinations became a high enough dimension that overfitting started to occur. Indeed, this is the pattern that our experiments show; however, before saturation occurs, state-of-the-art performance was obtained.

In total, we performed four experiments. In the first, we utilized the color histogram feature at global granularity. The resultant sensitivity and specificity were 0.675 and 0.9062, respectively, with an average precision at full depth of 0.743. In the second, we concatenated color and edge histograms at global granularities. Performance improved to 0.8 sensitivity and 0.9375 specificity, with an average precision at full depth of 0.88. In the third, we concatenated color, edge, and color LBP histograms (59 bins), all at global granularities. Performance capped at 0.9 sensitivity and 0.9 specificity, with an average precision of 0.927. Using a threshold where sensitivity is fixed to a value of 0.93 as reported in prior literature, this result improves the state of art by 4% in specificity (0.88 specificity vs. 0.84 in prior reports [209]).

In the fourth and final experiment, we continued to concatenate additional features, including both image type and image stats feature vectors. These features measure global image statistics, such as mean saturation, hue entropy, variance and switches, quantized color entropy and switches, variance, minimum value, maximum value, mean, median, standard deviation, central moments, average energy of the first level of 2D wavelet decomposition subbands, skin color, and number of unique colors in quantized color space. However, we found performance to decrease, likely due to overfitting of the small dataset from the feature vector becoming too large. Sensitivity and specificity reduced to 0.9 and 0.888, respectively, and Average Percision (AP) fell to 0.922.

10.4.3.2   Using Pattern Classifier on PH2

The goal of this section is to demonstrate that extracting dermatology features can improve the melanoma detection. In this section we have use ensemble modeling (which has been described in Section 10.3), leave-one-out cross-validation, and the 80%–20% setup for this experiment. The classification results are shown in Table 10.3.

We obtain 82% sensitivity (SEN) and 86% specificity (SPC) using the direct output of ensemble modeling on PH2. The classification result can be further improved by optimizing the threshold to obtain 90% SEN and 84% SPC, which is comparable to the original result published in the dataset [209]. This is achieved by setting up a mixed-cost function as in Equation 10.3, which

TABLE 10.3

Disease Classification Results

	Accuracy	SEN	SPC	Precision	F-Measure	AUC
PH2 ensemble	85%	82%	86%	60%	69%	93%
PH2 pattern classifier	91%	97%	65%	92%	94%	95%

is the weighted sum of the SEN and SPC, and finding the threshold that minimizes the cost.

$$C = \frac{c_{10}(1 - SEN) + c_{01}(1 - SPC)}{c_{10} + c_{01}} \tag{10.3}$$

The result indicates that the ensemble modeling approach works well for this PH2 dataset despite the fact that the training samples are very limited.

Then, we utilize the pattern classifier learned in Section 10.4.2 to predict the disease label. This is achieved by concatenating the 15 pattern prediction values (e.g., midlevel or semantic features) as features for the classifier. A linear SVM classifier is built based on those features. We also used leave-one-out cross-validation.

The result listed in Table 10.3 show the improvement of the pattern classifier over the result obtained from low-level features. The accuracy is improved from 85% to 91% and the AUC is improved from 0.93 to 0.95. Those pattern predication values can be considered middle-level features that have semantic meaning and have demonstrated high discriminative ability.

10.4.3.3 Using Ensemble Modeling on ISIC

As this dataset is an order of magnitude larger than the PH2 data, we changed back to the ensemble modeling algorithm. For our experiments, we studied two variants of the ISIC dataset. The first includes data from lesions that are clearly benign, and the second excludes data from clearly benign lesions, which may result in a more difficult task.

Experiments with clearly benign lesions involved 391 images of melanoma, 225 images of atypical lesions, and 2536 clearly benign lesions. The resultant AP at full depth was 0.967. At the cutoff threshold of 0.5 (logistically normalized SVM scores), we measured a sensitivity of 0.987 and specificity of 0.9482. At a threshold with fixed sensitivity values of 0.99, the experiment yielded a specificity value of 0.9445.

Excluding clearly benign lesions (391 melanoma, 225 atypical), the resultant AP at full depth was 0.983. At the cutoff threshold, trained models produced a sensitivity of 0.846 and specificity of 0.9375. At a threshold with fixed sensitivity values of 0.99, the experiment yielded a specificity value of 0.594.

To demonstrate the importance of the ensemble fusion involving multiple features, we reran the experiment excluding clearly benign lesions with the single top-performing feature in that scenario. The resultant threshold sensitivity was 0.872, with a specificity of 0.901. At a threshold a with sensitivity of 0.99, the specificity is reduced to 0.438.

In addition, we studied the ensemble modeling algorithms reviewed earlier for our experiments, under three different variations dealing with data imbalance:

1. For the first approach, we simply balanced the bags used for training such that an equal number of positive and negative examples were used in each bag. Enough bags were gathered to ensure complete coverage of the data. All bags were fed to the ensemble modeling approach, which then picked the bags that optimize performance on the validation dataset.
2. For the second approach, we trained models with a single bag per feature. Data imbalance was addressed by fitting a logistic function to probabilities that positive exemplars are observed over various windows of SVM scores, as determined by using balanced n-fold cross-validation training data. In this scheme, the value of 0.5 is used as the classifier decision threshold.
3. The third and final approach exactly mimics the second approach, except that unit models are retrained on 100% of the data after ensemble model parameters have been calculated.

Figure 10.5 shows the precision–recall plot on a 50% held-out test set. In summary, we observe that

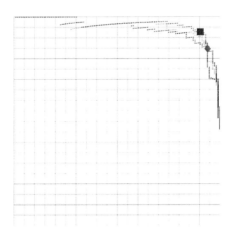

FIGURE 10.5 Precision/Recall plot on experimental dataset. The results of balanced bag, imbalanced bag and logisitc normalization approaches are printed. The graph highlights the trade of between percision and recall. The motivation here is to find the best spot to have a good balance of percision and recall. Dots on each plot has been picked to have this property. They show the threshold operating point (0 for raw SVM and 0.5 for logistic).

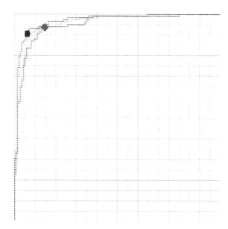

FIGURE 10.6 Receiver Operating Characteristic (ROC) plot on experimental dataset. The ROC curve demostrates the trade of true positive rate (TPR) against false positive rate (FPR) using various decision point tresholds. The plot depicts balanced bag, imbalanced bag and logisitic normalization approaches. The motivation of drawing the plot is to find the best spot to have a good balance of TPR and FPR.

- The line marked by a diamond denotes the balanced bag approach, and we set the threshold at 0. The accuracy obtained is 89.7%.
- The line marked by a circle denotes the imbalanced bag approach with ensemble logistic normalization, and we set the threshold at 0.5. The accuracy is 90.5%.
- The line marked by a square denotes the imbalanced bags with ensemble logistic normalization and unit model retraining, and we set the threshold at 0.5. The accuracy is 92.1%.

The improvement of the accuracy obtained clearly shows the effectiveness of the ensemble logistic normalization and unit model retraining. It improves the baseline performance step-by-step.

Figure 10.6 shows the corresponding ROC curve. The false positive rate $(1 - \text{specificity})$ is on the X-axis, with recall (sensitivity) on the Y-axis. As can be observed from the charts, training with single bags of all data and performing retraining after ensemble learning tends to produce slightly improved results. This makes sense, as additional examples are utilized in the unit models and subjected to the SVM hyperplane optimization.

10.5   CONCLUSION

Malignant melanoma is one of the most common and deadliest types of skin cancer worldwide. The survival rate depends highly on the stage and level of penetration: advanced and deeply penetrated melanoma is still difficult to treat, whereas early detection of superficial melanoma followed by immediate surgical excision of the lesion demonstrates good prognostic outcomes. A computer-based melanoma diagnostic system holds the potential to leverage massive amounts of experience and insight to provide more objective and quantitative analysis to help facilitate the diagnosis of melanoma in early stages. Toward this goal, this chapter presented an automatic dermoscopy image analysis system for classification of melanoma. Focusing on building a highly accurate and scalable classifier, the proposed approach extracted a variety of visual features from supplied training data, including low-level and midlevel or semantic features, which were then input to an ensemble learning pipeline to train classifiers at arbitrary scale (potentially millions of example images). Multilayer learning was performed to maximize the use of the most discriminant data patterns and features observed.

REFERENCES

1. American Cancer Society, Cancer facts and figures, available at http://www. cancer.org.
2. Australia skin cancer facts and figures, available at http://www.cancer.org.au.
3. A. C. Geller, S. M. Swetter, K. Brooks, M.-F. Demierre, and A. L. Yaroch, Screening, early detection, and trends for melanoma: Current status (2000–2006) and future directions, *Journal of the American Academy of Dermatology*, vol. 57, pp. 555–572, 2007.
4. R. P. Braun, L. E. French, and J. H. Saurat, Dermoscopy of pigmented lesions: A valuable tool in the diagnosis of melanoma, *Swiss Medical Weekly*, vol. 134, pp. 83–90, 2004.
5. C. M. Balch, A. C. Buzaid, S. Soong, M. B. Atkins, B. Michael, N. Cascinelli, D. G. Coit, I. D. Fleming et al., Final version of the American Joint Committee on Cancer staging system for cutaneous melanoma, *Journal of Clinical Oncology*, vol. 19, pp. 3635–3648, 2001.
6. C. M. Balch, S. J. Soong, J. E Gershenwald, J. F. Thompson, D. S. Reintgen, N. Cascinelli, M. Urist, K. M. McMasters, M. I. Ross, J. M. Kirkwood et al., Prognostic factors analysis of 17,600 melanoma patients: Validation of the American Joint Committee on Cancer melanoma staging system, *Journal of Clinical Oncology*, vol. 19, pp. 3622–3634, 2001.
7. R. Braun, H. Rabinovitz, M. Oliviero, A. Kopf, and J. Saurat, Dermoscopy of pigmented lesions, *Journal of the American Academy of Dermatology*, vol. 52, no. 1, pp. 109–121, 2005.
8. I. Maglogiannis and C. Doukas, Overview of advanced computer vision systems for skin lesions characterisation, *IEEE Transactions on Information Technology in Biomedicine*, vol. 13, no. 5, pp. 721–733, 2009.
9. R. J. Pariser and D. M. Pariser, Primary care physicians' errors in handling cutaneous disorders: A prospective survey, *Journal of the American Academy of Dermatology*, vol. 17, pp. 239–245, 1987.
10. H. Pehamberger, A. Steiner, and K. Wolff, In vivo epiluminescence microscopy of pigmented skin lesions. I. Pattern analysis of pigmented skin lesions, *Journal of the American Academy of Dermatology*, vol. 17, pp. 571–583, 1987.

11. W. Stolz, A. Riemann, A. B. Cognetta, L. Pillet, W. Abmayr, D. Holzel, P. Bilek, F. Nachbar, M. Landthaler, and O. Braun-Falco, ABCD rule of dermatoscopy: A new practical method for early recognition of malignant melanoma, *European Journal of Dermatology*, vol. 4, pp. 521–527, 1994.

12. S. W. Menzies, C. Ingvar, and W. H. McCarthy, A sensitivity and specificity analysis of the surface microscopy features of invasive melanoma, *Melanoma Research*, vol. 6, pp. 55–62, 1996.

13. G. Argenziano, G. Fabbrocini, P. Carli, V. D. Giorgi, E. Sammarco, and M. Delfino, Epiluminescence microscopy for the diagnosis of doubtful melanocytic skin lesions: Comparison of the ABCD rule of dermatoscopy and a new 7-point checklist based on pattern analysis, *Archives of Dermatology*, vol. 134, pp. 1563–1570, 1998.

14. J. Henning, S. Dusza, S. Wang, A. Marghoob, H. Rabinovitz, D. Polsky, and A. Kopf, The CASH (colour, architecture, symmetry, and homogeneity) algorithm for dermoscopy, *Journal of the American Academy of Dermatology*, vol. 56, no. 1, pp. 45–52, 2007.

15. C. Rosendahl, A. Cameron, I. McColl, and D. Wilkinson, Dermatoscopy in routine practice 'chaos and clues', *Australian Family Physician*, vol. 41, pp. 482–487, 2012.

16. P. Bourne, C. Rosendahl, J. Keir, and A. Cameron, BLINCK: A diagnostic algorithm for skin cancer diagnosis combining clinical features with dermatoscopy findings, *Dermatology Practical and Conceptual*, vol. 2, pp. 55–61, 2012.

17. M. Binder, M. Schwarz, A. Winkler, A. Steiner, A. Kaider, K. Wolff, Klaus, H. Pehamberger et al., Epiluminescence microscopy: A useful tool for the diagnosis of pigmented skin lesions for formally trained dermatologists, *Archives of Dermatology*, vol. 131, no. 3, pp. 286–291, 1995.

18. G. Argenziano, H. P. Soyer, S. Chimenti, R. Talamini, R. Corona, F. Sera, M. Binder et al., Dermoscopy of pigmented skin lesions: Results of a consensus meeting via the Internet, *Journal of the American Academy of Dermatology*, vol. 48, pp. 679–693, 2003.

19. J. Scharcanski and M. E. Celebi, *Computer Vision Techniques for the Diagnosis of Skin Cancer*, Springer, Berlin, Germany, 2013.

20. K. Korotkov and R. Garcia, Methodological review: Computerized analysis of pigmented skin lesions: A review, *Artificial Intelligence in Medicine*, vol. 56, pp. 69–90, 2012.

21. M. E. Celebi, W. V. Stoecker, and R. H. Moss, Advances in skin cancer image analysis, *Computerized Medical Imaging and Graphics*, vol. 35, no. 2, pp. 83–84, 2011.

22. V. Skladnev, A. Gutenev, S. S. W. Menzies, L. Bischof, G. Talbot, E. Breen, and M. Buckley, Diagnostic feature extraction in dermatological examination, patent number 10/478078, United States, 2004.

23. S. W. Menzies, L. Bischof, H. Talbot, A. Gutenev, M. Avramidis, W. Michelle, L. Livian, K. M. Sing et al., The performance of SolarScan. An automated dermoscopy image analysis instrument for the diagnosis of primary melanoma, *Archives of Dermatology*, vol. 141, pp. 1388–1397, 2005.

24. M. J. Jamora, B. D. Wainwright, S. A. Meehan, and J. C. Bystryn, Improved identification of potentially dangerous pigmented skin lesions by computerised image analysis, *Archives of Dermatology*, vol. 139, pp. 195–198, 2003.

25. P. Rubegni, M. Burroni, G. Cevenini, R. Perotti, G. Dell'Eva, P. Barbini, M. Fimiani, and L. Andreassi, Digital dermoscopy analysis and artificial neural network for the differentiation of clinically atypical pigmented skin lesions: A retrospective study, *Journal of Investigative Dermatology*, vol. 119, pp. 471–474, 2002.

26. K. Hoffmann, T. Gambichler, and A. Rick, Diagnostic and neural analysis of skin cancer (DANAOS): A multicentre study for collection and computer-aided analysis of data from pigmented skin lesions using digital dermoscopy, *British Journal of Dermatology*, vol. 149, pp. 801–809, 2003.

27. M. Elbaum, A. Kopf, H. Rabinovitz, R. Langley, and H. Kamino, Automatic differentiation of melanoma from melanocytic nevi with multispectral digital dermoscopy: A feasibility study, *Journal of the American Academy of Dermatology*, vol. 44, pp. 207–218, 2001.

28. M. Elbaum, Computer-aided melanoma diagnosis, *Dermatologic Clinics*, vol. 20, pp. 735–747, 2002.

29. D. Gutkowicz-Krusin, M. Elbaum, A. Jacobs, S. Keem, A. W. Kopf, H. Kamino, S. Wang, P. Rubin, H. Rabinovitz, M. Oliviero et al., Precision of automatic measurements of pigmented skin lesion parameters with a melaFind (TM) multispectral digital dermoscope, *Melanoma Research*, vol. 10, pp. 563–570, 2000.

30. M. Moncrieff, S. Cotton, E. Claridge, and P. Hall, Spectrophotometric intracutaneous analysis: A new technique for imaging pigmented skin lesions, *British Journal of Dermatology*, vol. 146, pp. 448–457, 2002.

31. S. Q. Wang, H. Rabinovitz, A. W. Kopf, and M. Oliviero, Current technologies for the in vivo diagnosis of cutaneous melanomas, *Clinics in Dermatology*, vol. 22, pp. 217–222, 2004.

32. W. Stoecker, R. Moss, J. Stanley, X. Chen, K. Gupta, R. Narayana, B. Shrestha, and P. Jella, Automatic detection of critical dermoscopy features for malignant melanoma diagnosis, patent number 11/421031, United States, 2006.

33. T. Schindewolf, R. Schiffner, W. Stolz, R. Albert, W. Abmayr, and H. Harms, Evaluation of different image acquisition techniques for a computer vision system in the diagnosis of malignant melanoma, *Clinics in Dermatology*, vol. 31, pp. 33–41, 1994.

34. J. Boldrick, C. Layton, J. Nguyen, and S. Swetter, Evaluation of digital dermoscopy in a pigmented lesion clinic: Clinician versus computer assessment of malignancy risk, *Journal of the American Academy of Dermatology*, vol. 56, no. 3, pp. 417–421, 2007.

35. H. Ganster, A. Pinz, R. Rohrer, E. Wildling, M. Binder, and H. Kittler, Automated melanoma recognition, *IEEE Transactions on Medical Imaging*, vol. 20, pp. 233–239, 2001.

36. S. Dreiseitl, L. Ohno-Machado, H. Kittler, S. Vinterbo, H. Billhardt, and M. Binder, A comparison of machine learning methods for the diagnosis of pigmented skin lesions, *Journal of Biomedical Informatics*, vol. 34, pp. 28–36, 2001.

37. M. E. Celebi, H. Kingravi, B. Uddin, H. Iyatomi, Y. A. Aslandogan, W. V. Stoecker, and R. H. Moss, A methodological approach to the classification of dermoscopy images, *Computerized Medical Imaging and Graphics*, vol. 31, pp. 362–373, 2007.

38. T. Hwanga, W. Leeb, S. Huad, and J. Fang, Cisplatin encapsulated in phosphatidylethanolamine liposomes enhances the in vitro cytotoxicity and in vivo intratumor drug accumulation against melanomas, *Journal of Dermatological Science*, vol. 46, pp. 11–20, 2007.

39. A. P. Dhawan, Early detection of cutaneous malignant melanoma by three dimensional nevoscopy, *Computer Methods and Programs in Biomedicine*, vol. 21, pp. 59–68, 1985.

40. S. V. Patwardhan, S. Dai, and A. P. Dhawan, Multi-spectral image analysis and classification of melanoma using fuzzy membership based partitions, *Computerized Medical Imaging and Graphics*, vol. 29, pp. 287–296, 2005.

41. X. Yuan, Z. Yang, G. Zouridakis, and N. Mullani, SVM-based texture classification and application to early melanoma detection, in *28th Annual International Conference of the IEEE Engineering in Medicine and Biology Society*, vol. 3, pp. 4775–4778, 2006.

42. R. G. B. Langley, M. Rajadhyaksha, P. J. Dwyer, A. J. Sober, T. J. Flotte, R. R. Anderson et al., Confocal scanning laser microscopy of benign and malignant melanocytic skin lesions in vivo, *Journal of the American Academy of Dermatology*, New York, NY, vol. 45, pp. 365–376, 2001.

43. K. J. Busam, K. Hester, C. Charles, D. L. Sachs, C. R. Antonescu, S. Gonzalez, A. C. Halpern et al., Detection of clinically amelanotic malignant melanoma and assessment of its margins by in vivo confocal scanning laser microscopy, *Archives of Dermatology*, vol. 137, pp. 923–929, 2001.

44. S. W. Menzies, Cutaneous melanoma: Making a clinical diagnosis, present and future, *Dermatologic Therapy*, vol. 19, pp. 32–39, 2006.

45. N. Lassau, A. Spatz, M. F. Avril, A. Tardivon, M. A. Anne, G. Mamelle, D. Vanel, L. J. Daniel et al., Value of high-frequency US for preoperative assessment of skin tumors, *Radiographics*, vol. 17, pp. 1559–1565, 1997.

46. C. C. Harland, S. G. Kale, P. Jackson, P. S. Mortimer, J. C. Bamber et al., Differentiation of common benign pigmented skin lesions from melanoma by high-resolution ultrasound, *British Journal of Dermatology*, vol. 143, pp. 281–289, 2000.

47. K. Hoffmann, J. Jung, S. Gammal, and P. Altmeyer, Malignant melanoma in 20-mhz b scan sonography, *Dermatology*, vol. 185, pp. 40–55, 1992.

48. J. Solomon, S. Mavinkurve, D. Cox, and R. M. Summers, Computer-assisted detection of subcutaneous melanomas, *Academic Radiology*, vol. 21, pp. 678–685, 2004.

49. C. Pleiss, J. Risse, H. Biersack, and H. Bender, Role of FDG-PET in the assessment of survival prognosis in melanoma, *Cancer Biotherapy and Radiopharmaceuticals*, vol. 22, pp. 740–747, 2007.

50. I. K. Daftari, E. Aghaian, J. O'Brien, W. Dillon, and T. L. Phillips, 3D MRI-based tumor delineation of ocular melanoma and its comparison with conventional techniques, *Medical Physics*, vol. 32, pp. 3355–3362, 2005.

51. P. Aberg, I. Nicander, J. Hansson, P. Geladi, U. Holmgren, and S. Ollmar, Skin cancer identification using multifrequency electrical impedance: A potential screening tool, *IEEE Transactions on Biomedical Engineering*, vol. 51, pp. 2097–2102, 2004.

52. S. Sigurdsson, P. A. Philipsen, L. K. Hansen, J. Larsen, M. Gniadecka, and H. C. Wulf, Detection of skin cancer by classification of Raman spectra, *IEEE Transactions on Biomedical Engineering*, vol. 51, pp. 1784–1793, 2004.

53. M. Sonka, V. Hlavac, and R. Boyle, *Image Processing, Analysis, and Machine Vision*, Cengage-Engineering, 2007.
54. R. Haralick and L. Shapiro, Image segmentation techniques, *Computer Vision, Graphics, and Image Processing*, vol. 29, pp. 100–132, 1985.
55. M. E. Celebi, H. Iyatomi, G. Schaefer, and W. V. Stoecker, Lesion border detection in dermoscopy images, *Computerised Medical Imaging and Graphics*, vol. 33, no. 2, pp. 148–153, 2009.
56. R. Garnavi, M. Aldeen, M. E. Celebi, S. Finch, and G. Varigos, Border detection in dermoscopy images using hybrid thresholding on optimised colour channels, *Computerized Medical Imaging and Graphics*, vol. 35, pp. 105–115, 2011.
57. H. Iyatomi, H. Oka, M. Saito, A. Miyake, M. Kimoto, J. Yamagami, S. Kobayashi et al., Quantitative assessment of tumour extraction from dermoscopy images and evaluation of computer-based extraction methods for an automatic melanoma diagnostic system, *Melanoma Research*, vol. 16, no. 2, pp. 183–190, 2006.
58. T. K. Lee, V. Ng, D. McLean, A. Coldman, and R. G. J. Sale, A multi-stage segmentation method for images of skin lesions, in *IEEE Pacific Rim Conference on Communications, Computers, and Signal Processing*, British Columbia, Canada, pp. 602–605, 1995.
59. M. Hintz-Madsen, L. K. Hansen, J. Larsen, and K. Drzewiecki, A probabilistic neural network framework for detection of malignant melanoma, in *Artificial Neural Networks in Cancer Diagnosis, Prognosis and Patient Management*, pp. 141–183, CRC Press, Boca Raton, FL, 2001.
60. A. Sbonera, E. Blanzieria, C. Ecchera, P. Bauerb, M. Cristofolinib, G. Zumianib, and S. Fortia, A knowledge based system for early melanoma diagnosis support, in *Proceedings of the 6th Intelligent Data Analysis in Medicine and Pharmacology (IDAMAP) Workshop*, London, UK, 2001.
61. G. Hance, S. Umbaugh, R. Moss, and W. V. Stoecker, Unsupervised colour image segmentation: With application to skin tumor borders, *IEEE Engineering in Medicine and Biology Magazine*, vol. 15, pp. 104–111, 1996.
62. P. Schmid, Segmentation of digitised dermatoscopic images by two-dimensional colour clustering, *IEEE Transactions on Medical Imaging*, vol. 18, no. 2, pp. 164–171, 1999.
63. R. Cucchiara, C. Grana, S. Seidenari, and G. Pellacani, Exploiting colour and topological features for region segmentation with recursive fuzzy c-means, *Machine Graphics and Vision*, vol. 11, pp. 169–182, 2002.
64. H. Galda, H. Murao, H. Tamaki, and S. Kitamura, Skin image segmentation using a self-organising map and genetic algorithms, *Transactions of the Institute of Electrical Engineers of Japan, Part C*, vol. 123, pp. 2056–2062, 2002.
65. P. Schmid-Saugeon, J. Guillod, and J. P. Thiran, Towards a computer-aided diagnosis system for pigmented skin lesions, *Computerized Medical Imaging and Graphics*, vol. 27, pp. 69–72, 2003.
66. R. Melli, C. Grana, and R. Cucchiara, Comparison of colour clustering algorithms for segmentation of dermatological images, in *Proceedings of the SPIE Medical Imaging Conference*, San Diego, CA, vol. 6144, pp. 3S1–3S9, 2006.
67. D. Delgado, C. Butakoff, B. K. Ersboll, and W. V. S. WV, Independent histogram pursuit for segmentation of skin lesions, *IEEE Transactions on Biomedical Engineering*, vol. 55, pp. 157–161, 2008.

68. H. Zhou, M. Chen, L. Zou, R. Gass, L. Ferris, L. Drogowski, and J. M. Rehg, Spatially constrained segmentation of dermoscopy images, in *5th IEEE International Symposium on Biomedical Imaging*, Paris, France, pp. 800–803, 2008.

69. W. E. Denton, A. W. G. Duller, and P. J. Fish, Boundary detection for skin lesions: An edge focusing algorithm, in *5th IEEE International Conference on Image Processing and Its Applications*, Edinburgh, Scotland, pp. 399–403, 1995.

70. Q. Abbas, M. E. Celebi, and I. F. Garcia, Skin tumor area extraction using an improved dynamic programming approach, *Skin Research and Technology*, vol. 18, no. 2, pp. 133–142, 2012.

71. Q. Abbas, M. E. Celebi, I. F. Garcia, and M. Rashid, Lesion border detection in dermoscopy images using dynamic programming, *Skin Research and Technology*, vol. 17, no. 1, pp. 91–100, 2011.

72. A. J. Round, A. W. Duller, and P. Fish, Colour segmentation for lesion classification, in *Proceedings of the 19th Annual International Conference of the IEEE Engineering in Medicine and Biology Society*, Chicago, IL, vol. 2, pp. 582–585, 1997.

73. J. Gao, J. Zhang, and M. G. Fleming, Segmentation of dermatoscopic images by stabilised inverse diffusion equations, in *IEEE International Conference on Image Processing (ICIP 1998)*, Chicago, IL, vol. 3, pp. 823–827, 1998.

74. M. E. Celebi, Y. A. Aslandogan, W. V. Stoecker, H. Iyatomi, H. Oka, and X. Chen, Unsupervised border detection in dermoscopy images, *Skin Research and Technology*, vol. 13, pp. 454–462, 2007.

75. M. E. Celebi, H. A. Kingravi, H. Iyatomi, Y. A. Aslandogan, W. V. Stoecker, R. H. Moss, J. M. Malters et al., Border detection in dermoscopy images using statistical region merging, *Skin Research and Technology*, vol. 14, pp. 347–353, 2008.

76. H. Wang, R. H. Moss, X. Chen, R. J. Stanley, W. V. Stoecker, M. E. Celebi, J. M. Malters et al., Modified watershed technique and post-processing for segmentation of skin lesions in dermoscopy images, *Computerized Medical Imaging and Graphics*, vol. 35, no. 2, pp. 116–120, 2011.

77. H. Wang, X. Chen, R. H. Moss, R. J. Stanley, W. V. Stoecker, M. E. Celebi, T. M. Szalapski et al., Segmentation of skin lesions in dermoscopy images using a watershed technique, *Skin Research and Technology*, vol. 16, pp. 378–384, 2010.

78. P. Schmid, Lesion detection in dermatoscopic images using anisotropic diffusion and morphological flooding, in *IEEE International Conference on Image Processing (ICIP 1999)*, Kobe, Japan, vol. 3, pp. 449–453, 1999.

79. H. Zhou, X. Li, G. Schaefer, M. E. Celebi, and P. Miller, Mean shift based gradient vector flow for image segmentation, *Computer Vision and Image Understanding*, vol. 117, no. 9, pp. 1004–1016, 2013.

80. H. Zhou, G. Schaefer, M. E. Celebi, F. Lin, and T. Liu, Gradient vector flow with mean shift for skin lesion segmentation, *Computerized Medical Imaging and Graphics*, vol. 35, no. 2, pp. 121–127, 2011.

81. Y. V. Haeghen, J. M. Naeyaert, and I. Lemahieu, Development of a dermatological workstation: Preliminary results on lesion segmentation in CIE l*a*b* colour space, in *International Conference on Colour in Graphics and Image Processing*, Saint-Etienne, France, vol. 1, pp. 6572–6575, 2000.

82. B. Erkol, R. Moss, R. Stanley, W. Stoecker, and E. Hvatum, Automatic lesion boundary detection in dermoscopy images using gradient vector flow snakes, *Skin Research and Technology*, vol. 11, pp. 17–26, 2005.

83. T. Mendonça, A. R. S. Marçal, A. Vieira, J. C. Nascimento, M. Silveira, J. S. Marques, and J. Rozeira, Comparison of segmentation methods for automatic diagnosis of dermoscopy images, in *Proceedings of the 29th Annual International Conference of the IEEE Engineering in Medicine and Biology Society*, Lyon, France, pp. 6572–6575, 2007.

84. T. Donadey and A. Giron, Boundary detection of black skin tumors using an adaptive radial-based approach, in *Proceedings of the SPIE Medical Imaging Conference*, San Diego, CA, vol. 3379, pp. 810–816, 2000.

85. A. R. Sadri, M. Zekri, S. Sadri, N. Gheissari, M. Mokhtari, and F. Kolahdouzan, Segmentation of dermoscopy images using wavelet networks, *IEEE Transactions on Biomedical Engineering*, vol. 60, no. 4, pp. 1134–1141, 2013.

86. P. Pagadala, Tumor border detection in epiluminescence microscopy images, Master's thesis, Department of Electrical and Computer Engineering, University of Missouri, Rolla, August 1998.

87. A. A. A. Al-abayechi, R. Logeswaran, W. H. Tan, and X. Guo, Lesion border detection in dermoscopy images using bilateral filter, in *2013 IEEE International Conference on Signal and Image Processing Applications*, Kuala Lumpur, Malaysia, pp. 365–368, 2013.

88. T. Donadey, C. Serruys, A. Giron, and W. Woelker, Image segmentation based on adaptive 3-D-analysis of the CIE-L*a*b colour space, in *Proceedings of the SPIE Visual Communications and Image Processing*, Orlando, FL, vol. 2727, pp. 1197–1203, 1996.

89. M. E. Celebi, Q. Wen, S. Hwang, H. Iyatomi, and G. Schaefer, Lesion border detection in dermoscopy images using ensembles of thresholding methods, *Skin Research and Technology*, vol. 19, no. 1, pp. e252–e258, 2013.

90. D. Ming, Q. Wen, J. Chen, and W. Liu, A generalized fusion approach for segmenting dermoscopy images using Markov random field, in *2013 6th International Congress on Image and Signal Processing (CISP)*, Hangzhou, China, vol. 1, pp. 532–537, 2013.

91. H. Zhou, G. Schaefer, A. Sadka, and M. E. Celebi, Anisotropic mean shift based fuzzy c-means segmentation of dermoscopy images, *IEEE Journal of Selected Topics in Signal Processing*, vol. 3, no. 1, pp. 26–34, 2009.

92. H. Iyatomi, H. Oka, M. E. Celebi, M. Hashimoto, M. Hagiwara, M. Tanaka, and K. Ogawa, An improved Internet-based melanoma screening system with dermatologist-like tumor area extraction algorithm, *Computerized Medical Imaging and Graphics*, vol. 32, no. 7, pp. 566–579, 2008.

93. N. Otsu, A threshold selection method from gray-level histograms, *IEEE Transactions on Systems, Man, and Cybernetics*, vol. 9, no. 1, pp. 62–66, 1979.

94. D. Ruiz, V. Berenguer, A. Soriano, and B. Sánchez, A decision support system for the diagnosis of melanoma: A comparative approach, *Expert Systems with Applications*, vol. 38, no. 12, pp. 15217–15223, 2011.

95. Y. D. Y and B. S. Manjunath, Unsupervised segmentation of colour-texture regions in images and video, *IEEE Transactions on Pattern Analysis and Machine Intelligence*, vol. 23, pp. 800–810, 2001.

96. T. Lee, V. Ng, R. Gallagher, A. Coldman, and D. McLean, DullRazor: A software approach to hair removal from images, *Computers in Biology and Medicine*, vol. 27, pp. 533–543, 1997.

97. A. Amelio and C. Pizzuti, Skin lesion image segmentation using a color genetic algorithm, in *Proceedings of the Fifteenth Annual Conference Companion*

on Genetic and Evolutionary Computation, Amsterdam, Netherlands, pp. 1471–1478, 2013.

98. Q. Wen, D. Ming, J. Chen, and W. Liu, A superpixel based post-processing approach for segmenting dermoscopy images, in *2013 Sixth International Conference on Advanced Computational Intelligence (ICACI)*, pp. 155–158, 2013.

99. X. Ren and J. Malik, Learning a classification model for segmentation, in *Proceedings of the Ninth IEEE International Conference on Computer Vision (ICCV '03)*, Hangzhou, China, vol. 2, pp. 10–17, 2003.

100. O. Sarrafzade, M. Baygi, and P. Ghassemi, Skin lesion detection in dermoscopy images using wavelet transform and morphology operations, in *2010 17th Iranian Conference of Biomedical Engineering (ICBME)*, Isfahan, Iran, pp. 1–4, 2010.

101. A. T. Beuren, R. Janasieivicz, G. Pinheiro, N. Grando, and J. Facon, Skin melanoma segmentation by morphological approach, in *Proceedings of the International Conference on Advances in Computing, Communications and Informatics*, Chennai, India, pp. 972–978, 2012.

102. W. Stolz, O. Braun-Falco, P. Bilek, M. Landthaler, W. H. C. Burgdorf, and A. B. Cognetta, *Colour Atlas of Dermatoscopy*, 2nd ed., vol. 1, Blackwell, 2002.

103. W. V. Stoecker, W. W. Li, and R. H. Moss, Automatic detection of asymmetry in skin tumors, *Computerized Medical Imaging and Graphics*, vol. 16, no. 3, pp. 191–197, 1992.

104. I. Maglogiannis and D. I. Kosmopoulos, Computational vision systems for the detection of malignant melanoma, *Oncology Reports*, vol. 15, pp. 1027–1032, 2006.

105. S. Seidenari, G. Pellacani, and C. Grana, Asymmetry in dermoscopic melanocytic lesion images: A computer description based on colour distribution, *Acta Dermato-Venereologica*, vol. 86, pp. 123–128, 2006.

106. Y. Chang, R. J. Stanley, R. H. Moss, and W. V. Stoecker, A systematic heuristic approach for feature selection for melanoma discrimination using clinical images, *Skin Research and Technology*, vol. 11, pp. 165–178, 2005.

107. Z. She, Y. Liu, and A. Damatoa, Combination of features from skin pattern and ABCD analysis for lesion classification, *Skin Research and Technology*, vol. 13, pp. 25–33, 2007.

108. K. Clawson, P. Morrow, B. Scotney, D. McKenna, and O. Dolan, Determination of optimal axes for skin lesion asymmetry quantification, in *IEEE International Conference on Image Processing (ICIP 2007)*, San Antonio, TX, vol. 2, pp. 453–456, 2007.

109. V. Ng, B. Fung, and T. K. Lee, Determining the asymmetry of skin lesion with fuzzy borders, *Computers in Biology and Medicine*, vol. 35, pp. 103–120, 2005.

110. L. Andreassi, R. Perotti, M. Burroni, G. Dell 'Eva, and M. Biagioli, Computerized image analysis of pigmented lesions, *Chronica Dermatologica*, vol. 5, pp. 11–24, 1995.

111. V. Ng and D. Cheung, Measuring asymmetries of skin lesions, in *IEEE International Conference on Systems, Man, and Cybernetics*, Orlando, FL, vol. 5, pp. 4211–4216, 1997.

112. K. M. Clawson, P. J. Morrow, B. W. Scotney, D. J. McKenna, and O. M. Dolan, Computerised skin lesion surface analysis for pigment asymmetry

quantification, in *IEEE International Conference on Machine Vision and Image Processing (IMVIP 2007)*, Kildare, Ireland, pp. 75–82, 2007.

113. A. G. Manousaki, A. G. Manios, E. I. Tsompanaki, Panayiotides, G. John, D. D. Tsiftsis, A. K. Kostaki, and A. D. Tosca, A simple digital image processing system to aid in melanoma diagnosis in an everyday melanocytic skin lesion unit: A preliminary report, *International Journal of Dermatology*, vol. 45, pp. 402–410, 2006.

114. T.-B. Holmstrom, A survey and evaluation of features for the diagnosis of malignant melanoma, Master's thesis, Department of Computing Science, Umea University, Umea, Sweden, 2005.

115. A. Bono, S. Tomatis, C. Bartoli, G. Tragni, G. Radaelli, A. Maurichi, and R. Marchesini, The ABCD system of melanoma detection: A spectrophotometric analysis of the asymmetry, border, colour, and dimension, *Cancer*, vol. 85, pp. 72–77, 1999.

116. H. Zabrodsky, S. Peleg, and D. Avnir, Symmetry as a continuous feature, *IEEE Transactions on Pattern Analysis and Machine Intelligence*, vol. 17, pp. 1154–1166, 1995.

117. E. Claridge, P. Hall, M. Keefe, and J. P. Allen, Shape analysis for classification of malignant melanoma, *Journal of Biomedical Engineering*, vol. 14, pp. 229–234, 1992.

118. S. Seidenari, G. Pellacani, and C. Grana, Pigment distribution in melanocytic lesion images: A digital parameter to be employed for computer-aided diagnosis, *Skin Research and Technology*, vol. 11, pp. 236–241, 2005.

119. G. R. Day, How blurry is that border? An investigation into algorithmic reproduction of skin lesion border cut-off, *Computerized Medical Imaging and Graphics*, vol. 24, pp. 69–72, 2000.

120. T. K. Lee, M. S. Atkins, R. Gallagher, C. E. Macaulay, A. Coldman, and D. I. McLean, Describing the structural shape of melanocytic lesions, in *Proceedings of the SPIE Medical Imaging Conference*, San Diego, CA, vol. 3661, pp. 1170–1179, 1999.

121. T. K. Lee and M. S. Atkins, New approach to measure border irregularity for melanocytic lesions, in *Proceedings of the SPIE Medical Imaging Conference*, San Diego, CA, vol. 3979, pp. 668–675, 2000.

122. T. K. Lee, D. I. McLean and M. S. Atkins, Irregularity index: A new border irregularity measure for cutaneous melanocytic lesions, *Medical Image Analysis*, vol. 7, pp. 47–64, 2003.

123. S. M. Chung and Q. Wang, Content-based retrieval and data mining of a skin cancer image database, in *International Conference on Information Technology: Coding and Computing (ITCC 2001)*, Las Vegas, NV, pp. 611–615, 2001.

124. Y. Cheng, R. Swamisai, S. E. Umbaugh, R. H. Moss, W. V. Stoecker, S. Teegala, and S. K. Srinivasan, Skin lesion classification using relative colour features, *Skin Research and Technology*, vol. 14, pp. 53–64, 2008.

125. T. K. Lee, Measuring border irregularity and shape of cutaneous melanocytic lesions, PhD thesis, School of Computing Science, Simon Fraser University, Burnaby, British Columbia, Canada, 2001.

126. I. Maglogiannis, S. Pavlopoulos, and D. Koutsouris, An integrated computer supported acquisition, handling, and characterisation system for pigmented skin lesions in dermatological images, *IEEE Transactions on Information Technology in Biomedicine*, vol. 9, pp. 86–98, 2005.

127. V. Ng and T. K. Lee, Measuring border irregularities of skin lesions using fractal dimensions, in *SPIE Electronic Imaging and Multimedia Systems Conference*, Beijing, China, vol. 2898, pp. 64–72, 1996.

128. B. S. Aribisala and E. Claridge, A border irregularity measure using a modified conditional entropy method as a malignant melanoma predictor, in *Image Analysis and Recognition*, vol. 3656 of *Lecture Notes in Computer Science*, pp. 914–921, Springer, Berlin, 2005.

129. S. Seidenari, G. Pellacani, and C. Grana, Computer description of colours in dermoscopic melanocytic lesion images reproducing clinical assessment, *British Journal of Dermatology*, vol. 149, pp. 523–529, 2003.

130. Y. Faziloglu, R. J. Stanley, R. H. Moss, W. V. Stoecker, and R. P. McLean, Colour histogram analysis for melanoma discrimination in clinical images, *Skin Research and Technology*, vol. 9, pp. 147–155, 2003.

131. S. E. Umbaugh, R. H. Moss, and W. V. Stoecker, Automatic colour segmentation of images with application to detection of variegated colouring in skin tumours, *IEEE Engineering in Medicine and Biology*, Atlanta, GA, vol. 8, pp. 43–52, 1989.

132. J. Chen, R. J. Stanley, R. H. Moss, and W. V. Stoecker, Colour analysis of skin lesion regions for melanoma discrimination in clinical images, *Skin Research and Technology*, vol. 9, pp. 94–104, 2003.

133. R. J. Stanley, R. H. Moss, W. V. Stoecker, and C. Aggarwal, A fuzzy-based histogram analysis technique for skin lesion discrimination in dermatology clinical images, *Computerized Medical Imaging and Graphics*, vol. 27, no. 27, pp. 387–396, 2003.

134. R. J. Stanley, W. V. Stoecker, and R. H. Moss, A relative colour approach to colour discrimination for malignant melanoma detection in dermoscopy images, *Skin Research and Technology*, vol. 13, pp. 62–72, 2007.

135. M. E. Celebi, H. Iyatomi, W. V. Stoecker, R. H. Moss, H. S. Rabinovitz, G. Argenziano, and H. P. Soyer, Automatic detection of blue-white veil and related structures in dermoscopy images, *Computerized Medical Imaging and Graphics*, vol. 32, no. 8, pp. 670–677, 2008.

136. I. Maglogiannis, E. Zafiropoulos, and C. Kyranoudis, Intelligent segmentation and classification of pigmented skin lesions in dermatological images, in *Advances in Artificial Intelligence*, vol. 3955 of *Lecture Notes in Computer Science*, pp. 214–223, Springer, Berlin, 2006.

137. C. Grana, R. Cucchiara, G. Pellacani, and S. Seidenari, Line detection and texture characterisation of network patterns, in *Proceedings of the 18th International Conference on Pattern Recognition (ICPR 2006)*, Hong Kong, China, vol. 2, pp. 275–278, 2006.

138. S. Fischer, P. Schmid, and G. Joe, Analysis of skin lesions with pigmented networks, in *Proceedings of International Conference on Image Processing*, Lausanne, Switzerland, vol. 1, pp. 323–326, 1996.

139. R. C. Gonzalez and P. Wintz, *Digital Image Processing*, Addison-Wesley, 1987.

140. M. Fleming, C. Steger, A. B. Cognetta, and J. Zhang, Analysis of the network pattern in dermatoscopic images, *Skin Research and Technology*, vol. 5, pp. 42–48, 1999.

141. A. Murali, W. V. Stoecker, and R. H. Moss, Detection of solid pigment in dermatoscopy images using texture analysis, *Skin Research and Technology*, vol. 6, pp. 193–198, 2000.

142. W. V. Stoecker, M. Wronkiewiecz, R. Chowdhury, R. J. Stanley, J. Xua, A. Bangert, B. Shrestha et al., Detection of granularity in dermoscopy images of malignant melanoma using colour and texture features, *Computerized Medical Imaging and Graphics*, vol. 35, pp. 144–147, 2011.

143. M. Sadeghi, M. Razmara, T. K. Lee, and M. Atkins, A novel method for detection of pigment network in dermoscopic images using graphs, *Computerized Medical Imaging and Graphics*, vol. 35, no. 2, pp. 137–143, 2011.

144. M. Sadeghi, T. Lee, D. Mclean, H. Lui, and M. Atkins, Detection and analysis of irregular streaks in dermoscopic images of skin lesions, *IEEE Transactions on Medical Imaging*, vol. 32, pp. 849–861, 2013.

145. C. Barata, J. Marques, and J. Rozeira, A system for the detection of pigment network in dermoscopy images using directional filters, *IEEE Transactions on Biomedical Engineering*, vol. 59, pp. 2744–2754, 2012.

146. J. L. García Arroyo and B. N. García Zapirain, Detection of pigment network in dermoscopy images using supervised machine learning and structural analysis, *Computers in Biology and Medicine*, vol. 44, pp. 144–157, 2014.

147. Q. Abbas, M. E. Celebi, C. Serrano, I. Fondón García, and G. Ma, Pattern classification of dermoscopy images: A perceptually uniform model, *Pattern Recognition*, vol. 46, pp. 86–97, 2013.

148. A. Saez, C. Serrano, and B. Acha, Model-based classification methods of global patterns in dermoscopic images, *IEEE Transactions on Medical Imaging*, vol. 33, pp. 1137–1147, 2014.

149. R. Amelard, A. Wong, and D. A. Clausi, Extracting high-level intuitive features (HLIF) for classifying skin lesions using standard camera images, in *9th Conference on Computer and Robot Vision*, Toronto, pp. 396–403, 2012.

150. R. Amelard, A. Wong, and D. A. Clausi, Extracting morphological high-level intuitive features (HLIF) for enhancing skin lesion classification, in *34th Annual International Conference of the IEEE Engineering in Medicine and Biology Society*, San Diego, CA, pp. 4458–4461, 2012.

151. R. Amelard, J. Glaister, A. Wong, and D. A. Clausi, *Melanoma Decision Support Using Lighting-Corrected Intuitive Feature Models*, Series in Bioengineering, pp. 193–219, Springer, Berlin, 2014.

152. R. Amelard, High-level intuitive features (HLIFs) for melanoma detection, Master of Applied Science thesis, Department of Systems Design Engineering, University of Waterloo, Waterloo, Ontario, Canada, 2013.

153. H. Liu and L. Yu, Toward integrating feature selection algorithms for classification and clustering, *IEEE Transactions on Knowledge and Data Engineering*, vol. 17, pp. 491–502, 2005.

154. M. Dash and H. Liu, Feature selection for classification, *Intelligent Data Analysis*, vol. 1, pp. 679–693, 1997.

155. H. Liu and H. Motoda, *Feature Selection for Knowledge Discovery and Data Mining*, Kluwer Academic, Boston, 1998.

156. P. Langley, Selection of relevant features in machine learning, in *AAAI Fall Symposium on Relevance*, New Orleans, Louisiana, pp. 140–144, 1994.

157. M. Dash, K. Choi, P. Scheuermann, and H. Liu, Feature selection for clustering: A filter solution, in *Second IEEE International Conference on Data Mining (ICDM '02)*, pp. 115–122, 2002.

158. M. A. Hall, Correlation-based feature selection for discrete and numeric class machine learning, in *17th International Conference on Machine Learning*, pp. 359–366, 2000.

159. L. Yu and H. Liu, Feature selection for high-dimensional data: A fast correlation-based filter solution, in *20th International Conference on Machine Learning*, pp. 856–863, 2003.

160. R. Kohavi and G. H. John, Wrappers for feature subset selection, *Artificial Intelligence*, vol. 97, pp. 273–324, 1997.

161. R. Caruana and D. Freitag, Greedy attribute selection, in *11th International Conference on Machine Learning*, pp. 28–36, 1994.

162. J. G. Dy and C. E. Brodley, Feature subset selection and order identification for unsupervised learning, in *17th International Conference on Machine Learning*, pp. 247–254, 2000.

163. Y. Kim, W. Street, and F. Menczer, Feature selection for unsupervised learning via evolutionary search, in *Sixth ACM SIGKDD International Conference on Knowledge Discovery and Data Mining*, pp. 365–369, 2000.

164. S. Das, Filters, wrappers and a boosting-based hybrid for feature selection, in *18th International Conference on Machine Learning*, pp. 74–81, 2001.

165. A. Y. Ng, On feature selection: Learning with exponentially many irrelevant features as training examples, in *15th International Conference on Machine Learning*, pp. 404–412, 1998.

166. E. Xing, M. Jordan, and R. Karp, Feature selection for high-dimensional genomic microarray data, in *18th International Conference on Machine Learning*, pp. 601–608, 2001.

167. R. Walvick, K. Patel, S. Patwardhan, and A. Dhawan, Classification of melanoma using wavelet-transform-based optimal feature set, in *Proceedings of the SPIE Medical Imaging Conference*, San Diego, CA, vol. 5370, pp. 944–951, 2004.

168. T. Roß, H. Handels, J. Kreusch, H. Busche, H. Wolf, and S. Pöppl, Automatic classification of skin tumours with high resolution surface profiles, in *Computer Analysis of Images and Patterns* (V. Hlavac and R. Sara, eds.), vol. 970 of *Lecture Notes in Computer Science*, pp. 368–375, Springer, Berlin, 1995.

169. A. Nimunkar, A. Dhawan, P. Relue, and S. Patwardhan, Wavelet and statistical analysis for melanoma, in *Proceedings of the SPIE Medical Imaging Conference*, San Diego, CA, vol. 4684, pp. 1346–1352, 2002.

170. M. E. Celebi, H. A. Kingravi, B. Uddin, H. Iyatomi, Y. A. Aslandogan, W. V. Stoecker, and R. H. Moss, A methodological approach to the classification of dermoscopy images, *Computerized Medical Imaging and Graphics*, vol. 31, pp. 362–373, 2007.

171. H. Iyatomi, H. Oka, M. E. Celebi, M. Tanaka, and K. Ogawa, Parameterisation of dermoscopic findings for the Internet-based melanoma screening system, in *IEEE Symposium on Computational Intelligence in Image and Signal Processing (CIISP 2007)*, Honolulu, HI, pp. 189–193, 2007.

172. R. Garnavi, M. Aldeen, and J. Bailey, Computer-aided diagnosis of melanoma using border and wavelet-based texture analysis, *IEEE Transactions on Information Technology in Biomedicine*, vol. 16, no. 6, pp. 1239–1252, 2012.

173. A. Green, N. Martin, J. Pfitzner, MO'Rourke, and N. Knight, Computer image analysis in the diagnosis of melanoma, *Journal of the American Academy of Dermatology*, vol. 31, pp. 958–964, 1994.

174. G. Pellacani, M. Martini, and S. Seidenari, Digital videomicroscopy with image analysis and automatic classification as an aid for diagnosis of Spitz nevus, *Skin Research and Technology*, vol. 5, pp. 266–272, 1999.

175. M. Burroni, R. Corona, G. Dell'Eva, F. Sera, R. Bono, P. Puddu, R. Perotti, F. Nobile, L. Andreassi, and P. Rubegni, Melanoma computer-aided diagnosis: Reliability and feasibility study, *Clinical Cancer Research*, vol. 10, pp. 1881–1886, 2004.

176. K. V. Mardia, J. T. Kent, and J. Bibby, *Multivariate Analysis*, Academic Press, London, 1979.

177. S. E. Umbaugh, R. H. Moss, and W. V. Stoecker, Applying artificial intelligence to the identification of variegated colouring in skin tumors, *IEEE Engineering in Medicine and Biology Magazine*, vol. 10, pp. 57–62, 1991.

178. B. D. Ripley, Neural networks and related methods for classification, *Journal of the Royal Statistical Society B*, vol. 56, no. 3, pp. 409–456, 1994.

179. C. M. Bishop, *Neural Networks for Pattern Recognition*, Oxford University Press, 1995.

180. C. Barata, M. Ruela, M. Francisco, T. Mendonca, and J. S. Marques, Two systems for the detection of melanomas in dermoscopy images using texture and color features, *IEEE Systems Journal*, vol. PP, no. 99, pp. 1–15, 2013.

181. B. V. Dasarathy, *Nearest Neighbor (NN) Norms: NN Pattern Classification Techniques*, IEEE Computer Society Press, 1991.

182. T. Tommasi, E. L. Torre, and B. Caputo, Melanoma recognition using representative and discriminative kernel classifiers, in *Computer Vision Approaches to Medical Image Analysis*, vol. 4241 of *Lecture Notes in Computer Science*, pp. 1–12, Springer, Berlin, 2006.

183. M. Amico, M. Ferri, and I. Stanganelli, Qualitative asymmetry measure for melanoma detection, in *IEEE International Symposium on Biomedical Imaging: Nano to Macro*, Arlington, VA, vol. 2, pp. 1155–1158, 2004.

184. C. J. C. Burges, A tutorial on support vector machines for pattern recognition, *Data Mining and Knowledge Discovery*, vol. 2, no. 2, pp. 121–167, 1998.

185. A. Kjoelen, M. J. Thompson, S. E. Umbaugh, R. H. Moss, and W. V. Stoecker, Performance of AI methods in detecting melanoma, *IEEE Engineering in Medicine and Biology Magazine*, vol. 14, pp. 411–416, 1995.

186. M. Wiltgen, A. Gergerb, and J. Smolle, Tissue counter analysis of benign common nevi and malignant melanoma, *International Journal of Medical Informatics*, vol. 69, pp. 17–28, 2003.

187. M. Zorman, M. M. Stiglic, P. Kokol, and I. Maltic, The limitations of decision trees and automatic learning in real world medical decision making, *Journal of Medical Systems*, vol. 21, no. 6, pp. 403–415, 1997.

188. D. E. Clark, Computational methods for probabilistic decision trees, *Computers and Biomedical Research*, vol. 30, pp. 19–33, 1997.

189. X.-Y. Liu, J. Wu, and Z.-H. Zhou, Exploratory undersampling for class-imbalance learning, *IEEE Transactions on Systems, Man, and Cybernetics, Part B: Cybernetics*, vol. 39, pp. 539–550, 2009.

190. Y. Liu, A. An, and X. Huang, Boosting prediction accuracy on imbalanced datasets with SVM ensembles, in *Proceedings of the 10th Pacific-Asia Conference on Knowledge Discovery and Data Mining, 2006*, Singapore, pp. 107–118, 2007.

191. R. Akbani, S. Kwek, and N. Japkowicz, Applying support vector machines to imbalanced datasets, in *Proceedings of the 15th European Conference on Machine Learning (ECML)*, Pisa, Italy, pp. 39–50, 2004.

192. H. He and E. Garcia, Learning from imbalanced data, *IEEE Transactions on Knowledge and Data Engineering*, vol. 21, pp. 1263–1284, 2009.

193. G. Wu and E. Y. Chang, Class-boundary alignment for imbalanced dataset learning, in *In ICML 2003 Workshop on Learning from Imbalanced Data Sets*, Washington, DC, pp. 49–56, 2003.

194. Y. Tang, Y.-Q. Zhang, N. Chawla, and S. Krasser, SVMs modeling for highly imbalanced classification, *IEEE Transactions on Systems, Man, and Cybernetics, Part B: Cybernetics*, vol. 39, pp. 281–288, 2009.

195. R. Yan, J. Tesic, and J. Smith, Model-shared subspace boosting for multi-label classification, *ACM KDD*, San Jose, CA, vol. 13, pp. 86–91, 2007.

196. N. C. F. Codella, A. Natsev, G. Hua, M. Hill, L. Cao, L. Gong, and J. R. Smith, Video event detection using temporal pyramids of visual semantics with kernel optimization and model subspace boosting, in *2012 IEEE International Conference on Multimedia and Expo (ICME)*, Melbourne, Victoria, pp. 747–752, 2012.

197. N. C. F. Codella, G. Hua, L. Cao, M. Merler, L. Gong, M. Hill, and J. R. Smith, Large-scale video event classification using dynamic temporal pyramid matching of visual semantics, in *2013 20th IEEE International Conference on Image Processing (ICIP)*, Quebec, Canada, pp. 2877–2881.

198. L. Cao, L. Gong, J. R. Kender, N. C. F. Codella, and J. R. Smith, Learning by focusing: A new framework for concept recognition and feature selection, in *2013 IEEE International Conference on Multimedia and Expo*, pp. 1–6, 2013.

199. M. Abedini, L. Cao, N. Codella, J. H. Connell, R. Garnavi, A. Geva, M. Merler, Q.-B. Nguyen, S. U. Pankanti, J. R. Smith, X. Sun, and A. Tzadok, IBM research at ImageCLEF 2013 medical tasks, in *ImageCLEFmed 2013 AMIA Medical Image Retrieval Workshop*, Portland, OR, 2013.

200. T. Ahonen, A. Hadid, and M. Pietikainen, Face recognition with LBP, *Lecture Notes in Computer Science*, vol. 32, pp. 469–481, 2004.

201. C. Zhu, C. Bichot, and L. Chen, Multi-scale color local binary patterns for visual object classes recognition, *International Conference on Pattern Recognition (ICPR)*, vol. 32, pp. 469–481, 2010.

202. Y. Liu, A. An, and X. Huang, Boosting prediction accuracy on imbalanced datasets with SVM ensembles, in *Advances in Knowledge Discovery and Data Mining* (W.-K. Ng, M. Kitsuregawa, J. Li, and K. Chang, eds.), vol. 3918 of *Lecture Notes in Computer Science*, pp. 107–118, Springer, Berlin, 2006.

203. P. Kang and S. Cho, EUS SVMs: Ensemble of under-sampled SVMs for data imbalance problems, in *Neural Information Processing* (I. King, J. Wang, L.-W. Chan, and D. Wang, eds.), vol. 4232 of *Lecture Notes in Computer Science*, pp. 837–846, Springer, Berlin, 2006.

204. N. C. F. Codella, G. Hua, A. Natsev, and J. R. Smith, Towards large scale land-cover recognition of satellite images, in *2011 8th International Conference on Information, Communications and Signal Processing (ICICS)*, Singapore, pp. 1–5, 2011.

205. L. Brown, L. Cao, S.-F. Chang, Y. Cheng, A. Choudhary, N. Codella, C. Cotton, D. Ellis, Q. Fan, R. Feris et al., IBM research and Columbia University TRECVID-2013 multimedia event detection (med), multimedia event

recounting (mer), surveillance event detection (sed), and semantic indexing (sin) systems, in *NIST TRECVID Workshop*, Gaithersburg, MD, 2013.

206. A. Vedaldi and A. Zisserman, Efficient additive kernels via explicit feature maps, *IEEE Transactions on Pattern Analysis and Machine Intelligence*, vol. 34, pp. 480–492, 2012.

207. J. R. Kender, Separability and refinement of hierarchical semantic video labels and their ground truth, in *2008 IEEE International Conference on Multimedia and Expo*, Hannover, Germany, pp. 673–676, 2008.

208. R. Yan, M.-O. Fleury, M. Merler, A. Natsev, and J. R. Smith, Large-scale multimedia semantic concept modeling using robust subspace bagging and MapReduce, in *Proceedings of the First ACM Workshop on Large-Scale Multimedia Retrieval and Mining (LS-MMRM '09)*, New York, pp. 35–42, 2009.

209. T. Mendonca, P. M. Ferreira, J. Marques, A. R. S. Marcal, and J. Rozeira, Ph2: A dermoscopic image database for research and benchmarking, in *35th International Conference of the IEEE Engineering in Medicine and Biology Society*, Osaka, Japan, pp. 5437–5440, 2013.

210. The International Skin Imaging Collaboration (ISIC), Melanoma Project. http://www.isdis.net/.

11 Early Detection of Melanoma in Dermoscopy of Skin Lesion Images by Computer Vision–Based System

Hoda Zare
Mashhad University of Medical Sciences
Mashhad, Iran

Mohammad Taghi Bahreyni Toossi
Mashhad University of Medical Sciences
Mashhad, Iran

CONTENTS

11.1   INTRODUCTION

Melanoma is a very serious form of cancer that occurs most often in the skin; it is also known as cutaneous melanoma. The word *melanoma* is derived from the Greek words *melas* (black) and *-oma* (tumor). Melanoma is initiated in melanocyte cells that produce a pigment called melanin. The major environmental risk factor for melanoma is overexposure to the sun's harmful rays, known as ultraviolet (UV) radiation. Melanoma is the least common of all skin cancers, but is the most deadly type. According to the American Cancer Society, melanoma accounts for only about 4% of all skin cancer cases but is responsible for 79% of all skin cancer–related deaths [1]. Melanoma is now the seventh most frequent cancer in Canada and the fifth most common malignancy in the United States [2]. The good news is that when melanoma is diagnosed in its early stages, it can be treated and cured without complications and the chances for long-term, disease-free survival are excellent. Nevertheless, the early diagnosing of melanoma is not always trivial even for experienced dermatologists and more probably for primary care physicians or less experienced dermatologists [3, 4].

However, it is highly desirable and advantageous for dermatologists to have a diagnostic system that provides quantitative and objective evaluation of the skin lesion, versus the subjective clinical assessment. Due to improvements in skin imaging technology and image processing techniques in recent decades, there have been significant increases in interest in the area of computer-aided diagnosis of melanoma. The aim of such systems is to remove subjectivity and uncertainty from the diagnostic process, provide a reliable second opinion to dermatologists, and overcome the low reproducibility found in clinical diagnosis. Therefore, advances in computer-aided diagnostic methods can aid self-examination approaches and reduce the mortality significantly [4–11].

Dermoscopy, also known as epiluminescence microscopy, is a noninvasive skin imaging technique that makes subsurface structures more easily visible than conventional clinical images. Close examination of pigmented skin lesions by this technique increases the effectiveness of clinical diagnostic tools by providing new morphological criteria to distinguish melanoma from other melanocytic and nonmelanocytic pigmented skin lesions [12].

However, it has been demonstrated that dermoscopy may actually lower the diagnostic accuracy in the hands of inexperienced dermatologists. Therefore, due to the lack of reproducibility and subjectivity of human interpretation, the development of computerized image analysis techniques is of paramount importance [13]. Computer-aided diagnosis of dermoscopy images has proven to be a promising technique in developing a quantitative and objective way of classifying skin lesions. A noninvasive computer-aided diagnostic system typically consists of five main components: image preprocessing, image segmentation, feature extraction, feature selection, and classification.

11.1.1   PREPROCESSING: REMOVAL OF ARTIFACTS

The image preprocessing step includes calibration, image enhancement, and removal of artifacts such as illumination, dermoscopic gel, hair, skin lines, and ruler markings. Presence of hair in dermoscopic images is a challenge in an automated diagnostic system for the early diagnosis of melanoma. Hair pixels usually present in dermoscopy images and occlude some of the specifications of the lesion, such as its boundary and texture. Hence, the removal of hair pixels is an important preprocessing step in such systems. Ineffective hair removal algorithms lead to weak segmentation and poor pattern analysis of dermoscopy images. Hair removal can be divided into two distinct steps: (1) detection and removal of the hair pixels in the image and (2) estimation of the color and texture of skin beneath the detected hairs and replacement of the hair pixels by estimated skin pixels [12].

Numerous methods have been developed for hair removal in dermoscopy images. The first method in digitally removing hairs from dermoscopic images is proposed by Lee et al.: a freely available program called DullRazor. The goal of DullRazor's method is to remove dark thick hairs; thus, it cannot remove light-colored or thin hairs [14].

Schmid-Saugeon et al. used a similar approach, but the morphological closing operator was applied to the three components of the Luv color space. It has similar applicability limitations as DullRazor [2].

Zhou et al. implemented automatic hair and ruler marking detection using curvilinear structure analysis and performed explicit curve fitting to increase the robustness of their detection algorithm. Finally, the artifact pixels were replaced by a feature-guided exemplar-based inpainting method. This algorithm is applicable to dark hair only [15].

Xie et al. used the morphological closing top hat operator to enhance hair and a statistical threshold to detect the hair regions. Then, they used an inpainting method based on partial differential equation (PDE) to remove hairs. This study focuses mainly on dark hair [16].

Abbas et al. presented a comparative study on hair removal methods that indicate that a hair repair algorithm based on the fast marching method achieves an accurate result [17]. Abbas et al. proposed a novel hair detection and repair algorithm. Hairs are detected using a matched filtering with the first derivative of the Gaussian method and subsequently enhanced by a morphological technique that is inpainted by a fast marching method [18].

11.1.2 SKIN LESION SEGMENTATION

Image segmentation is the process of dividing an image into disjoint and homogeneous partitions with respect to some characteristics, such as color, texture, and so forth, or in other words, it is the process of locating the boundaries between the regions [19, 20]. The accuracy of the detected border is crucial, as exclusion of any part of the lesion may lead to loss of dermoscopic patterns, color, and texture-based information that can be extracted from the interior of the lesion. Moreover, the geometric shape of the lesion and structural properties of the border have diagnostic importance, all of which depend on the detected border [21].

In recent decades, numerous methods have been developed for automated border detection in dermoscopy images. As suggested by Celebi et al. [13], segmentation methods can be categorized in the following classes of techniques: histogram thresholding [2, 3, 22–28], color clustering methods [2, 29–35], edge and region-based methods [13, 27, 36–40], morphological methods [37, 41], model-based methods [38, 42], active contour [43–46], and soft computing methods [47].

The combination of some of these methods provided different border detection methods. For example, Iyatomi et al. described a method called the dermatologist-like tumor extraction algorithm (DTEA), which is based on thresholding followed by iterative region growing [48].

In the J-image segmentation algorithm (JSEG), which is suggested by Celebi et al., the computational time is reduced by incorporating approximate lesion localization and searching the border neighborhood rather than the whole image [49].

Melli et al. combined an unsupervised clustering component with a supervised classification module to automatically extract the boundary of the skin lesion. In the clustering phase, they employed and compared four major clustering algorithms: median cut, k-means, fuzzy c-means, and mean shift. The comparison, which was performed in terms of sensitivity, specificity, and the average of these two parameters, revealed that the best results were obtained from the mean-shift algorithm [34].

11.1.3 FEATURE EXTRACTION

Feature extraction is the process of extracting certain characteristic attributes and generating a set of meaningful descriptors from an image. The purpose of the feature extraction component in a computer-aided diagnosis system of melanoma is to extract various features from a given skin image that best characterize a given lesion as benign or malignant. The features employed by the computer-based system must have high sensitivity (high correlation of the feature with malignancy and high probability of true positive response) and high specificity (high probability of true negative response) [4].

Numerous methods for extracting features from skin lesion images have been proposed in the literature. These methods analyze various components, like shape, color, and texture features.

Several studies have proven the efficiency of shape descriptors for the detection of melanoma. Simple parameters such as lesion area and perimeter are extracted in [3, 25]. Other shape features include aspect ratio [25, 50]; lesion asymmetry with respect to a lesion symmetry axis [51–55]; circularity [55–57] and bulkiness index [58] to investigate the asymmetry; border irregularity [59–61]; and calculation of circularity and compactness [25, 62, 63], smoothness [57], and fractal dimension [56, 58] to represent border irregularity.

Color features are mainly statistical parameters calculated from different color channels. Typical color images consist of the three-color channels red, green, and blue (RGB). The color features are based on measurements on these color channels, or other color channels, such as cyan, magenta, yellow (CMY); hue, saturation, value (HSV); and Y luminance and U-V chrominance components (YUV); or various combinations of them [4].

In the literature, minimum, maximum, mean, and standard deviation statistical parameters over the three channels of different color spaces have been measured [25, 28, 46]. Other color features used in different studies include color asymmetry [46, 52–54, 64], centroid distance as a distance between the geometric and the brightness centroid, Luv histogram distance to determine the color similarity of two regions [25], and relative color histogram analysis [53, 65, 66].

In order to quantify the texture present in a lesion, some researchers used a set of statistical texture features of Haralick et al. [67], which are derived from a gray-level co-occurrence matrix (GLCM) [25, 67–69].

Few researchers used dermoscopic structural features for the diagnosis of melanoma [70, 71]. These dermoscopic structures include atypical pigment networks [11, 69, 72–76], streaks [77, 78], globules/dots/blotches [74, 79–82], and blue–white veil [83, 84].

11.1.4   FEATURE SELECTION

Feature selection is an important step in computer-aided diagnosis of melanoma. The purpose of this step is to select a reasonable reduced number of useful features and eliminate redundant, irrelevant, or noisy features. Feature selection algorithms can be categorized in two classes: (1) filter-based methods that rely on general characteristics of the data to select a subset of features with no classification or learning algorithm and (2) wrapper methods that use the prediction performance of a predetermined learning algorithm to evaluate the goodness of a feature subset [25].

In the research that has been performed in the field of computer diagnosis of melanoma, some feature selection algorithms are used, for example, sequential forward selection (SFS) algorithm [85], statistical feature selection method (unpaired t-test for normally distributed and Wilcoxon rank-sum test for nonnormally distributed features), statistical approaches of sequential floating forward selection (SFFS), sequential floating backward selection (SFBS), leave one out (LOO) [2, 53], correlation-based feature selection (CFS) [25, 86], and relief algorithm [25].

11.1.5   CLASSIFICATION

Classification is the process of distributing items into classes of similar types. In computerized analysis of dermoscopy images, lesions are classified as melanomas or nonmelanomas according to their extracted features. The classification process is divided into training and testing phases. In order to determine the performance of the system, a set of images with known labels is given to the classifier and the accuracy of the classification is affected by the size of the training set.

The most popular classification methods that have been employed in computer-based melanoma diagnostic systems in the literature include the discriminant analysis method [24, 28, 81, 87], k-nearest neighborhood (KNN) algorithm [3, 85, 87, 88], decision trees [4, 28, 88, 89], support vector machine (SVM) [4, 25, 88, 90], and artificial neural network (ANN) [85, 88, 91]. In the rest of this chapter we present a computer-aided diagnostic system of melanoma with the aim of improving some of the existing methods and developing new techniques.

11.2 PROPOSED SYSTEM

11.2.1 HAIR REMOVAL ALGORITHM [12]

The proposed hair removal algorithm consists of two steps: (1) hair detection with the use of adaptive canny edge detector and refinement by morphological operators and (2) hair repair by multiresolution coherence transport inpainting technique.

11.2.1.1 Hair Detection from Dermoscopy Images

In the first step, the principal component analysis (PCA) transform is applied to the image to facilitate the hair segmentation process by enhancing its contrast, followed by a Wiener filter with a mask size of 3*3 for noise removal. Next, an improved canny edge detection method is used for detection of hair boundaries. In this method, autoselection of the dual threshold is performed by the gradient magnitude histogram concavity analysis [92]. The method is based on obtaining the convex hull of the gradient magnitude histogram and analyzing the concavities of the convex hull. Therefore, the deepest concavity points become candidates as high threshold (Th) for the canny operator, and the low threshold is equal to 0.4*Th. Then, the hairs are segmented by applying the morphological dilation operator on the edge-detected image. It can be noticed that segmented images contain misclassified objects with shorter lengths than normal hairs. Therefore, special labeling and morphological operations are utilized to detect them. Morphological opening is performed by line structuring elements oriented in different directions. Finally, to obtain smooth hair lines, dilation and filling operators are applied to the hair mask. Figure 11.1 shows the multiple stages of hair mask extraction in a dermoscopy image. The hair segmentation result for sample images is obtained as illustrated in Figure 11.2.

11.2.1.2 Hair Repair

Image inpainting is used to remove and repair the unnecessary elements, such as hairs. Bornemann and März proposed the fast image inpainting based on coherence transport. It traverses the inpainting domain by the fast marching method just once while transporting, along the way, image values in a coherence direction robustly estimated by means of the structure tensor [93]. We proposed a multiresolution coherence transport inpainting for dermoscopy images. This method combines the simple coherence transport inpainting with a wavelet decomposition/reconstruction method in an iterative and multi-resolution structure. A set of instructions is performed in each iteration until the maximum number of iterations is reached. The pseudocode of the proposed inpainting algorithm is presented in Figure 11.3.

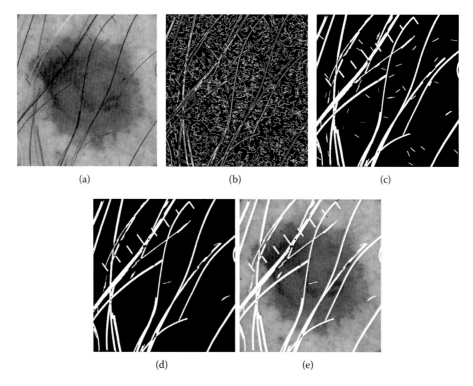

FIGURE 11.1 (a) Original dermoscopy image. (b) Edge-detected image using adaptive canny edge detector. (c) Hair extraction in different directions. (d) Hair mask. (e) Hair removal from image.

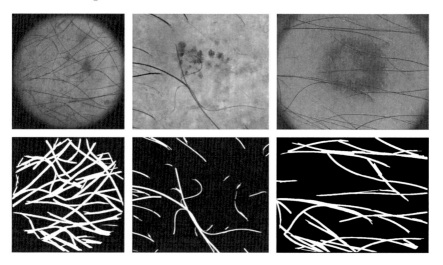

FIGURE 11.2 The results of the hair segmentation algorithm. (From Bahreyni Toossi, M. T. et al., *Skin Research and Technology*, vol. 19, no. 3, pp. 230–235, 2013.)

$Image_{inpainted} \leftarrow$ IterativeInpainting ($Image, Mask, MaxIteration$)
input: $Image, Mask, MaxIteration$;
output: $Image_{inpainted}$;
parameter: $WaveletName, InpaintingParameter$;

$Image^1_{inpainted} \leftarrow$ CoherenceTransportInpainting ($Image, Mask, InpaintingParameter$);
if $MaxIteration = 0$
  $Image_{inpainted} = Image^1_{inpainted}$;
  return $Image_{inpainted}$;
$(Approximation, Detail^{Horizontal}, Detail^{Vertical}, Detail^{Diagonal}) \leftarrow$ DWT2D ($Image, WaveletName$);
$Mask_2 \leftarrow$ resize($Mask, 0.5$);
$Approximation_{inpainted} \leftarrow$ IterativeInpainting ($Approximation, Mask_2, MaxIteration - 1$);
$Detail^{Horizontal}_{inpainted} \leftarrow$ IterativeInpainting ($Detail^{Horizontal}, Mask_2, MaxIteration - 1$);
$Detail^{Vertical}_{inpainted} \leftarrow$ IterativeInpainting ($Detail^{Vertical}, Mask_2, MaxIteration - 1$);
$Detail^{Diagonal}_{inpainted} \leftarrow$ IterativeInpainting ($Detail^{Diagonal}, Mask_2, MaxIteration - 1$);
$Image^2_{inpainted} \leftarrow$ IDWT2D ($Approximation_{inpainted}, Detail^{Horizontal}_{inpainted}, Detail^{Vertical}_{inpainted}, Detail^{Diagonal}_{inpainted}$);
$Image_{inpainted} = (Image^1_{inpainted} + Image^2_{inpainted})/2$;
return $Image_{inpainted}$;

FIGURE 11.3 The pseudocode of the proposed multiresolution iterative coherence transport inpainting algorithm. (From Bahreyni Toossi, M. T. et al., *Skin Research and Technology*, vol. 19, no. 3, pp. 230–235, 2013.)

11.2.2 LESION BORDER DETECTION IN DERMOSCOPY IMAGES

Active contour models are widely used in image segmentation problems, especially for medical images with a lot of noise and intensity inhomogeneity. These models can be categorized into edge-based and region-based models. The region-based models have many advantages over the edge-based ones. They are less sensitive to noise as well as the location of the initial contour. Also, they provide better performance for images with weak edges.

In this research, we used a novel region-based active contour model in a level-set framework for skin lesion segmentation in dermoscopy images. In the mentioned model, a new region-based signed pressure function (SPF) and novel level-set model are proposed by Zhang et al. [94]. SPF is introduced using statistical information inside and outside the contour and has opposite signs around the lesion boundary, so that the contour can shrink or expand when it is outside or inside the object, respectively. The level-set function is initialized to a binary function and a Gaussian filter is applied to regularize the level-set function and avoid reinitialization. Computational complexity analysis shows that this method is more efficient than the traditional level-set methods [94]. The procedure of the algorithm consists mainly of the following steps:

1. Convert the RGB color image ($I(x)$) to grayscale using a PCA transform.

2. Initialize the level-set function φ into a binary function (initialize a contour C containing the objects that are of interest, iteration index $k = 0$):

$$\varphi = \begin{cases} 1 & outside\ C \\ 0 & C \\ -1 & inside\ C \end{cases} \tag{11.1}$$

3. Compute the values of C_1 and C_2 using Equations 11.2 and 11.3, respectively:

$$C_1(\varphi) = \frac{\int I(x).H(\varphi)dx}{\int H(\varphi)dx} \tag{11.2}$$

$$C_2(\varphi) = \frac{\int I(x).(1 - H(\varphi))dx}{\int (1 - H(\varphi))dx} \tag{11.3}$$

where

$$H(\varphi) = \begin{cases} 1 & \varphi \geq 0 \\ 0 & otherwise \end{cases} \tag{11.4}$$

4. Calculate the SPF function using the values of C_1 and C_2 as follows:

$$SPF(I(x)) = \frac{I(x) - \frac{C_1 + C_2}{2}}{\max(|I(x) - \frac{C_1 + C_2}{2}|)} \tag{11.5}$$

5. Update the level-set function with iteration number:

$$\frac{\partial \varphi}{\partial t} = SPF(T(x)).\alpha|\nabla \varphi| \tag{11.6}$$

where α is a factor to increase the segmentation speed.
6. Regularize the level-set function with a Gaussian filter ($\varphi = \varphi * G_\sigma$).
7. Reestimate C_1 and C_2 for the $(k+1)$ iteration; then compare the results between the kth and $(k+1)$th iterations. Check whether the evolution of the level-set function has converged. If not, return to step 3.

Figure 11.4 demonstrates the segmentation results of the level-set active contour algorithm on a dermoscopy image.

11.2.3   FEATURE EXTRACTION

In this study we propose a comprehensive and effective feature extraction method with a combination of different types of features, including geometric, color, texture, and wavelet-based textures.

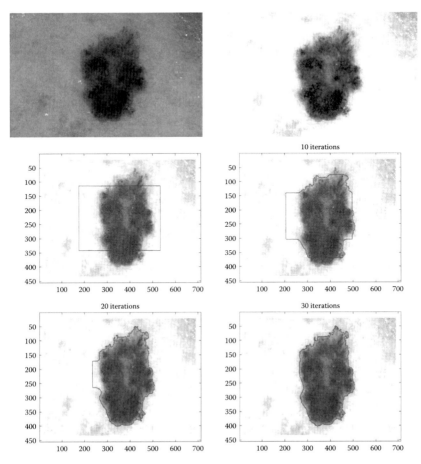

FIGURE 11.4 Segmentation results of the level-set active contour algorithm in a dermoscopy image. (Reprinted with permission from Argenziano, G. et al., *Dermoscopy: A Tutorial*, EDRA Medical Publishing and New Media, Milan, Italy, 2002.)

11.2.3.1 Geometric Features

The main requisite for extracting geometric features is the segmentation step where the lesion is separated from the background, normal skin. The output of the segmentation step is a binary image and the following three geometric features are extracted from this image:

Irregularity index reflects the irregularity of the lesion border and is calculated as

$$Irregularity = \frac{P^2}{4\pi A} \tag{11.7}$$

where p and A are the perimeter and area of the lesion, respectively.

Aspect ratio is defined as the eccentricity of the skin lesion and describes the proportional relationships between its length of the major axis (L_1) and its length of the minor axis (L_2):

$$Aspect\ ratio = \frac{L_1}{L_2} \tag{11.8}$$

Asymmetry is defined as the area difference between the two halves of the lesion. In order to evaluate this feature, the major axis orientation of the lesion (θ) is calculated. Then the lesion is rotated ($\theta°$) in the opposite direction, to align the lesion symmetry axes with the image axes (x and y). To determine the lesion symmetry axes, the smallest bounding box of the lesion is estimated. Symmetry axes for calculated the bounding rectangle are used as the symmetry axes (major and minor axes) for the lesion. Finally, the lesion is hypothetically folded along the symmetry axes and the region on one side of the axis is subtracted from the reflected region on the other side. Then, two asymmetry measures A_x and A_y are calculated about the axes. Asymmetry indices were calculated as shown in Equations 11.9 and 11.10 [25]. Figure 11.5 represents the different steps of asymmetry measurements.

$$A_1 = \frac{\min(A_x, A_y)}{A} \times 100\% \tag{11.9}$$

$$A_2 = \frac{A_x + A_y}{A} \times 100\% \tag{11.10}$$

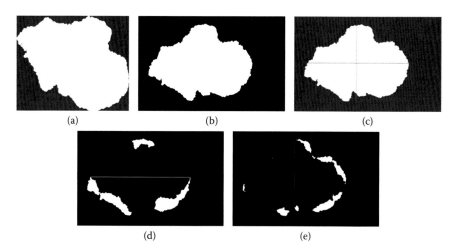

(a)   (b)   (c)

(d)   (e)

FIGURE 11.5 (a) Lesion binary mask. (b) Rotation of the lesion mask. (c) Bounding box and estimated symmetry axis. (d, e) Asymmetry around the symmetry axes.

11.2.3.2   Color Features

The analysis of the lesion colors is crucial in the classification of dermoscopic images. In this study eight different color spaces are used to extract color features. The eight color spaces are RGB, rgb (normalized RGB), HSV, $I_1/I_2/I_3$ (Ohta space), $L_1/L_2/L_3$, CIELuv, CIELab, and yCbCr. According to the color criteria, such as decoupling of chrominance and luminance, invariance to illumination intensity, and perceptual uniformity, none of the color spaces satisfy all of the criteria [25]. Thus, consideration of several color spaces that complement each other is necessary. Figure 11.6 represents an example of melanoma lesion in different color spaces.

In order to quantify the color features of the lesion, various statistical parameters are calculated (e.g., ratio of the standard deviation to the mean, skewness, and centroidal distance).

Ratio of the standard deviation to the mean: The mean and standard deviation represent the average color and color variegation over each color channel, respectively. This feature is calculated for all three channels of eight color spaces. The total number of color features in this stage is 24.

Skewness: Describes asymmetry from the normal distribution in a set of statistical data. Skewness can come in the form of negative or positive, depending on whether data points are skewed to the left (negative skew) or to the right (positive skew) of the data average. This parameter is defined as follows:

$$Skewness = \frac{E(x - \mu)^3}{\sigma^3} \tag{11.11}$$

where μ is the mean of x samples, σ is the standard deviation, and E is the expectation operator. Skewness is calculated in eight color spaces for each color channel (the total number of 24 features).

Centroidal distance: The centroidal distance for a color channel is defined as the distance between the mask and the brightness centroid of that channel. In the brightness centroid calculation the moments were weighted by the pixel values. In homogenous lesions, the centroidal distance is small. In order to achieve scaling invariability, the centroidal distance is divided by the lesion diameter [25]. Figure 11.7 illustrates the centroidal distance in a sample of melanoma and benign lesions. This feature is calculated for all channels of the eight color spaces. The total number of color features in this category is 24.

11.2.3.3   Texture Features

In order to quantify the texture present in a skin lesion, we implement 13 of the statistical texture features of Haralick et al., which are derived from

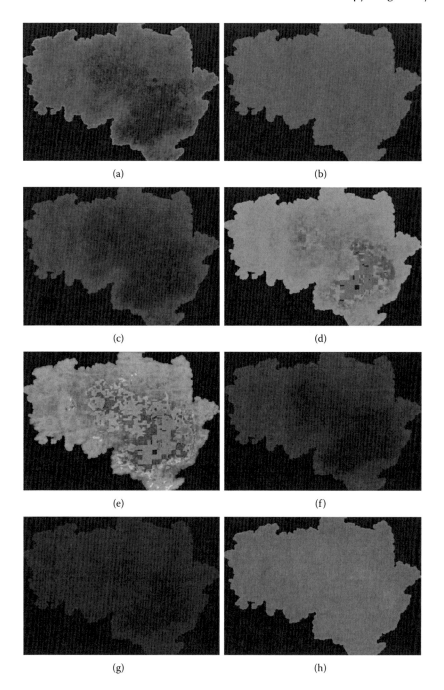

FIGURE 11.6 (**See color insert.**) Dermoscopy image of melanoma lesion in eight color spaces. (a) RGB; (b) rgb; (c) $I_1/I_2/I_3$; (d) $L_1/L_2/L_3$; (d) hsv; (e) Luv; (f) Lab; (g) yCbCr.

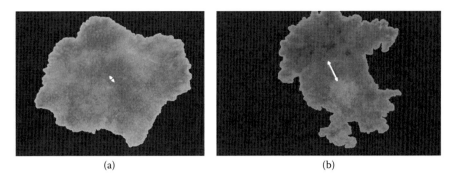

FIGURE 11.7 Centroidal distance in two lesions: (a) nonmelanoma lesion and (b) melanoma lesion.

a gray-level co-occurrence matrix (GLCM) [95]. These texture features are summarized in Equations 11.12 through 11.24.

$$Energy = \sum_{i,j} p(i,j)^2 \tag{11.12}$$

$$Entropy = -\sum_{i,j} p(i,j)\log(p(i,j)) \tag{11.13}$$

$$Contrast = \sum_{i,j} |i-j|^2 p(i,j) \tag{11.14}$$

$$Variance = \sum_{i,j} (i-\mu)^2 p(i,j) \tag{11.15}$$

$$Homogenity = \sum_{i,j} \frac{p(i,j)}{1+|i-j|} \tag{11.16}$$

$$Correlation = \sum_{i,j} \frac{(i-\mu_i)(j-\mu_j)p(i,j)}{\sigma_i\sigma_j} \tag{11.17}$$

$$Sum\ average = \sum_{i=2}^{2N_g} i p_{x+y}(i) \tag{11.18}$$

$$Sum\ variance = \sum_{i=2}^{2N_g} (i-SA)^2 i p_{x+y}(i) \tag{11.19}$$

$$Sum\ entropy = -\sum_{i=2}^{2N_g} p_{x+y}(i)\log(p_{x+y}(i)) \tag{11.20}$$

$$Difference\ variance = \sum_{i=0}^{N_g-1} (i-\mu_{x-y})^2 p_{x-y}(i) \tag{11.21}$$

$$Difference\ entropy = -\sum_{i=0}^{N_g-1} p_{x-y}(i) \log(p_{x-y}(i)) \qquad (11.22)$$

$$Information\ of\ correlation\ 1 = \frac{Ent - H_{xy1}}{\max(H_x - H_y)} \qquad (11.23)$$

$$Information\ of\ correlation\ 2 = (1 - \exp[-0.2(H_{xy2} - Ent)])^{1/2} \qquad (11.24)$$

where $p(i,j)$ is the matrix element of GLCM, μ is the mean value of P, N_g is the number of gray levels, μ_x, μ_y, σ_x, and σ_y are the means and standard deviations of P_x and P_y, and

$$p_{x+y}(k) = \sum_{i,j} p(i,j) \quad for\ i+j = k = 2,3,\ldots,2N_g$$

$$p_{x-y}(k) = \sum_{i,j} p(i,j) \quad for\ |i-j| = k = 2,3,\ldots,N_g-1$$

$$\mu_{x_y} = \sum_{i=0}^{N_g-1} i p_{x-y}(i) \quad p_x(i) = \sum_{j=1}^{N_g} p(i,j) \quad p_y(j) = \sum_{j=1}^{N_g} p(i,j)$$

$$H_{XY1} = -\sum_{i,j} p(i,j) \log(p_x(i)p_y(j))$$

$$H_{XY2} = -\sum_{i,j} p_x(i)p_y(j) \log(p_x(i)p_y(j))$$

Co-occurrence matrices, introduced by Haralick et al. [67], are statistical descriptors that both measure the grayscale distribution in an image and consider the spatial interactions between pixels. Let N be the total number of gray levels in the image; the GLCM is a square matrix G of order N, where the (i,j)th entry of G represents the number of occasions a pixel with intensity i is adjacent to a pixel with intensity j. We construct GLCM matrices in the four directions of $0°$, $45°$, $90°$, and $135°$ within the distance of 2 pixels using 64 gray levels. In order to obtain rotation-invariant features, the statistics calculated from four directions are averaged. Then, normalized GLCM is calculated. Finally, 13 texture features are calculated for grayscale images in eight color spaces. Therefore, the total number of texture features extracted from each image is 104.

11.2.3.4 Wavelet-Based Texture Features

Wavelet-based texture analysis provides a multiresolution analytical platform that enables us to characterize an image in multiple spatial/frequency spaces. Tree-structured wavelet analysis provides low-, middle-, and high-frequency decompositions by decomposing both approximate (low-frequency) and detailed (high-frequency) coefficients [96]. In dermoscopy images analysis, the lower-frequency decomposition gives information about the general properties (shape) of the skin lesion, which is clinically important, and the higher-frequency components provide information about the textural details and internal patterns of the lesion, which are also significant in the diagnosis. In this study we implement one-level decomposition of the tree-structured wavelet transform. The method applies wavelet transform on three color channels of red, green, and blue, and also on the eight images in different color spaces. Note that in each color space, the color image is converted to a grayscale image using the PCA method. For each image, 13 statistical texture features of Haralick et al. are applied on both the original image and wavelet coefficients of each subimage of the wavelet tree. In total, 572 features are extracted from each image.

11.2.4 FEATURES NORMALIZATION

Features that are extracted from the images are numerically in different ranges. Normalization of features is used to standardize the range of independent features. Many classifiers require that the features be normalized in a specified range. For this purpose, a Z-score transformation is used. This method is one of the most common procedures in feature normalization and is given by [25]

$$Z_{ij} = \frac{((x_{ij} - \mu_j)/(3\sigma_j) + 1)}{2} \tag{11.25}$$

where x_{ij} represents the value of the jth feature of the ith sample, and μ_j and σ_j are the mean and standard deviation of the jth feature, respectively.

11.2.5 FEATURE SELECTION

In this study, due to the high dimension of the feature vector, the filter-based model is adopted for feature selection. So, in order to select the optimal model, three methods of filter-based feature selection are implemented.

11.2.5.1 Correlation-Based Feature Selection

The correlation feature selection (CFS) measure evaluates subsets of features on the basis of the following hypothesis: good feature subsets contain features highly correlated with the classification, yet uncorrelated to each other. The correlation criterion measures the predictability of one variable by another variable and is defined as follows:

$$C_s = \frac{k\overline{r_{cf}}}{\sqrt{k + k(k-1)\overline{r_{ff}}}} \tag{11.26}$$

where S is a feature subset consisting of k features, $\overline{r_{cf}}$ is the average value of all feature–class correlations, and $\overline{r_{ff}}$ is the average value of all feature–feature correlations.

11.2.5.2 Relief-Based Feature Selection

Relief is a feature selection strategy that chooses instances randomly and changes the weights of the feature relevance based on the nearest neighbor. By selecting a sample, the relief algorithm searches for its two nearest neighbors: one from the same class and the other from a different class. Then the values of their features are compared and the relevance scores for each feature are updated accordingly. The key idea is to estimate the quality of attributes according to how well their values distinguish between samples that are near to each other [97].

11.2.5.3 T-Test Feature Selection

The t-test assesses statistically the difference between the means of two independent groups. This method is performed by calculating T:

$$T = \frac{(\mu_1 - \mu_2)}{\sqrt{\left(\frac{1}{n_1} + \frac{1}{n_2}\right)\left(\frac{(n_1-1)\sigma_1^2 + (n_2-1)\sigma_2^2}{n_1 + n_2 - 2}\right)}} \qquad (11.27)$$

where μ_i, σ_i, and n_i are the mean, standard deviation, and number of samples in class i. The larger T is, the larger the difference of feature values between two classes. As that difference will be critical in classification, features with higher T are selected.

11.2.6 CLASSIFICATION

Classification is the final step in the diagnosis process, wherein the optimal feature set determined in the feature selection process is utilized to differentiate melanoma from benign lesions. Image classification analyzes the numerical properties of selected features and organizes data into categories. Classification algorithms typically employ two phases of processing: training and testing. In the initial training phase, characteristic properties of typical features are isolated, and based on these, a unique description of each classification category, that is, training class, is created. In the subsequent testing phase, these feature–space partitions are used to classify image features. In this study, three methods of classification are employed: k-nearest neighbor, support vector machine, and artificial neural network. A brief introduction of each classifier is now provided.

11.2.6.1 k-Nearest Neighbor

KNN is one of the simplest but widely used machine learning algorithms. In this method a skin lesion is classified by a majority vote of its neighbors, with the lesion being assigned to the class that is most common among its k-nearest neighbors. The motivation for this classifier is that patterns that are close to each other in the feature space are likely to belong to the same pattern class. The neighbors are taken from a set of samples for which the correct classification is known. It is common to use the Euclidean distance. Choosing an appropriate k is essential to make the classification more successful. In a two-class classification problem (our examination), it is helpful to choose k to be an odd number, as this avoids draw votes. Therefore, in this work, a good value for k is determined by considering a range of k ($k = 1, 3, 5, 7,$ and 9).

11.2.6.2 Support Vector Machine

The support vector machine (SVM), as proposed by Vapnik, is a linear and a machine learning paradigm based on statistical learning theory [98]. SVM performs classification by constructing a set of N-dimensional hyperplanes that optimally separate the given data into classes, using the largest possible margin. Margin is the distance between the optimal hyperplane and the nearest training data points of any class, and the larger the margin, the lower the generalization error of the classifier. Boser et al. proposed an approach to create nonlinear classifiers by applying kernel functions [99]. Some common kernels include linear, polynomial, Gaussian or radial basis function (RBF), and Sigmoid [100]. In this study, different kernel functions are used, and the function with the highest accuracy in classification is selected.

11.2.6.3 Artificial Neural Network

In an artificial neural network (ANN), simple artificial nodes, called neurons, are connected together to form a network that mimics a biological neural network. A neural network consists of a set of connected cells or neurons. The neurons receive impulses from either input cells or other neurons and perform some kind of transformation of the input and transmit the outcome to other neurons or to output cells. The neural networks are built from layers of neurons connected so that one layer receives input from the preceding layer of neurons and passes the output on to the subsequent layer. The most popular form of neural network architecture is the multilayer perceptron (MLP) used in our study. MLP is a feed forward neural network with one or more layers between the input and the output layer. Feed forward means that data flows in one direction from the input to the output layer (forward). This type of network is trained with the back propagation learning algorithm. With back propagation, the input data are repeatedly presented to the neural network. With each presentation, the output of the neural network is compared to the desired output and an error is computed. This error is then fed back (back propagated) to the neural network and used to adjust the weights such that the error decreases with each iteration and the neural model gets closer and closer to producing the desired output. This process is known as training.

In this work three layers are defined: input, hidden, and output. The number of neurons in the input layer is equal to the number of features selected in the previous sections. The optimum number of hidden layers and the number of neurons in each layer are found by using trial-and-error techniques.

11.3 EXPERIMENTAL RESULTS AND DISCUSSION

The proposed computer vision-based system was developed in MATLAB® version 7_12_0_635-R2011a (Mathworks, Inc., Natick, Massachusetts). All computations were performed on a personal computer with a 3.2 GHz AMD Phenom II X4 955 processor (AMD, Inc., Sunnyvale, California) and 4 GB RAM with Microsoft Windows 7, 32 bits, as the operating system.

11.3.1 HAIR REMOVAL

The proposed algorithm was tested on a set of 50 dermoscopy images acquired from an atlas of dermoscopy [101]. These were images obtained from different sources and stored in the RGB color format with dimensions ranging from 520×340 pixels to 1600×1200 pixels. Manual hair segmentation given by dermatologist is used as ground truth for the performance evaluation.

11.3.1.1 Assessment of the Proposed Hair Detection Method

To estimate the accuracy of the proposed algorithm and to quantify the automatic hair detection error, quantitative evaluations were performed using three statistical metrics: true detection rate (TDR), false positive rate (FPR), and diagnostic accuracy (DA).

TDR measures the rate of pixels that were classified as hair by both the automatic algorithm and the medical expert, and FPR measures the rate of pixels that were classified as hair by the automatic segmentation and were not classified as hair by the medical expert. These metrics are calculated as follows:

$$\text{True detection rate (TDR)} = \frac{TP}{TP + FN} \times 100\% \tag{11.28}$$

$$\text{False positive rate (FPR)} = \frac{FP}{TP + FN} \times 100\% \tag{11.29}$$

$$\text{Diagnostic accuracy (DA)} = \frac{TP}{TP + FP + FN} \times 100\% \tag{11.30}$$

where TP, FP, and FN stand for the number of true positive, false positive, and false negative, respectively. Figure 11.8 shows the result of manual and automatic hair detection with the proposed method. These metrics are computed to compare the proposed hair detection algorithm with the DullRazor hair removal software [14] that identifies the dark hair locations by a generalized grayscale morphological closing operation. The results of hair detection

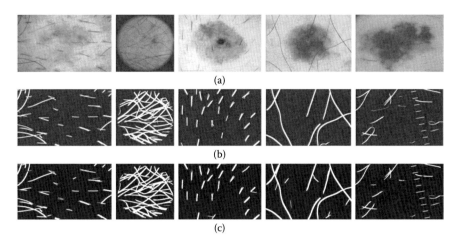

FIGURE 11.8 (a) The original images. (b) Manual hair segmentation. (c) Automatic hair detection using adaptive canny edge detector.

using two methods show that DullRazor is not suitable for the light and thin hairs. Moreover, this software selects parts of the lesion structure as hair, so the lesion pattern is destroyed (Figure 11.9). The quantitative results of the proposed algorithm and DullRazor software are presented in Table 11.1.

11.3.1.2 Assessment of the Proposed Hair Repair Method

The original images without hair pixels (white pixels in Figure 11.10) are repaired with the proposed multi-resolution coherence transport inpainting method. To evaluate the performance of the proposed algorithm, three statistical metrics—entropy, standard deviation, and co-occurrence matrix—are used to compare the texture of original images (without hair pixels) and the images inpainted by the proposed multiresolution method. Normalized difference of entropy (NDE), normalized difference of standard deviation (NDSD), and mean normalized difference of co-occurrence matrix (MNDCOM) are calculated between the two types of images. Lesser differences are expected for a better inpainting method. Table 11.2 shows the comparative results between our proposed method and the coherence transport algorithm [16] on 50 dermoscopy images. It can be noticed that our proposed multiresolution coherence transport inpainting method achieves better results than the simple coherence transport method.

11.3.2 LESION SEGMENTATION

The proposed segmentation method is tested on a set of 100 dermoscopy images (30 malignant melanoma and 100 benign) obtained from the EDRA *Interactive Atlas of Dermoscopy* [101] and three private dermatology practices [13]. The benign lesions include nevocellular and dysplastic nevi. The

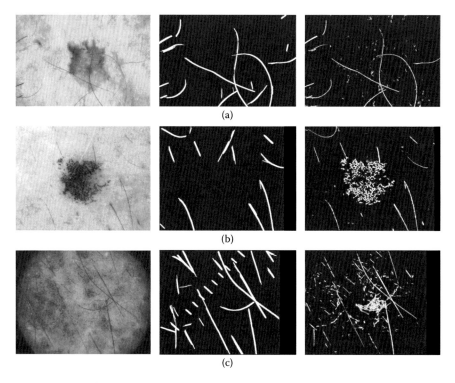

FIGURE 11.9 (a) The original images. (b) The results of hair detection using the proposed algorithm. (c) The results of hair detection using DullRazor. (From Bahreyni Toossi, M. T. et al., *Skin Research and Technology*, vol. 19, no. 3, pp. 230–235, 2013.)

TABLE 11.1

Comparison of the Hair Detection Algorithms for 50 Dermoscopy Images

Hair Detection Method	DA (%)	TDR (%)	FPR (%)
Proposed algorithm	88.3	93.2	4
DullRazor [62]	48.6	70.2	33.4

Source: Bahreyni Toossi, M. T. et al., *Skin Research and Technology*, vol. 19, no. 3, pp. 230–235, 2013.

images are 24-bit RGB color type with dimensions ranging from 512×768 pixels to 2556×1693 pixels. As a ground truth for the evaluation of the border detection error, manual borders are determined by three dermatologists: Dr. William Stoecker, Dr. Joseph Malters, and Dr. James Grichnik,

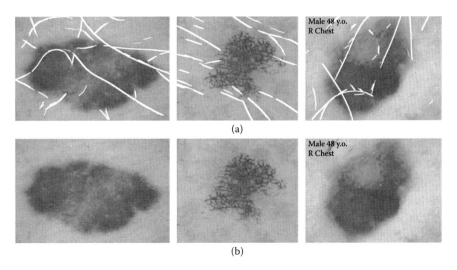

(a)

(b)

FIGURE 11.10 The results of the proposed multiresolution coherence transport inpainting for hair repair. (a) The images without hair pixels (white pixels). (b) Repaired images.

TABLE 11.2

Comparative Results between the Simple Coherence Transport and the Proposed Multiresolution Coherence Transport Inpainting for Hair Repair

Hair Repair Method	NDE (%)	NDSD (%)	MNDCOM (%)
Multiresolution coherence transport inpainting (proposed algorithm)	0.72	2.1	0.40
Coherence transport inpainting algorithm [93]	0.95	2.5	0.42

Source: Bahreyni Toossi, M. T. et al., *Skin Research and Technology*, vol. 19, no. 3, pp. 230–235, 2013.

---

using the second-order B-spline method [13]. Figure 11.11 shows the results of the level-set active contour segmentation algorithm on typical images.

To compare the automatic borders (generated by the proposed level-set active contour segmentation method) with the manual borders (drawn by three dermatologists), in order to evaluate the goodness of the detected borders, various metrics are used: sensitivity, specificity, accuracy, segmentation error, and similarity [102–104]. Sensitivity represents the percentage of actual lesion that has been truly detected. Specificity shows the percentage of actual background skin that has been truly detected. Accuracy shows the degree of closeness of the detected border to the actual border, which takes both background skin and lesion pixels into account. The segmentation error metric provides a good indication of the overall segmentation performance, and the

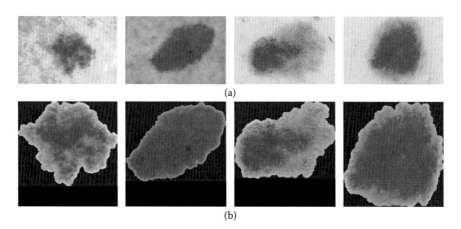

(a)

(b)

FIGURE 11.11 Results of the level-set active contour segmentation method. (a) The original images. (b) Segmented images. (Reprinted with permission from Argenziano, G. et al., *Dermoscopy: A Tutorial*, EDRA Medical Publishing and New Media, Milan, Italy, 2002.)

similarity indicates the degree of likeness between two automatic and manual borders. These metrics are defined by

$$Sensitivity = \frac{TP}{TP + FN} \times 100\% \tag{11.31}$$

$$Specificity = \frac{TN}{TN + FP} \times 100\% \tag{11.32}$$

$$Accuracy = \frac{TP + TN}{TP + FP + FN + TN} \times 100\% \tag{11.33}$$

$$Segmentation\ error = \frac{FP + FN}{TP + FN} \times 100\% \tag{11.34}$$

$$Similarity = \frac{2TP}{2TP + FP + FN} \times 100\% \tag{11.35}$$

where TP and TN represent the number of pixels that are detected correctly as part of the lesion and background skin, respectively, in both the manual and automatic borders. FP represents the number of pixels that are identified as part of the lesion in the automatic border, but are labeled as part of the background skin in the manual border. FN represents the number of pixels that are identified as part of the background skin in the automatic border, but are labeled as part of the lesion in the manual border. To evaluate the variabilities among the three dermatologists (that drew the manual borders), a similarity metric is used to quantify the degree of similarity between any two borders, without taking either of them as the ground truth [7]. Table 11.3 demonstrates the mean and standard deviation values of similarity between the borders drawn by the three dermatologists. The similarity values indicate

TABLE 11.3

Mean ± Standard Deviation for Similarity (%) between Dermatologists

Dermatologists	Mean Similarity (%)	Std Similarity (%)
D1-D2	95.26	3.47
D1-D3	94.85	3.36
D2-D3	95.73	1.88

TABLE 11.4

Mean and Standard Deviation Values of Various Metrics for the Proposed Segmentation

Segmentation Method	Dermatologist	Statistic	Sensitivity	Specificity	Accuracy	Similarity	Seg. Error
Active contour algorithm (AC)	D1	Mean	92.10	98.79	97.29	93.30	12.15
		Std	6.94	1.21	1.6	3.02	5.34
	D2	Mean	95.03	98.73	97.89	94.83	9.78
		Std	5.15	1.09	1.19	2.15	3.22
	D3	Mean	95.12	97.93	97.19	94.28	10.85
		Std	6.25	1.79	1.93	2.76	4.48

that there are higher similarities between the dermatologists, which indicate the reliability of the ground truth.

Segmentation results (mean and standard deviation) are quantitatively evaluated by comparing automated results (our proposed segmentation method) to manual borders independently drawn by the three dermatologists. The comparison is done with respect to five different metrics: sensitivity, specificity, accuracy, segmentation error, and similarity (Table 11.4).

11.3.2.1 Comparison with Other Automated Segmentation Methods

Table 11.5 indicates the mean and standard deviation of segmentation error for the five automated methods [40] and the proposed method. The lowest error value in each row is shown in bold. It can be seen that the results vary significantly across the border sets, highlighting the subjectivity of human experts in the border determination procedure. According to dermatologists 2 and 3, the proposed method in this study (AC) shows better results than the other methods. However, according to dermatologist 1, the SRM method achieves the better results of our study. It should be noted that all studies have used the images from the same set (100 images), but in the evaluation of SRM, only 90 images have been selected.

TABLE 11.5

Segmentation Error Results (Mean and Standard Deviation) for Several Methods

Dermatologist	Statistics	OSFCM	DTEA	Mean-Shift	JSEG	SRM	Proposed AC Method (This Study)
D1	Mean	27.52	12.24	12.21	12.55	10.52	12.15
	Std	13.54	5.65	7.37	6.77	5.31	5.34
D2	Mean	25.84	10.50	11.26	11.37	10.27	9.78
	Std	12.43	4.10	6.57	5.57	6.35	3.22
D3	Mean	24.35	10.86	11.98	11.58	11.11	10.85
	Std	13.45	5.08	9.19	6.78	6.12	4.48

Note: DTEA, dermatologist-like tumor extraction algorithm; JSEG, J-image segmentation algorithm; OSFCM, orientation-sensitive fuzzy c-means; SRM, statistical region merging.

11.3.2.2 Effect of Proposed Hair Removal Method on Lesion Segmentation

Hair artifacts in a dermoscopy image can reduce the accuracy of the segmentation of skin lesions. Figure 11.12 demonstrates the results of the lesion segmentation in sample dermoscopy images before and after hair removal. Thereby, using the hair removal algorithm, the segmentation veracity is improved. Table 11.6 shows the segmentation error on the images before and after hair removal. It can be seen that the segmentation error is effectively reduced after hair removal. Specially, skin lesion segmentation after our proposed hair detection and hair repair algorithm has minimum error with respect to other cases.

11.3.3 FEATURE EXTRACTION, FEATURE SELECTION, AND CLASSIFICATION

In this section, 322 digital dermoscopy images were collected from two dermoscopy atlases [101, 106]. These images were gathered from different sources and stored in the RGB color format with dimensions ranging from 712×454 to 2000×1500 pixels. Among the 322 images, 102 were melanoma and 220 were benign. The diagnosis distribution of melanomas includes: 18 melanomas in situ, 12 superficial spreading melanomas, 10 lentigo malignas, 22 nodular melanomas, and 40 invasive melanomas (24 lesions with Breslow thickness less than 0.5 mm, 12 lesions with thickness between 0.5 and 1 mm, and 4 lesions with thickness more than 1 mm). The distribution of benign cases includes 55 Clark (dysplastic) nevi, 42 combined nevi, 38 seborheic keratosis,

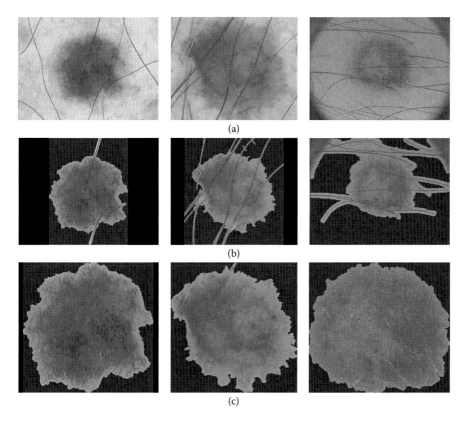

FIGURE 11.12 Lesion segmentation before and after hair removal. (a) The original images. (b) Lesion segmentation before hair removal. (c) Lesion segmentation after hair removal.

TABLE 11.6

Quantitative Results of Skin Lesion Segmentation before and after Hair Removal Algorithms

Hair Detection Method	Hair Repair Method	Segmentation Error (%)
None	None	16.26
DullRazor [105]	DullRazor [105]	12.11
Proposed hair detection method	Coherence transport method [93]	10.74
Proposed hair detection method	Proposed multiresolution coherence transport method	9.9

Source: Bahreyni Toossi, M. T. et al., *Skin Research and Technology*, vol. 19, no. 3, pp. 230–235, 2013.

25 Reed/Spitz nevi, 25 junctional nevi, 10 blue nevi, 10 basal cell carcinoma (BCC), 10 congenital nevi, and 5 dermatofibromas. The type of lesions was specified by histopathological examinations in cases where significant risk for melanoma was present; otherwise, they were diagnosed by follow-up examinations.

11.3.3.1 Selection of Optimal Features

In the feature extraction phase, a feature vector with dimensions of 755×1 is obtained for each image. This vector is created from geometric (4), color (75), texture (104), and wavelet-based texture (572) features. The number of features selected by the feature selection algorithm is an important parameter that needs to be considered in order to determine a good classification performance. For this purpose, extracted features were ranked by the three feature selection algorithms: CFS, relief, and t-test. Then the first 100 highest-ranked features by each feature selection method were used for classification by quadratic discriminant analysis (QDA). We computed the misclassification error (MCE) for various numbers of features. MCE is defined as the number of misclassified observations divided by the number of observations. In order to reasonably estimate the performance of the classifier, the 226 training samples were used to fit the QDA model and the MCE was computed on 96 test observations. Figure 11.13 shows the plot of MCE as a function of the number of features for various feature selection methods. The results demonstrate the superiority of the t-test feature selection over the other methods.

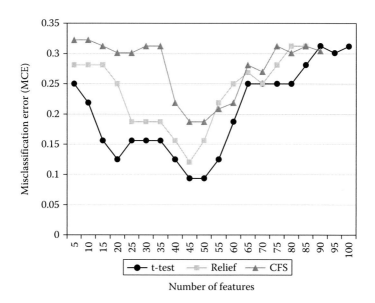

FIGURE 11.13 MCE vs. the number of features for various feature selection algorithms.

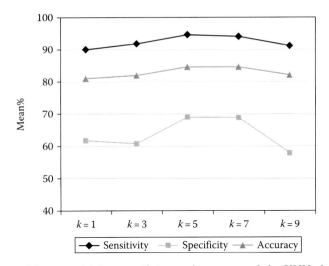

FIGURE 11.14 Mean sensitivity, specificity, and accuracy of the KNN classifier with different values of k.

11.3.3.2 Evaluation of KNN Classification Algorithm

In order to select training and test sets in the KNN classifier, leave-one-out cross-validation (LOOCV) is used. LOOCV involves using a single observation from the original sample as the validation data, and the remaining observations as the training data. This is repeated such that each observation in the sample is used once as the validation data. Due to the fact that optimal k has to be estimated experimentally, different odd values were tested ($k = 1, 3, 5, 7, 9$), in order to conclude which k achieved higher performance measures in terms of sensitivity, specificity, and accuracy in the classification based on two classes. The best results were obtained for $k = 5$, which achieved a sensitivity of 94.6%, specificity of 69%, and accuracy of 84.6% (Figure 11.14). In order to assess the optimal number of features using the KNN classifier, KNN algorithms were analyzed with different numbers of features (Figure 11.15). The best results were obtained for 45 features by the t-test feature selection method.

11.3.3.3 Evaluation of SVM Classification Algorithm

To assess the SVM, this classifier with linear, quadratic, polynomial, and RBF kernel functions is utilized to classify the images. Similar to the KNN algorithm, leave-one-out cross-validation is carried out on the training set to determine the optimal kernel parameters. The corresponding results for different kernel functions are presented in Table 11.7. As the results show, the linear and RBF kernels yield a higher diagnostic accuracy. So, the accuracy metric is evaluated by linear and RBF kernels for different numbers of features in Table 11.8.

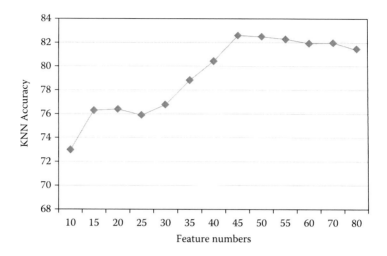

FIGURE 11.15   Classification accuracy in different number of features.

TABLE 11.7
Results of SVM Classification for Different Kernel Functions

	Linear	Quadratic	Polynomial	RBF
Sensitivity	90	73.33	88.6	84.09
Specificity	86.36	77.27	69.61	85.29
Accuracy	87.5	76.04	82.61	84.47

In order to assess the variability of results between the training and the test set, all classification algorithms in this study were repeated 10 times and mean values of the parameters were obtained.

11.3.3.4   Evaluation of ANN Classification Algorithm

Based on 45 selected features by the t-test method, we used a back propagation ANN to classify dermoscopy images in two classes. The classifier network consists of 45 input neurons (equal to selected features) and one output neuron (melanoma or benign). Feed forward neural networks can have one or more hidden layers. Sometimes adding a second hidden layer can enhance the processing power of a neural network. Adding too many layers or hidden neurons can also detract from the trainability of the neural network. In addition to the number of hidden layers, we must also consider the number of neurons in each hidden layer. The optimum number of hidden neurons was found out by a trial-and-error approach. Table 11.9 shows the statistical results of the ANN classifier algorithm in different numbers of hidden layers and neurons.

TABLE 11.8

Results of SVM Classification for Linear and RBF Kernel Functions in Different Numbers of Features

Number of Features	10	20	30	40	45	50	60	70	80
Accuracy_RBF	73	75.8	74.5	85.4	84.5	82.6	77.6	71.1	71.1
Accuracy_Linear	70.8	71.7	73.9	84.8	87.5	87.5	87.3	86.9	86.7

TABLE 11.9

ANN Classifier Performance in Different Numbers of Hidden Layers and Neurons

Number of Neurons in Hidden Layer 1	Number of Neurons in Hidden Layer 2	Sensitivity	Specificity	Accuracy
5	—	79	92	88
15	—	82	94	91
25	—	83	94	92
5	5	85	93	90
5	15	87	93	93
5	25	90	96	95
15	5	87	96	93
25	**5**	**93**	**96**	**95**
10	5	87	94	90
10	15	88	93	90
10	25	88	94	91
25	10	92	95	93
15	10	90	94	91

The best results were obtained from two hidden layers with 25 neurons in the first layer and 5 neurons in the second. In addition to determining the optimum network structure for the classification, the ANN classifier was evaluated with the number of different features (Figure 11.16). The best results were obtained for 50 features by the t-test feature selection method.

11.3.3.5 Comparison of Different Classification Methods

In this study, we implemented different classification algorithms, namely, KNN, SVM, and ANN; in all classification systems, the same set of images were used. Figure 11.17 presents a comparison of the best results achieved by each classification method. The best performance is obtained by the ANN classification algorithm (for 50 features), with an accuracy of 95.9%, sensitivity of 94.7%, and specificity of 96.7%. A variety of statistical and machine learning approaches are used for the classification of dermoscopic images in the literature. Different classification results may be obtained depending on the

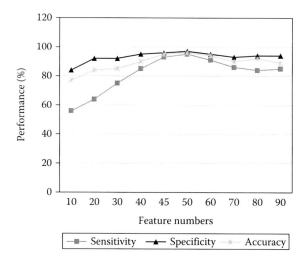

FIGURE 11.16 ANN algorithm performance in different number of features.

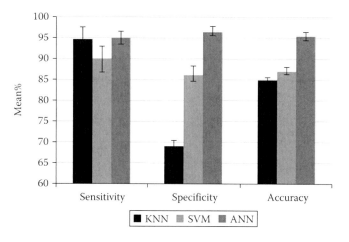

FIGURE 11.17 Comparative results of classification methods used in this study.

classifier chosen; differences in sample size and percentage of melanoma, dysplastic nevi, and benign lesions in the samples; and the number of features used for discrimination.

11.4 CONCLUSION

Malignant melanoma is the deadliest form of skin cancer and its early diagnosis is of extreme importance for the reduction of mortality rates. Computer-based melanoma diagnosis has become a major research area in recent years, with the aim of assisting physicians through the provision of quantitative reproducible analysis of the skin lesion. In this chapter we presented a computer-based diagnostic system for early detection of melanoma. This system involves several components, including image preprocessing, image segmentation (border detection), feature extraction, feature selection, and classification. In the preprocessing step, the proposed approach involves hair detection using the adaptive canny edge detector and hair repair using multiresolution coherence transport inpainting. The results indicate that the proposed algorithm is highly accurate and able to detect and inpaint the hair pixels with few errors. Therefore, the proposed method is an efficient approach to process the hairy dermoscopy images before diagnosing the skin lesions. In the segmentation step, an automatic and unsupervised border detection algorithm according to the region-based active contour method is presented to separate the lesion from the background skin. The proposed algorithm with 94% sensitivity and 98% specificity has achieved much better results than other automated methods available so far. Furthermore, multiple feature sets, including geometric (4), color (75), texture (104), and wavelet-based texture (572) features, are extracted from the images. Overall, the number of features extracted from each image is 755. The next step includes feature selection and optimal integration of features, wherein the relief, t-test, and correlation-based feature selection methods are applied. Therefore, 50 features from the total are selected by means of optimal method (t-test). Selected features include aspect ratio and asymmetry from geometric features; ratio of the standard deviation to the mean in YCbCr color space from color features; and energy, entropy, sum entropy, and information of correlation in HSV, $I_1/I_2/I_3$, $L_1/L_2/L_3$, CIELuv, and CIELab color spaces from texture and wavelet-based texture features. Finally, three methods of classification—KNN, SVM, and ANN—are employed, and the best results are obtained with the ANN classification algorithm. Overall, the results reveal that our computer-based diagnostic system gives high performance. Further improvements along this study include applying pattern recognition techniques to extract certain differential structures (high-level features), such as blue–white veil, pigmented network, globules, and dots.

REFERENCES

1. Melanoma Center, Melanoma Basics, http://www.melanomacenter.org/basics/index.html.
2. P. Schmid-Saugeon, J. Guillod, and J.-P. Thiran, Towards a computer-aided diagnosis system for pigmented skin lesions, *Computerized Medical Imaging and Graphics*, vol. 27, no. 1, pp. 65–78, 2003.
3. H. Ganster, A. Pinz, R. Rohrer, E. Wildling, M. Binder, and H. Kittler, Automated melanoma recognition, *IEEE Transactions on Medical Imaging*, vol. 20, no. 3, pp. 233–239, 2001.
4. I. Maglogiannis and C. N. Doukas, Overview of advanced computer vision systems for skin lesions characterization, *IEEE Transactions on Information Technology in Biomedicine*, vol. 13, no. 5, pp. 721–733, 2009.

5. R. P. Braun, H. S. Rabinovitz, M. Oliviero, A. W. Kopf, and J.-H. Saurat, Dermoscopy of pigmented skin lesions, *Journal of the American Academy of Dermatology*, vol. 52, no. 1, pp. 109–121, 2005.

6. R. J. Pariser and D. M. Pariser, Primary care physicians' errors in handling cutaneous disorders: a prospective survey, *Journal of the American Academy of Dermatology*, vol. 17, no. 2, pp. 239–245, 1987.

7. R. Garnavi, M. Aldeen, M. E. Celebi, G. Varigos, and S. Finch, Border detection in dermoscopy images using hybrid thresholding on optimized color channels, *Computerized Medical Imaging and Graphics*, vol. 35, no. 2, pp. 105–115, 2011.

8. J. Scharcanski and M. E. Celebi, *Computer Vision Techniques for the Diagnosis of Skin Cancer*, Springer, Berlin, 2013.

9. K. Korotkov and R. Garcia, Computerized analysis of pigmented skin lesions: a review, *Artificial Intelligence in Medicine*, vol. 56, no. 2, pp. 69–90, 2012.

10. M. E. Celebi, W. V. Stoecker, and R. H. Moss, Advances in skin cancer image analysis, *Computerized Medical Imaging and Graphics*, vol. 35, no. 2, pp. 83–84, 2011.

11. M. Sadeghi, Towards prevention and early diagnosis of skin cancer: computer-aided analysis of dermoscopy images, PhD thesis, Applied Science: School of Computing Science, Vancouver, Canada, 2012.

12. M. T. B. Toossi, H. R. Pourreza, H. Zare, M. H. Sigari, P. Layegh, and A. Azimi, An effective hair removal algorithm for dermoscopy images, *Skin Research and Technology*, vol. 19, no. 3, pp. 230–235, 2013.

13. M. E. Celebi, Y. Alp Aslandogan, W. V. Stoecker, H. Iyatomi, H. Oka, and X. Chen, Unsupervised border detection in dermoscopy images, *Skin Research and Technology*, vol. 13, no. 4, pp. 454–462, 2007.

14. T. Lee, V. Ng, R. Gallagher, A. Coldman, and D. McLean, Dullrazor: A software approach to hair removal from images, *Computers in Biology and Medicine*, vol. 27, no. 6, pp. 533–543, 1997.

15. H. Zhou, M. Chen, R. Gass, J. M. Rehg, L. Ferris, J. Ho, and L. Drogowski, Feature-preserving artifact removal from dermoscopy images, in *Proceedings of the SPIE Medical Imaging Conference*, San Diego, CA, vol. 6914, p. 69141B, 2008.

16. F.-Y. Xie, S.-Y. Qin, Z.-G. Jiang, and R.-S. Meng, PDE-based unsupervised repair of hair-occluded information in dermoscopy images of melanoma, *Computerized Medical Imaging and Graphics*, vol. 33, no. 4, pp. 275–282, 2009.

17. Q. Abbas, M. E. Celebi, and I. F. García, Hair removal methods: a comparative study for dermoscopy images, *Biomedical Signal Processing and Control*, vol. 6, no. 4, pp. 395–404, 2011.

18. Q. Abbas, I. F. Garcia, M. E. Celebi, and W. Ahmad, A feature-preserving hair removal algorithm for dermoscopy images, *Skin Research and Technology*, vol. 19, no. 1, pp. e27–e36, 2013.

19. M. Sonka, V. Hlavac, and R. Boyle, *Image Processing, Analysis, and Machine Vision*, PWS Publishing Company, 1998.

20. R. M. Haralick and L. G. Shapiro, Image segmentation techniques, *Computer Vision, Graphics, and Image Processing*, vol. 29, no. 1, pp. 100–132, 1985.

21. M. E. Celebi, H. Iyatomi, G. Schaefer, and W. V. Stoecker, Lesion border detection in dermoscopy images, *Computerized Medical Imaging and Graphics*, vol. 33, no. 2, pp. 148–153, 2009.

22. T. Lee, V. Ng, D. McLean, A. Coldman, R. Gallagher, and J. Sale, A multistage segmentation method for images of skin lesions, in *Proceedings of the IEEE Pacific Rim Conference on Communications, Computers, and Signal Processing*, Victoria, British Columbia, pp. 602–605, 1995.

23. Y. Deng and B. Manjunath, Unsupervised segmentation of color-texture regions in images and video, *IEEE Transactions on Pattern Analysis and Machine Intelligence*, vol. 23, no. 8, pp. 800–810, 2001.

24. A. Green, N. Martin, J. Pfitzner, M. O'Rourke, and N. Knight, Computer image analysis in the diagnosis of melanoma, *Journal of the American Academy of Dermatology*, vol. 31, no. 6, pp. 958–964, 1994.

25. M. E. Celebi, H. A. Kingravi, B. Uddin, H. Iyatomi, Y. A. Aslandogan, W. V. Stoecker, and R. H. Moss, A methodological approach to the classification of dermoscopy images, *Computerized Medical Imaging and Graphics*, vol. 31, no. 6, pp. 362–373, 2007.

26. L. Xu, M. Jackowski, A. Goshtasby, D. Roseman, S. Bines, C. Yu, A. Dhawan, and A. Huntley, Segmentation of skin cancer images, *Image and Vision Computing*, vol. 17, no. 1, pp. 65–74, 1999.

27. Q. Abbas, M. E. Celebi, I. F. Garcia, and M. Rashid, Lesion border detection in dermoscopy images using dynamic programming, *Skin Research and Technology*, vol. 17, no. 1, pp. 91–100, 2011.

28. A. Sboner, E. Blanzieri, C. Eccher, P. Bauer, M. Cristofolini, G. Zumiani, and S. Forti, A knowledge based system for early melanoma diagnosis support, in *Proceedings of the 6th IDAMAP Workshop: Intelligent Data Analysis in Medicine and Pharmacology*, London, pp. 30–35, 2001.

29. D. D. Gómez, C. Butakoff, B. K. Ersboll, and W. Stoecker, Independent histogram pursuit for segmentation of skin lesions, *IEEE Transactions on Biomedical Engineering*, vol. 55, no. 1, pp. 157–161, 2008.

30. G. A. Hance, S. E. Umbaugh, R. H. Moss, and W. V. Stoecker, Unsupervised color image segmentation: with application to skin tumor borders, *IEEE Engineering in Medicine and Biology Magazine*, vol. 15, no. 1, pp. 104–111, 1996.

31. P. Schmid, Segmentation of digitized dermatoscopic images by two-dimensional color clustering, *IEEE Transactions on Medical Imaging*, vol. 18, no. 2, pp. 164–171, 1999.

32. R. Cucchiara, C. Grana, S. Seidenari, and G. Pellacani, Exploiting color and topological features for region segmentation with recursive fuzzy c-means, *Machine Graphics and Vision*, vol. 11, no. 2–3, pp. 169–182, 2002.

33. H. Galda, H. Murao, H. Tamaki, and S. Kitamura, Skin image segmentation using a self-organizing map and genetic algorithms, *IEEJ Transactions on Electronics, Information and Systems*, vol. 123, pp. 2056–2062, 2003.

34. R. Melli, C. Grana, and R. Cucchiara, Comparison of color clustering algorithms for segmentation of dermatological images, in *Proceedings of the SPIE Medical Imaging Conference*, San Diego, CA, Vol. 6144, p. 61443S, 2006.

35. H. Zhou, M. Chen, L. Zou, R. Gass, L. Ferris, L. Drogowski, and J. M. Rehg, Spatially constrained segmentation of dermoscopy images, in *Proceedings of the 5th IEEE International Symposium on Biomedical Imaging: From Nano to Macro*, pp. 800–803, 2008.

36. W. Denton, A. Duller, and P. Fish, Boundary detection for skin lesions: an edge focusing algorithm, in *Proceedings of the 5th International Conference on Image Processing and Its Applications*, pp. 399–403, 1995.

37. A. Round, A. Duller, and P. Fish, Colour segmentation for lesion classification, in *Proceedings of the 19th Annual International Conference of the IEEE*, pp. 582–585, 1997.

38. J. Gao, J. Zhang, M. G. Fleming, I. Pollak, and A. B. Cognetta, Segmentation of dermatoscopic images by stabilized inverse diffusion equations, in *Proceedings of the International Conference on Image Processing*, Chicago, IL, Vol. 3, pp. 823–827, 1998.

39. Q. Abbas, M. E. Celebi, and I. F. Garcia, Skin tumor area extraction using an improved dynamic programming approach, *Skin Research and Technology*, vol. 18, no. 2, pp. 133–142, 2012.

40. M. E. Celebi, H. A. Kingravi, H. Iyatomi, Y. Alp Aslandogan, W. V. Stoecker, R. H. Moss, J. M. Malters, J. M. Grichnik, A. A. Marghoob, and H. S. Rabinovitz, Border detection in dermoscopy images using statistical region merging, *Skin Research and Technology*, vol. 14, no. 3, pp. 347–353, 2008.

41. S. B. Forman, T. C. Ferringer, S. J. Peckham, S. R. Dalton, G. T. Sasaki, L. F. Libow, and D. M. Elston, Is superficial spreading melanoma still the most common form of malignant melanoma? *Journal of the American Academy of Dermatology*, vol. 58, no. 6, pp. 1013–1020, 2008.

42. S. W. Menzies, Cutaneous melanoma: making a clinical diagnosis, present and future, *Dermatologic Therapy*, vol. 19, no. 1, pp. 32–39, 2006.

43. Y. Vander Haeghen, J. Naeyaert, and I. Lemahieu, Development of a dermatological workstation: preliminary results on lesion segmentation in CIE LAB color space, in *Proceedings of the International Conference on Color in Graphics and Image Processing*, Saint-Etienne, France, pp. 328–333, 2000.

44. B. Erkol, R. H. Moss, R. Joe Stanley, W. V. Stoecker, and E. Hvatum, Automatic lesion boundary detection in dermoscopy images using gradient vector flow snakes, *Skin Research and Technology*, vol. 11, no. 1, pp. 17–26, 2005.

45. T. Mendonça, A. R. S. Marçal, A. Vieira, J. C. Nascimento, M. Silveira, J. S. Marques, and J. Rozeira, Comparison of segmentation methods for automatic diagnosis of dermoscopy images, in *Proceedings of the 29th Annual International Conference of the IEEE Engineering in Medicine and Biology Society*, Lyon, France, pp. 6572–6575, 2007.

46. A. G. Manousaki, A. G. Manios, E. I. Tsompanaki, J. G. Panayiotides, D. D. Tsiftsis, A. K. Kostaki, and A. D. Tosca, A simple digital image processing system to aid in melanoma diagnosis in an everyday melanocytic skin lesion unit: a preliminary report, *International Journal of Dermatology*, vol. 45, no. 4, pp. 402–410, 2006.

47. T. Donadey, C. Serruys, A. Giron, G. Aitken, J. P. Vignali, R. Triller, and B. Fertil, Boundary detection of black skin tumors using an adaptive radial-based approach, in *Proceedings of the SPIE Medical Imaging Conference*, San Diego, CA, Vol. 3979, pp. 810–816, 2000.

48. H. Iyatomi, H. Oka, M. E. Celebi, M. Hashimoto, M. Hagiwara, M. Tanaka, and K. Ogawa, An improved Internet-based melanoma screening system with dermatologist-like tumor area extraction algorithm, *Computerized Medical Imaging and Graphics*, vol. 32, no. 7, pp. 566–579, 2008.

49. M. E. Celebi, Y. A. Aslandogan, W. V. Stoecker, H. Iyatomi, H. Oka, and X. Chen, Unsupervised border detection in dermoscopy images, *Skin Research and Technology*, vol. 13, no. 4, pp. 454–462, 2007.

50. D. Ruiz, V. Berenguer, A. Soriano, and B. Sánchez, A decision support system for the diagnosis of melanoma: a comparative approach, *Expert Systems with Applications*, vol. 38, no. 12, pp. 15217–15223, 2011.

51. W. V. Stoecker, W. W. Li, and R. H. Moss, Automatic detection of asymmetry in skin tumors, *Computerized Medical Imaging and Graphics*, vol. 16, no. 3, pp. 191–197, 1992.

52. S. Seidenari, G. Pellacani, and C. Grana, Asymmetry in dermoscopic melanocytic lesion images: a computer description based on colour distribution, *Acta Dermato-Venereologica*, vol. 86, no. 2, pp. 123–128, 2006.

53. Y. Chang, R. J. Stanley, R. H. Moss, and W. V. Stoecker, A systematic heuristic approach for feature selection for melanoma discrimination using clinical images, *Skin Research and Technology*, vol. 11, no. 3, pp. 165–178, 2005.

54. K. Clawson, P. Morrow, B. Scotney, D. McKenna, and O. Dolan, Determination of optimal axes for skin lesion asymmetry quantification, in *Proceedings of the IEEE International Conference on Image Processing*, San Antonio, TX, vol. 2, pp. 453–456, 2007.

55. V. T. Y. Ng, B. Y. M. Fung, and T. K. Lee, Determining the asymmetry of skin lesion with fuzzy borders, *Computers in Biology and Medicine*, vol. 35, no. 2, pp. 103–120, 2005.

56. V. Ng, and D. Cheung, Measuring asymmetries of skin lesions, in *Proceedings of the IEEE International Conference on Computational Cybernetics and Simulation, Systems, Man, and Cybernetics*, Orlando, Vol. 5, pp. 4211–4216, 1997.

57. A. Bono, S. Tomatis, C. Bartoli, G. Tragni, G. Radaelli, A. Maurichi, and R. Marchesini, The ABCD system of melanoma detection, *Cancer*, vol. 85, no. 1, pp. 72–77, 1999.

58. E. Claridge, P. Hall, M. Keefe, and J. Allen, Shape analysis for classification of malignant melanoma, *Journal of Biomedical Engineering*, vol. 14, no. 3, pp. 229–234, 1992.

59. T. Lee, S. Atkins, R. Gallagher, C. MacAulay, A. Coldman, and D. Mclean, Describing the structural shape of melanocytic lesions, in *Proceedings of the SPIE Medical Imaging Conference*, pp. 1170–1179, 1999.

60. T. K. Lee and M. S. Atkins, A new approach to measure border irregularity for melanocytic lesions, in *Proceedings of the SPIE Medical Imaging Conference*, pp. 668–675, 2000.

61. T. K. Lee, D. I. McLean, and M. Stella Atkins, Irregularity index: a new border irregularity measure for cutaneous melanocytic lesions, *Medical Image Analysis*, vol. 7, no. 1, pp. 47–64, 2003.

62. S. M. Chung and Q. Wang, Content-based retrieval and data mining of a skin cancer image database, in *Proceedings of the IEEE International Conference on Information Technology: Coding and Computing*, pp. 611–615, 2001.

63. Y. I. Cheng, R. Swamisai, S. E. Umbaugh, R. H. Moss, W. V. Stoecker, S. Teegala, and S. K. Srinivasan, Skin lesion classification using relative color features, *Skin Research and Technology*, vol. 14, no. 1, pp. 53–64, 2008.

64. T. Holmstrom, A survey and evaluation of features for the diagnosis of malignant melanoma, Master's thesis, Umeå University, 2005.

65. Y. Faziloglu, R. J. Stanley, R. H. Moss, W. Van Stoecker, and R. P. McLean, Colour histogram analysis for melanoma discrimination in clinical images, *Skin Research and Technology*, vol. 9, no. 2, pp. 147–156, 2003.

66. J. Chen, R. J. Stanley, R. H. Moss, and W. Van Stoecker, Colour analysis of skin lesion regions for melanoma discrimination in clinical images, *Skin Research and Technology*, vol. 9, no. 2, pp. 94–104, 2003.

67. R. M. Haralick, K. Shanmugam, and I. H. Dinstein, Textural features for image classification, *IEEE Transactions on Systems, Man and Cybernetics*, no. 6, pp. 610–621, 1973.

68. J. Kontinen, J. Röning, and R. M. MacKie, Texture features in the classification of melanocytic lesions, in *Proceedings of the 9th International Conference on Image Analysis and Processing*, Florence, Italy, pp. 453–460, 1997.

69. M. Sadeghi, M. Razmara, T. K. Lee, and M. S. Atkins, A novel method for detection of pigment network in dermoscopic images using graphs, *Computerized Medical Imaging and Graphics*, vol. 35, no. 2, pp. 137–143, 2011.

70. J. L. García Arroyo and B. García Zapirain, Detection of pigment network in dermoscopy images using supervised machine learning and structural analysis, *Computers in Biology and Medicine*, vol. 44, pp. 144–157, 2014.

71. A. Sáez, C. Serrano, and B. Acha, Model-based classification methods of global patterns in dermoscopic images, in *IEEE Transactions on Medical Imaging*, vol. 33, no. 5, pp. 1137–1147, 2014.

72. C. Barata, J. S. Marques, and J. Rozeira, A system for the detection of pigment network in dermoscopy images using directional filters, *IEEE Transactions on Biomedical Engineering*, vol. 59, no. 10, pp. 2744–2754, 2012.

73. Q. Abbas, M. E. Celebi, C. Serrano, I. Fondón García, and G. Ma, Pattern classification of dermoscopy images: a perceptually uniform model, *Pattern Recognition*, vol. 46, no. 1, pp. 86–97, 2013.

74. M. G. Fleming, C. Steger, J. Zhang, J. Gao, A. B. Cognetta, and C. R Dyer, Techniques for a structural analysis of dermatoscopic imagery, *Computerized Medical Imaging and Graphics*, vol. 22, no. 5, pp. 375–389, 1998.

75. G. Di Leo, C. Liguori, A. Paolillo, and P. Sommella, An improved procedure for the automatic detection of dermoscopic structures in digital ELM images of skin lesions, in *Proceedings of the IEEE Conference on Virtual Environments, Human-Computer Interfaces and Measurement Systems*, pp. 190–194, 2008.

76. B. Shrestha, J. Bishop, K. Kam, X. Chen, R. H. Moss, W. V. Stoecker, S. Umbaugh, R. J. Stanley, M. E. Celebi, and A. A. Marghoob, Detection of atypical texture features in early malignant melanoma, *Skin Research and Technology*, vol. 16, no. 1, pp. 60–65, 2010.

77. H. Mirzaalian, T. K. Lee, and G. Hamarneh, Learning features for streak detection in dermoscopic color images using localized radial flux of principal intensity curvature, in *Proceedings of the IEEE Workshop on Mathematical Methods in Biomedical Image Analysis*, pp. 97–101, 2012.

78. M. Sadeghi, T. K. Lee, D. I. McLean, H. Lui, and M. S. Atkins, Detection and analysis of irregular streaks in dermoscopic images of skin lesions, *IEEE Transactions on Medical Imaging*, vol. 32, no. 5, pp. 849–861, 2013.

79. A. Khan, K. Gupta, R. J. Stanley, W. V. Stoecker, R. H. Moss, G. Argenziano, H. P. Soyer, H. S. Rabinovitz, and A. B. Cognetta, Fuzzy logic techniques for blotch feature evaluation in dermoscopy images, *Computerized Medical Imaging and Graphics*, vol. 33, no. 1, pp. 50–57, 2009.

80. W. V. Stoecker, K. Gupta, R. J. Stanley, R. H. Moss, and B. Shrestha, Detection of asymmetric blotches (asymmetric structureless areas) in dermoscopy images

of malignant melanoma using relative color, *Skin Research and Technology*, vol. 11, no. 3, pp. 179–184, 2005.

81. G. Pellacani, C. Grana, R. Cucchiara, and S. Seidenari, Automated extraction and description of dark areas in surface microscopy melanocytic lesion images, *Dermatology*, vol. 208, no. 1, pp. 21–26, 2004.

82. S. Skrovseth, T. R. Schopf, K. Thon, M. Zortea, M. Geilhufe, K. Mollersen, H. M. Kirchesch, and F. Godtliebsen, A computer aided diagnostic system for malignant melanomas, in *Proceedings of the 3rd International Symposium on Applied Sciences in Biomedical and Communication Technologies*, pp. 1–5, 2010.

83. A. Madooei, M. S. Drew, M. Sadeghi, and M. S. Atkins, Automatic detection of blue-white veil by discrete colour matching in dermoscopy images, in *Proceedings of the Medical Image Computing and Computer-Assisted Intervention Conference*, Nagoya, Japan, pp. 453–460, 2013.

84. M. E. Celebi, H. Iyatomi, W. V. Stoecker, R. H. Moss, H. S. Rabinovitz, G. Argenziano, and H. P. Soyer, Automatic detection of blue-white veil and related structures in dermoscopy images, *Computerized Medical Imaging and Graphics*, vol. 32, no. 8, pp. 670, 2008.

85. T. Roß, H. Handels, J. Kreusch, H. Busche, H. Wolf, and S. Pöppl, Automatic classification of skin tumours with high resolution surface profiles, in *Proceedings of the Computer Analysis of Images and Patterns Conference*, pp. 368–375, 1995.

86. H. Iyatomi, H. Oka, M. E. Celebi, M. Tanaka, and K. Ogawa, Parameterization of dermoscopic findings for the Internet-based melanoma screening system, in *Proceedings of the IEEE Symposium on Computational Intelligence in Image and Signal Processing*, pp. 189–193, 2007.

87. M. Burroni, R. Corona, G. Dell'Eva, F. Sera, R. Bono, P. Puddu, R. Perotti, F. Nobile, L. Andreassi, and P. Rubegni, Melanoma computer-aided diagnosis reliability and feasibility study, *Clinical Cancer Research*, vol. 10, no. 6, pp. 1881–1886, 2004.

88. S. Dreiseitl, L. Ohno-Machado, H. Kittler, S. Vinterbo, H. Billhardt, and M. Binder, A comparison of machine learning methods for the diagnosis of pigmented skin lesions, *Journal of Biomedical Informatics*, vol. 34, no. 1, pp. 28–36, 2001.

89. M. Wiltgen, A. Gerger, and J. Smolle, Tissue counter analysis of benign common nevi and malignant melanoma, *International Journal of Medical Informatics*, vol. 69, no. 1, pp. 17, 2003.

90. K. Tabatabaie, A. Esteki, and P. Toossi, Extraction of skin lesion texture features based on independent component analysis, *Skin Research and Technology*, vol. 15, no. 4, pp. 433–439, 2009.

91. S. E. Umbaugh, R. H. Moss, and W. V. Stoecker, Applying artificial intelligence to the identification of variegated coloring in skin tumors, *IEEE Engineering in Medicine and Biology Magazine*, vol. 10, no. 4, pp. 57–62, 1991.

92. A. Rosenfeld and P. De La Torre, Histogram concavity analysis as an aid in threshold selection, *IEEE Transactions on Systems, Man and Cybernetics*, vol. 13, no. 2, pp. 231–235, 1983.

93. F. Bornemann and T. März, Fast image inpainting based on coherence transport, *Journal of Mathematical Imaging and Vision*, vol. 28, no. 3, pp. 259–278, 2007.

94. K. Zhang, L. Zhang, H. Song, and W. Zhou, Active contours with selective local or global segmentation: a new formulation and level set method, *Image and Vision Computing*, vol. 28, no. 4, pp. 668–676, 2010.

95. D. A. Clausi, An analysis of co-occurrence texture statistics as a function of grey level quantization, *Canadian Journal of Remote Sensing*, vol. 28, no. 1, pp. 45–62, 2002.

96. T. Chang and C.-C. Kuo, Texture analysis and classification with tree-structured wavelet transform, *IEEE Transactions on Image Processing*, vol. 2, no. 4, pp. 429–441, 1993.

97. I. Kononenko and E. Simec, Induction of decision trees using RELIEFF, in *Proceedings of the ISSEK94 Workshop on Mathematical and Statistical Methods in Artificial Intelligence*, Udine, Italy, pp. 199–220, 1995.

98. V. N. Vapnik, *Statistical Learning Theory*, John Wiley and Sons, 1998.

99. B. E. Boser, I. M. Guyon, and V. N. Vapnik, A training algorithm for optimal margin classifiers, in *Proceedings of the 5th Annual Workshop on Computational Learning Theory*, ACM Press, Pittsburgh, PA, pp. 144–152, 1992.

100. V. Vapnik, *The Nature of Statistical Learning Theory*, Springer, Berlin, 1999.

101. *Dermoscopy Atlas*, Skin Cancer Society of Australia, 2007.

102. M. E. Celebi, G. Schaefer, H. Iyatomi, W. V. Stoecker, J. M. Malters, and J. M. Grichnik, An improved objective evaluation measure for border detection in dermoscopy images, *Skin Research and Technology*, vol. 15, no. 4, pp. 444–450, 2009.

103. E. Peserico and A. Silletti, Is (N) PRI suitable for evaluating automated segmentation of cutaneous lesions? *Pattern Recognition Letters*, vol. 31, no. 16, pp. 2464–2467, 2010.

104. R. Garnavi, M. Aldeen, and M. E. Celebi, Weighted performance index for objective evaluation of border detection methods in dermoscopy images, *Skin Research and Technology*, vol. 17, no. 1, pp. 35–44, 2011.

105. T. Lee, V. Ng, R. Gallagher, A. Coldman, and D. McLean, DullRazor: a software approach to hair removal from images, *Computers in Biology and Medicine*, vol. 27, no. 6, pp. 533–543, 1997.

106. S. W. Menzies, K. A. Crotty, C. Ingvar, and W. H. McCarthy, *An Atlas of Surface Microscopy of Pigmented Skin Lesions: Dermoscopy*, McGraw-Hill, 2003.

12 From Dermoscopy to Mobile Teledermatology

Luís Rosado
Fraunhofer Portugal AICOS
Porto, Portugal

Maria João M. Vasconcelos
Fraunhofer Portugal AICOS
Porto, Portugal

Rui Castro
Fraunhofer Portugal AICOS
Porto, Portugal

João Manuel R. S. Tavares
Universidade do Porto
Porto, Portugal

CONTENTS

12.1 INTRODUCTION

Skin cancer constitutes nowadays the most common malignancies in the Caucasian population, with incidences that are reaching epidemic proportions [1]. According to the American Cancer Society, one in every three cancers diagnosed is a skin cancer.

Although malignant melanoma (MM) accounts for only a small percentage of skin cancer, it is far more dangerous than other skin cancers and causes most skin cancer deaths. If detected during the early stages of its development, the success rates of recovery are very high, so early diagnosis of MM is extremely important. According to the World Health Organization [1], the global annual occurrences of nonmelanoma and melanoma skin cancers are estimated to be between 2 million and 3 million and 132,000, respectively.

Malignant melanoma is the fastest-growing form of cancer and, if not detected early, is the deadliest form, accounting for nearly 37,000 annual deaths. Despite the huge number of visual inspections (60 million to 70 million) performed annually, melanoma-based mortality rates are as high as 23%, mainly due to missed or late diagnosed melanomas. This could be attributed to the limitations of the traditional visual inspection, which gives subjective results and is prone to uncertain diagnosis. In addition to missing melanomas, it may also give rise to false positives, resulting in unnecessary biopsies.

It is estimated that only 3% out of the 6 million to 7 million excisions performed annually turn out to be malignant melanoma. Also, the treatment for melanoma alone costs €1.18 billion a year. This explains the criticality of the need for early detection of melanoma.

As an example, the skin cancer corresponds approximately to 25% of all malignant tumors detected each year in Portugal, affecting one in every five persons throughout life. MM represents 10% of all skin cancer, but it is responsible for around 80% of all skin cancer–related deaths registered in Portugal [2]. Each year there are about 700 new cases of MM in Portugal. A recent study presented by the Portuguese Health Central Administration [3] shows an inadequate distribution of dermatologists in the country. The clearly inadequate distribution of the human resources of the dermatology services comes from two main factors: (1) there is a clear uneven regional distribution of dermatologists, with overallocation of specialists near the big urban centers, and (2) the number of dermatologists currently working in the healthcare system represents only 60% of the required resources estimated.

With increasing aging population globally, there is a growing incidence of skin cancer. But the percentage of population participating in skin cancer screening versus the incidence is alarmingly low. Late detection leads to a rise in skin cancer mortalities, especially melanomas. As such, there is a need for complementing existing technologies in order to check out the malignancy level of a mole. In addition, given the current need to decrease the costs of the healthcare providers and the new lightweight monitoring systems that can be carried around easily and used regularly by patients. It is considered crucial to find new ways of making better decisions on treatment without having to meet the patients face-to-face. The search for new "personal health systems" is, in fact, one of the major priorities of the European Union current eHealth program [4]. In this context, teledermatology has the potential to improve efficiency and quality aspects of care at lower costs and has proven to have similar accuracy and reliability as face-to-face dermatology [5, 6]. Moreover, mobile teledermatology (MT) appears to be a promising tool for personal dermatology data acquisition [7, 8], with the potential of not only becoming an easily applicable tool that empowers patients to adopt an active role in managing their own health status and facilitates the early diagnosis of skin cancers, but also offering the opportunity to make available consultations with experts in critical areas. Besides, an automated MT triage framework would not only have the purpose of delivering dermatologic expertise to those critical zones, but also be important to prevent the overloading of the already scarce resources. A recent study [9] focused on the importance of MT in the developing world, which confirmed the added value of using a system that amplifies the access to dermatologic expertise in underserved regions.

A detailed review of the computerized analysis of pigmented skin lesions and skin cancer images can be seen in [10, 11], where the authors present an extensive review of this research topic to microscopic (dermoscopic) and macroscopic (clinical) images. More recently, in [12] the state of the art in the utilization of computer vision techniques in the diagnosis of skin cancer is given, covering also microscopic and macroscopic images.

In Section 12.2, a summary about the available dermatological databases and atlases is presented. Afterwards, in Section 12.3, we discuss the stages related to medical imaging applied in melanoma diagnosis. Starting with image acquisition types used and passing through the preprocessing inherent challenges, such as uneven illumination, color correction, contrast enhancement, hair removal, and image restoration, giving a brief review of these challenges and also presenting self-developed methodologies used to overcome problems like reflection or blur detection. In Section 12.4, a physical and information architecture is proposed that is suitable for a patient-oriented system of skin lesion analysis using smart devices. In Section 12.5, a review of the existing smart device–adaptable dermoscopes is given, together with a discussion on their differences, in terms of color reproduction, image area and distortion, illumination, sharpness, and differential structure visibility. This chapter ends with conclusions about the topics discussed.

12.2 DERMATOLOGICAL DATABASES

To be able to develop a reliable and robust system for melanoma detection, it is crucial to have a complete set of images as diverse as possible and correctly annotated.

The available dermatological databases and atlases are indicated in Table 12.1, where details like the total number of images or melanoma images; the score information of asymmetry, border, color, and differential structure (ABCD) [13]; and the type of images are specified. Although there already exist enough dermoscopic database images with medical annotation, there is only one medical annotated database with images acquired via mobile device.

The construction of a complete dataset with different image types (acquired using dermoscopic, macroscopic, or mobile imaging devices like mobile phones), conveniently annotated by experts for research and benchmarking purposes, would be of extreme importance in order to allow comparative studies in the near future. It would not only facilitate the development of computer-aided diagnosis systems, but also be useful for patient knowledge about this subject. This is confirmed by [12], which states that the absence of

TABLE 12.1

Dermatological Datasets

Databases	Total Images	Melanoma Images	ABCD Score	Type
IPO Mobile [15]	90	NA	Yes	MP
IPO [15]	217	12	Yes	D/M
Interactive Dermoscopy Atlas [16]	729	219	Yes	D/M
PH² [17]	200	40	Yes	D
Menzies Atlas [18]	320	NA	NA	D
Dermnet Skin Disease Atlas [19]	23,000	190	No	M
Danderm [20]	3000	49	No	M/C
MED M Heenen [21]	1207	51	No	M/C
Dermatology Atlas [22]	8084	80	No	M/C
Dermatlas Net [23]	1000	32	No	M/C
Dermoscopy Atlas [24]	NA	153	No	D/M/C
DermIS [25]	NA	300	No	D/M/C
DermQuest [26]	NA	312	No	D/M/C

Note: Type: D, dermoscopic; M, macroscopic; C, clinical; MP, mobile phone; NA, not available.

benchmark datasets for standardized algorithm evaluation is a barrier to more dynamic development in this area. In fact, according to a recent study [14] on the impact of visual images on patient skin self-examination (SSE) knowledge, attitudes, and accuracy, images positively affect knowledge and self-efficacy related to SSE.

12.3 DERMATOLOGY DIGITAL IMAGING

Along the years different imaging techniques were used for melanoma diagnosis, which is detailed next. In the following subsection, a review of existing techniques is presented, and in the last subsection, self-developed methodologies to overcome some of the problems of dealing with these kinds of images are also described.

12.3.1 IMAGE ACQUISITION

In the 1960s and 1970s the diagnosis of melanoma was simply based on symptoms, such as bleeding, itching, and ulceration, and at the time of diagnosis the prognosis was poor. Later, the introduction of the asymmetry, border, color, and diameter (ABCD) rule by Friedman et al. [27] allowed the early detection of a high number of melanomas, and it has been adopted worldwide since then. This rule is based on simple clinical morphological features of melanoma, and the inclusion of a fifth criterion, E, for evolution concerning morphological changes of the lesion over time, brought improvement to the existent rule. Because the clinical diagnosis based on the ABCD rule fails to recognize small melanomas and some benign melanocytic nevi may mimic melanoma from a clinical point of view, new imaging techniques were developed to overcome these problems. More specifically, in [13] Stolz et al. addresses the ABCD dermoscopy rule that quantifies if the selected melanocytic lesion is benign, suspicious, or malignant according to the score information of asymmetry, border, color, and differential structures.

A number of studies had shown that medium-resolution microscopic views using skin surface microscopy (dermoscopy) provided a new level of clinical morphology linking clinical morphology and histopathology. Dermoscopy (epiluminescence microscopy, dermatoscopy, skin surface, incident light microscopy) has been established in the last three decades as the preferred imaging method for improving early detection of MM and for reducing unnecessary excision of benign nevi. It is a noninvasive, in vivo examination with a microscope that uses incident light and oil immersion to make subsurface structures of the skin accessible to visual examination. This method allows the observer to look not only onto but also into the superficial skin layers, permitting a more detailed inspection of pigmented skin lesions. More recently, new handheld devices using polarized light have been introduced, which renders the epidermis translucent, making the use of oil for visualizing the subsurface structures unnecessary [28]. Moreover, it is important to note that some of these handheld dermoscopes are already capable of adapting to smartphones, as is explored in Section 12.5. According to [29], dermoscopy improves the diagnostic accuracy for melanoma in comparison with inspection by the unaided eye, but only for experienced examiners. In addition, study [30] indicates that analysis by either a trained dermatologist or a trained artificial neural network can improve the diagnostic accuracy of melanoma compared with that of an inexperienced clinician, and that computational diagnosis might represent a useful tool for the screening of melanoma, particularly at centers not experienced in dermoscopy.

Medium-resolution clinical images of lesions (macros) are usually acquired using oblique modeling lighting and at close distances to best represent the view that a physician would see under a detailed skin inspection regime in an ideal clinic setting. These macroscopic views could be the best indicators of suspicious lesions [31]. Another possibility that is less expensive and easier to spread is to obtain images from mobile devices such as smartphones. This alternative allows both clinicians in general and patients in particular to obtain several images of suspicious moles to be further analyzed by experienced examiners. The same procedure can be adapted using smartphone-adaptable dermoscopes, obtaining the same image quality as regular dermoscopes, with the added value of image storage and associated benefits, such as being possible to discuss the high-quality image with specialists worldwide in the short term or analyzing the mole evolution in the long term.

Finally, clinical images consist of general imaging of the body with the intent to show the skin condition, the number of lesions, the amount of sun damage, and other clinical identifiers that are also important for the relative assessment of the overall risk of the patient. In [31] a comparative study between a personal device such as a smartphone and clinical photography in monitoring skin lesions is made. Although the quality of images produced using clinical photography is superior, personal device technology still provides useful clinical information, as well as offering a relatively inexpensive alternative.

When professional applications for skin imaging rely on high-quality image acquisition devices, the resulting image quality is supposed to be optimal for skin cancer detection purposes. And when compared to dermoscopy or smartphone-adaptable dermoscopes, these images may contain several additional artifacts that could have impact in terms of image quality. Because of that, new challenges appear regarding preprocessing of macroscopic images acquired with cameras of mobile devices.

12.3.2 IMAGE PREPROCESSING CHALLENGES

12.3.2.1 Color Spaces

The Commission Internationale de L'Éclairage (CIE) has defined a system that classifies color according to the human visual system. CIE RGB (red–green–blue) and CIE XYZ (Y closely matches luminance, while X and Z give color information) were the first mathematically defined color spaces, where CIE RGB is a set of CIE color-matching curves based on many experiments with average observers and pure light sources at specific RGB wavelengths where the resulting spectral curves are called the CIE standard primaries, and CIE XYZ is based on and derived from the first, where XYZ are extrapolations of RGB created to avoid negative numbers and are called tristimulus values [32].

In an attempt to linearize the perceptibility of color differences, the CIE proposed two other color spaces, CIE L*a*b* and CIE L*u*v*, where L* represents the lightness of the color; a* and b* represent the color differences in terms of redness–greenness and yellowness–blueness, respectively; and u* and v* represent differences in the chromaticity coordinates, but are not associated with color names as are a* and b*. These color spaces are device independent, since they are based on the CIE system; however, they suffer from being quite unintuitive [32, 33]. Since CIE L*u*v* and CIE L*a*b* are absolute color spaces, they define color exactly and thus include more color than other color spaces (even more than the human eye can see).

The most known color space is RGB, which is three primary additive colors and is represented by a three-dimensional Cartesian coordinate system [32–34]. This system is commonly used in computational applications since no transform is required to display information on common computer screens. RGB is a device-dependent color space because the values depend on the specific sensitivity function of the imaging acquisition device. The main disadvantage of this color space in applications with natural images is a high correlation between its components. The chromaticity variables (rgb) are the normalized RGB color variables in order to reduce the dependence of lightning intensities changes in space [32, 34].

The hue, saturation, and lightness color space (HSL) or similar ones, like HSI (intensity), HSV (value), or HCI (chroma), are based on linear transformations from RGB and are device dependent [32–35]. The advantage of these systems lies in the intuitive manner of specifying color, making them a good choice in user interfaces and, more importantly, the small correlation between the three components [36].

The luminance–chrominance color spaces like YC_bC_r (Y is the luma component; C_b and C_r are the blue-difference and red-difference chroma components, respectively) separate RGB into luminance and chrominance information and are used in compression applications and digital video encoding [32, 34]. The advantage of converting an original RGB image into luminance–chrominance color space is that the components are pairwise uncorrelated. Furthermore, the chrominance channels contain much redundant information and can easily be subsampled without sacrificing any visual quality for the reconstructed image.

In order to overcome sensitivity against various imaging conditions, Gevers and Smeulders proposed $c_1c_2c_3$, $l_1l_2l_3$, and $m_1m_2m_3$ color spaces [37]. $c_1c_2c_3$ was proposed to achieve independency of color illumination and discount

TABLE 12.2

Sensitivity of Different Color Spaces

Color Space	Color of Illuminant	Illumination Intensity	Highlight	Shadow
RGB	−	−	−	−
rgb	−	+	−	+
H	−	+	+	+
S	−	+	−	+
YC_bC_r	+ (only Y)	−	−	−
$c_1c_2c_3$	−	+	−	+
$l_1l_2l_3$	+	+	+	+
$m_1m_2m_3$	+	+	−	+

Source: Gevers, T., and Smeulders, A. W. M., *Pattern Recognition*, vol. 32, no. 3, pp. 453–464, 1999.

the object's geometry, $l_1l_2l_3$ was proposed to determine the direction of the triangular color plane in RGB space, and $m_1m_2m_3$ achieved a constant color model considering a change in spectral power distribution of the illumination [33, 34, 38]. Nevertheless, it should be noted that the former color spaces were built assuming dichromatic reflectance and white illumination.

Because of separation of luminance and chrominance components, the YC_bC_r color space is one of the most popular choices for skin detection. In [39], the authors use YC_bC_r to model skin and further segment the human face in color from images; other examples that use this color space are found in [40–43]. Recently, in [44], a comparison of skin color segmentation results using the YC_bC_r and CIE L*a*b* color spaces, experimental results showed that CIE L*a*b* performs better because it gives more information than the other color space model.

Different color spaces are better for different applications, since some colors are perceptually linear or just more intuitive to use. Also, some color spaces are tied to a specific imaging equipment, while others are equally valid on whatever device is used. Taking into account the referenced studies, Table 12.2 was built considering different color spaces and their sensitivity to color illuminant, illumination intensity, highlight, and shadows. In the table + means invariance and − no variance to the criteria.

12.3.2.2 Illumination

The correction of uneven illumination is considered crucial to prevent segmentation errors in several skin lesion analysis methodologies. The authors in [45] realized that the uneven illumination corresponded to a low-frequency spatial component of the image, while the information about the skin texture and the pigmented lesion was enclosed in the high spatial frequency component of the image. Thus, they proposed a correction of the illumination by simply removing the low-frequency spatial component of the image. Although this method can be efficient for some images, it requires specific parameters that are not unique for different images, and the authors do not detail how to obtain them automatically.

New techniques to improve the processing of skin images acquired with standard imaging cameras were also proposed in [46], such as a data-driven shading attenuation stage to improve the robustness of the skin lesion segmentation. It starts by converting the input image from the original RGB color space to the HSV color space and retaining the V channel value; then a pixel set of the four corners of the image is extracted in order to estimate a quadratic function, and this information is used to relight the image itself. This method is adequate to model and attenuate the global illumination variation; however, it tends to have limited effect on local cast shadows and also tends to fail on surface shapes that are not locally smooth, since the quadratic function is not able to capture the local illumination variation. The approach of [47] follows the previous method and uses the entropy minimization technique, succeeding in removing or strongly attenuating shading and intensity falloffs.

Homomorphic filtering (HF) [48] is a generalized technique for nonlinear image enhancement; it normalizes the brightness of a dermoscopic image. A later improvement of the former technique to human perception is presented in [49], where HF is performed in both spatial and frequency domains, by processing the J plane of the JCh color space, followed by a contrast adjustment in this color space.

Wang et al. [39], in contrast, use a three-step brightness adjustment procedure to minimize the vignetting effect (darkened image corners due to position-dependent loss of brightness in the output of an optical system) in dermoscopic images. After defining a set of concentric circular regions, the brightness of the next circular region, starting at the image center, is adjusted so that the average intensity is equal at the center.

Recently, a multistage illumination modeling algorithm [50] was proposed to correct illumination variation in dermatological skin lesion images. It first determines a nonparametric model of illumination using Monte Carlo sampling and a parametric model assuming a quadratic surface model is used to determine the final illumination estimate based on a subset of pixels from the first step. Finally, by using the final illuminate estimate, the reflectance component of the image is calculated and a new image is built that is corrected for illumination.

12.3.2.3 Color Correction

Different illumination or different imaging devices will lead to distinct image colors of the same lesion and so can also compromise further steps.

In [51], an algorithm for automatic color correction of digital skin images in teledermatology was proposed. For that, the widely known principle that skin color is one of the basic colors of human color perception was considered. A different method to assess skin tones and retrieve color information from uncalibrated images consists of imaging a skin region with a calibration target and extracting its color values to compute a color correction transform [52].

Another approach capable of addressing this problem is based on the automatic color equalization technique [53], which consists of two main stages: chromatic/spatial adjustment and dynamic tone reproduction scaling. Iyatomi et al. [54] also described a color correction method for dermoscopy images based on the HSV color model where a multiple linear regression model is built for each channel using low-level features extracted from a training image set. Then, through the use of these regression models, the method automatically adjusts the hue and saturation of a previously unseen image. In [55], the authors describe a two-stage color normalization scheme where color variations are removed and the contrast of the images is enhanced by combining Grayworld and MaxRGB normalization techniques.

The authors [56] suggest selecting judicious colors from an image database to design a customized pattern before applying usual color correction. Also, a comparative study was conducted, concluding that the approach ensures a stronger constancy of the color of interest and provides a more robust automatic classification of skin tissues.

12.3.2.4   Contrast Enhancement

Histogram equalization is commonly used contrast adjustment by allowing for areas with lower contrast to gain a higher contrast by spreading out the most frequent intensity values. Generalizations of this method use multiple histograms to emphasize local contrast, rather than overall contrast. Examples of such methods include adaptive histogram equalization (AHE) [57] and contrast limited adaptive histogram equalization (CLAHE) [58]. Another method to perform histogram analysis in order to enhance contrast was proposed in [59], where a scale–space filter is applied.

A smart contrast enhancement technique that also uses histogram equalization is shown in [60]. It is capable of classifying global and local histogram equalizations.

A technique known as independent histogram pursuit [61] consists of finding a combination of spectral bands that enhance the contrast between healthy skin and lesions. Another method used in dermoscopic images consists in determining the optimal weights and converting them by maximizing Otsu's histogram bimodality measure [62, 63]. Alternatively, in [64], an adaptive histogram equalization step is presented that uses processing blocks instead of the entire image, which implies that each block's contrast is enhanced independent of the dominant image information.

In [55], the authors also consider the problems of poor contrast, which make accurate border detection difficult [65] and address this problem by applying the automatic color equalization technique. Recently, a software tool for contrast enhancement and segmentation of melanoma was described in [66] by using intensity remapping and Gaussian filter techniques.

In order to enhance the edges in the original images and facilitate the segmentation process, it is common to apply the Karhunen–Loève transform (KLT) in pigmented skin lesions [61, 67–69].

12.3.2.5 Hair Removal

Hair pixels, usually present in skin images, occlude some of the information of the lesion, such as its boundary and texture. Therefore, in melanoma recognition these hair artifacts should be removed, preferentially preserving all the lesion features while keeping the computational cost low. Common disadvantages associated with hair removal algorithms are oversegmentation, undesirable blurring, alteration of the tumor texture, and color bleeding.

In 1997, Lee et al. [70] proposed the DullRazor hair removal algorithm for dermoscopic images. It consists of three basic steps: identifying the dark hair locations using morphological operations, replacing the hair pixels with the nearby nonhair pixels through bilinear interpolation, and smoothing the final result using an adaptive median filter. This algorithm, however, tends to erase important details of the original images by making the pigmented network unclear, and it cannot remove light-colored or thin hairs.

The median filter is one of the most commonly used smoothing filter in the literature and it has proven capable of eliminating most of the artifacts in dermoscopy images [71, 72]. To attenuate the influence of hair, Celebi et al. [72] proposed to smooth the input image by applying a median filter with a mask of an appropriate size. Similarly, the works of Saugeon et al. [73] and Fleming et al. [74] detect and remove hair using morphological operations and thresholding in CIE L*u*v* color space. In these techniques, a hair mask is generated by a fixed thresholding procedure on these thin structures based on their luminosity, and at the end, each masked pixel is replaced by an average of its neighboring nonmasked pixels.

She et al. [75] proposed an alternative method to estimate the underlying color of hair pixels based on a band-limited signal interpolation technique. This method takes the Fourier transform of the image, sets the response outside of a defined region to zero, takes the inverse Fourier transform and updates the pixels within the mask region accordingly, and repeats the previous process until convergence.

Inpainting is a technique originally used to restore films and photographs; however, it has also been used to unocclude hair from dermoscopic images of skin lesions. First, the entire image is analyzed to give guidance on how the specific areas should be filled. The inpainting process then involves: continuing structural elements into the gaps, filling the gaps with the color of the boundaries, and adding texture [76]. In [77], the authors compare inpainting to the conventional software DullRazor [70] and She et al.'s [75] results. Inpainting performed on average of 32.7% better than the linear interpolation of DullRazor, and it was also more stable under heavy occlusion. The results implied that DullRazor and inpainting perform more consistent estimations.

Xie et al. [78] proposed an automated hair removal algorithm based on partial differential equation (PDE). The algorithm includes three steps: (1) the melanoma images with hairs are enhanced by a morphologic closing-based top-hat operator and then segmented through a statistic threshold, (2) the hairs are extracted based on the elongate of the connected region, and (3) the hair-occluded information is repaired by the PDE-based image inpainting. The advantage of using this approach is that it utilizes neighborhood-based information in a natural manner while maintaining a sharp boundary; however, the main drawback is that the diffusion process introduces some blur.

Most existing methods for dermoscopic hair segmentation overlook the case of hair lighter than the background and the skin. So, [79] uses a universal kernel that is capable of segmenting both dark and light hair of constant width, without prior knowledge of the hair color. Its limitation, however, lies in the cases of fine hairs and hairs with many intersections.

In [80], the authors use an automatic hair removal algorithm that consists of hair detection and image inpainting. The hair removal algorithm [70] used was previously described. As for inpainting, state-of-the-art algorithms were explored [81] and the authors presented a novel algorithm for removing large objects from digital images. The approach employs an exemplar-based texture synthesis technique modulated by a unified scheme for determining the fill order of the target region where pixels maintain a confidence value, which, together with image isophotes, influences their fill priority.

A comparative study of the state of the art of hair repair methods for dermoscopic images was performed in [49], and a new method was proposed. The new method starts to do hair detection with the use of a derivative of the Gaussian filter, applies morphological techniques for the refinement, and achieves hair repair using fast marching image inpainting. A similar methodology was presented at the same time, designated VirtualShave [82], where individual hairs are identified by a top-hat filter followed by morphological postprocessing and then replaced through PDE-based inpainting.

An improved DullRazor algorithm, known as E-shaver [83], was presented years later. It starts to detect the predominant orientation of hairs in the original image by using radon transform, followed by filtering the image with Prewitt filters using the orientation of existing hairs. Afterwards, nonhair structures and noise are removed from the image by thresholding-average-thresholding, followed by smoothing. More recently, [64] described two hair removal algorithms: one using a closing morphological operation and another, more robust, that consists of a combination of bicubic interpolation and top-hat transform.

12.3.2.6 Image Restoration

Image restoration techniques are oriented toward the reconstruction of the original image from a degraded observation. This degradation can be due to many forms, such as motion blur, noise, or even an out-of-focus camera.

Classical image restoration techniques are inverse filtering and Wiener filter. Inverse filtering was developed by Nathan in 1966 [84] to restore images and is also known as deconvolution; it has the advantage of requiring only the point spread function as a priori knowledge, but the drawback that the noise is amplified. Improved restoration quality became possible with Wiener filter techniques, which incorporate a priori statistical knowledge of the noise field. The constrained least-squares filter [85] is another approach for overcoming some of the difficulties of the inverse filter and Wiener filter, while still retaining the simplicity of a spatially invariant linear filter. Studies such as the ones presented in [69, 86, 87] use the Wiener filter as a preprocessing step in skin cancer image-based analysis.

When no a priori knowledge about the image degradation is available, the required information should be extracted from the original image either explicitly or implicitly; this technique is named blind image restoration [88–90]. Therefore, it is necessary to simultaneously estimate both the original image and point spread function using partial information about the image processing and possibly even about the original image. In [91], the blind algorithm is proposed where a number of vector quantization codebooks are designed by using bandpass-filtered prototype images and calculating the distortion between the given image and each codebook, and then the one with the minimum average distortion is selected. In [92], a Bayesian model with priors for both the image and the point spread function is addressed based on a variation approach.

In [93], a total variation methodology is presented where the image blur and the hyperparameters are estimated simultaneously by using a hierarchical Bayesian model. Recently, a novel blind image deconvolution algorithm [94] was developed within a Bayesian framework utilizing a nonconvex quasi-norm-based sparse prior on the image and a total variation prior on the unknown blur.

12.3.3 IMAGING PREPROCESSING ALGORITHMS

Algorithms capable of performing image quality assessment for dermatological images acquired via mobile devices, in particular mobile phones, are of extreme importance to ensure the proper success of further image analysis for skin cancer prevention. Therefore, we should not diminish the significance of the development of preprocessing algorithms specifically for that purpose.

12.3.3.1 Reflection Detection

In [95], a new methodology to detect reflections on dermatological images acquired by mobile phones is presented. In this work, the authors start to

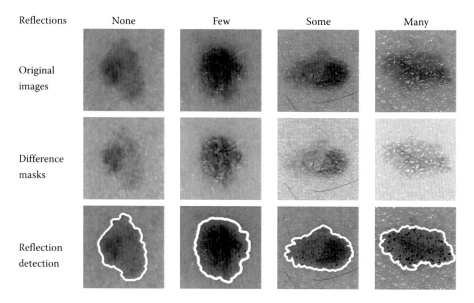

FIGURE 12.1 Results obtained in each step of the reflection detection algorithm described in [95] for images classified as having no, few, some, and many reflections: original images, difference masks, and final results (reflections in black and signal contours in white).

apply a filter to the original RGB image to attenuate the mean luminance and enhance the contours and use the difference between the L channel and a variation from the H channel, from the L*a*b* and HSV color spaces, respectively, to enhance the reflection regions. This choice of the color spaces came from the fact that the L channel is considered dependent on highlights, while the H channel is invariant to highlights [37]. Afterwards, the difference image is smoothed through a Gaussian filter to remove small variations and the segmentation of the reflection regions is obtained based on the difference image histogram.

The methodology was applied to 75 images previously classified according to their level of reflections and the results confirmed the good quality of the suggested algorithm (some examples are shown in Figure 12.1).

12.3.3.2 Blur Detection

Another study [96] was developed regarding image quality assessment that focuses on blur distortion level. Briefly, the authors collected a set of features related to blur detection and analyzed each feature's discriminatory ability concerning two dermatological image datasets. The authors tested the capability to detect blur artificially induced in dermoscopic images from the public database PH^2 [17] and also the blur resulting from the normal image acquisition process using a mobile phone from the Institute of Portuguese

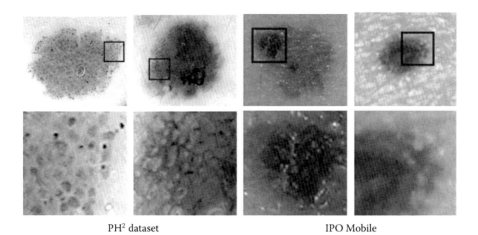

PH^2 dataset   IPO Mobile

FIGURE 12.2 Examples of two images from the PH^2 dataset on the left and focused and blurred images from the IPO Mobile dataset on the right (original images in the first row and detailed image regions [identified by the blue squares in the original images] in the second row). (Adapted from Vasconcelos, M. J. M. and L. Rosado, No-reference blur assessment of dermatological images acquired via mobile devices, in *International Conference on Image and Signal Processing 2014*, Cherbourg, France, pp. 350–357, 2014.)

Oncology (IPO) Mobile database [15] (see Figure 12.2). Here, the usage of no reference objective methods is explored for blur detection purposes (i.e., methods capable of reporting the image quality without human involvement, and where the absolute value is based on the characteristics of the image itself). Therefore, a set of features previously referred in the literature for blur detection, as well as some others not yet tested for this purpose, were implemented, and attributes like sum, mean, and standard deviation were calculated for each feature. Those features were grouped according to their working principle: gradient based, Laplacian based, statistical based, DCT/DFT based, and other principles, gathering a total of 78 features (see Table 12.3). The Mann–Whitney U statistic divided by the product of the two distributions (focus and blurred) was obtained for each feature, in order to compare their individual discriminatory abilities. The results demonstrated that the collected features are capable of successfully discriminating between focused and blurred images. Additionally, it was possible to conclude that the subset of features with the best discriminatory ability considerably depended on the nature of the blur distortion in the used images. When using the PH^2 dataset, with dermoscopic images, best discriminatory results came from the DCT/DFT family, followed by the Laplacian family. For the IPO Mobile dataset, with mobile images, the best results came from the Laplacian family as well as the gradient family. So far, this is a ongoing work where the authors are also evaluating the impact of feature selection methods, as well as the application of different

TABLE 12.3

Summary of the Features Extracted for Blur Detection

Group	Name	Attributes
Gradient based	Energy image gradient	Sum, mean, std, max
	Squared gradient	Sum, mean, std, max
	Tenengrad	Sum, mean, std, max, var
Laplacian based	Energy of Laplacian	Sum, mean, std, max
	Sum modified Laplacian	Sum, mean, std, max
	Diagonal Laplacian	Sum, mean, std, max
	Variance of Laplacian	Mean, std, max, var
	Laplacian and Gaussian	Sum, mean, std, max
Statistical based	Gray-level variance	Sum, mean, std, min, max, var
	Normalized gray-level variance	Normalized variance
	Histogram entropy	Sum (R, G, B, gray)
	Histogram range	Range (R, G, B, gray)
DCT/ DFT	DCT	Sum, mean, std, min, max
	DFT	Sum, mean, std, min, max
Other principles	Brenner's measure	Sum, mean, std
	Image curvature	Sum, mean, std, min, max
	Spatial Frequency measure	Sum, mean, std, max
	Vollath's autocorrelation	Sum, mean, std, max
	Perceptual blur	Count and mean (horizontal and vertical)

Source: With kind permission from Springer Science+Business Media: Lecture Notes in Computer Science, No-reference blur assessment of dermatological images acquired via mobile devices, 8509, 2014, 350–357, Vasconcelos, M., and Rosado, L.

classification methodologies, to achieve a final robust methodology for the automatic detection of blurred images.

12.4   MOBILE TELEDERMATOLOGY: TOWARD A PATIENT-ORIENTED DESIGN APPROACH

The practicality of a mobile teledermatology (MT) system equipped with mobile phone cameras was already reported and confirmed in some studies [97–100]. Another recent study [9] focused on the importance of MT in the developing world, confirming the aided value of using a system that amplifies access to dermatologic expertise in underserved regions.

The study in [101] proved that the usage of a store-and-forward teledermatology (SFTD) system was beneficial in aiding a triage system for potentially malignant skin lesions, helping to improve patients' prioritization, service efficiency and clinical outcomes. The authors of [102, 103] foresee that mobile dermatology might become a triage system for skin cancer, with patients themselves capturing images and sending them to a referring center to be evaluated. In [104], two studies of the SFTD system were analyzed regarding the relation cost-effectiveness when compared to conventional consult processes. In the first case, considering the costs born only from the department, the results showed that SFTD yielded greater costs, but also greater effectiveness; however, if the economic perspective of the society was taken into account, the SFTD was considered to be potentially cost saving. In the second case, the societal economic perspective was taken into account, and SFTD incurred less cost and yielded greater effectiveness. Long-term studies of TD working as a routine tool for the daily practice of skin cancer clinics at public hospitals are still lacking; however, this approach has been recently associated with better service efficiency and high patient satisfaction and is cheaper than conventional care [105, 106].

The traditional clinical diagnosis of MM ranges between 65% and 80% [107], but the usage of dermoscopy was described as a technique capable of improving the diagnostic accuracy [29]. In [8], the first study performing MT using cellular phones with in-built cameras is presented. In this work, the authors used a close-up clinical image and a dermoscopic image by applying the mobile phone on a pocket dermoscopy device to investigate the feasibility of teleconsultation using a mobile phone. The images were acquired with a Sony Ericcson K 750i with a built-in 2-megapixel camera with autofocus, macro mode, and zoom, and the dermoscopy device was a Dermlite II Pro HR with a 25 mm 10× lens. The images were reviewed by two teleconsultants and compared to face-to-face diagnoses, obtaining correct scores of 89% and 91.5% for clinical and dermoscopic images, respectively. However, face-to-face consultation is considered superior to SFTD as a clinical assessment method due to its benefits in terms of lesion palpation and additional inquiry and examination [105, 106].

Summarizing, there is strong evidence that skin cancer triage services should be integrated with a community of dermatological expertises, simultaneously ensuring that teleconsultants (TCs) must always feel able to invite patients to attend for a face-to-face assessment whenever necessary [108].

So far, the great majority of the proposed methodologies in the literature are based on dermoscopic image analysis, usually aiming for dermatology specialist's usage as decision support systems. From a patient perspective, instead, one can identify different needs and implementation strategies. Patients with a clinical or family history of skin cancer should regularly consult their dermatologists for physical skin examinations, for instance, once a year. Between these appointments the patients are usually advised by their doctors to check for relevant changes in their skin moles, and to anticipate the consultation in case of detecting something suspicious. Unfortunately, the patients typically do not have enough dermatological expertise to perform this kind of risk assessment. Because of that, patient-oriented approaches are new paradigms for skin lesion analysis, trying not only to motivate and educate the patients, but also to empower them in terms of dermatological expertise, which can lead to a significant impact in the early diagnosis of skin mole malignancies.

In Section 12.4.1, a physical and information architecture suitable for a patient-oriented system of skin lesion analysis based on smart mobile devices with image cameras is proposed [109].

12.4.1 PATIENT-ORIENTED SYSTEM

12.4.1.1 Physical Architecture

A physical architecture (Figure 12.3) for a patient-oriented system of skin lesion analysis is formed by three main blocks:

1. *Front-end device (the user's smart device)*: Used to acquire or load an image of a skin lesion and send it to the server for analysis. The application that allows the communication between the smartphone and the server is the HTTP communication protocol.
2. *Server*: The server side consists of a RESTFul web service implemented in Java using the Jersey library [110] and deployed on an Apache Tomcat 7.0 web server. The image processing module (IPM) can be implemented in C++ using the OpenCv library [111], which will be executed as an external program when an image is received in the server. The IPM will receive as input the original skin lesion image and return a quantitative analysis of the image, in addition to a visual output of the segmentation and feature extraction steps.
3. *Back-end device*: The device that will receive the outputs generated by the IPM analysis. From the user's perspective, the results can be directly returned to one's own smart device. Moreover, the IPM analysis information can also be provided to dermatology specialists through a web interface.

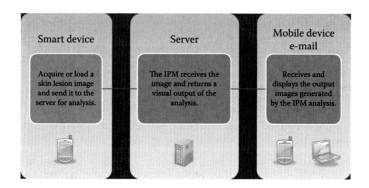

FIGURE 12.3 Physical diagram architecture.

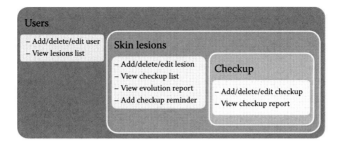

FIGURE 12.4 Diagram of the information architecture proposed. (Reprinted with permission from Rosado, L. et al., *International Journal of Online Engineering*, vol. 9, pp. 27–29, 2013.)

12.4.1.2 Information Architecture

In the proposed patient-oriented solution, the information flows along three main groups: users, skin lesions, and checkups (see Figure 12.4). The application may have several users, and one user may have several skin lesions; one skin lesion has one or more checkups. Each user has the following information: (1) name, (2) gender, and (3) age. Each skin lesion has the following information: (1) location on the body and (2) list of checkups. Each checkup has the following information: (1) skin lesion image, (2) checkup date, (3) four ABCD feature scores (generated by the IPM), and (4) skin lesion size (in mm).

12.5 SMART DEVICE–ADAPTABLE DERMOSCOPES

This section gives a review of the existing smart device–adaptable dermoscopes, together with a study regarding their differences in terms of color reproduction, image area and distortion, illumination, sharpness, and differential structure visibility. Here, we used two different smartphones: the Samsung Galaxy S4 and the iPhone 5, which are currently top-range devices of the Android and iOS operating systems, respectively. Table 12.4 presents the camera specifications of each smartphone used.

By the time of our study, there were two different brands of dermoscopes with adaptability to smartphones on the market: the pocket Dermlite line [112] of 3Gen from the United States and the Handyscope dermoscope of FotoFinder from Germany [113]. The pocket Dermlite line allows stand-alone usability, meaning that it can work without a camera and the adaptation of the DL1, DL2, and DL3 dermoscopes; also, to test this line, we selected two dermoscopes from different ranges: the Dermlite DL1 (bottom range) and the Dermlite DL3 (top range). Regarding the FotoFinder line, we selected the Handyscope for iPhone 5. The prices of the considered adaptable dermoscopes ranged between €400 and €800 at the time of this study, and we used a magnification of 10× in all dermoscopes. Table 12.5 shows the specifications of the three considered smart devices–adaptable dermoscopes.

TABLE 12.4

Camera Specifications of the Two Considered Smartphones

	Samsung Galaxy S4	iPhone 5
Camera	13 megapixels	8 megapixels
Flash	LED	LED
Aperture size	F2.2	F2.4
Focal length	31 mm	—
Sensor size	1/3.06 in.	1/3.2 in.

TABLE 12.5

Specifications of the Three Considered Smart Device–Adaptable Dermoscopes

	Dermlite DL1	Dermlite DL3	Handyscope
Number of LEDS	4	– 21 (Cross-polarization) – 7 (Nonpolarization)	– 6 (Cross-polarization) – 6 (Nonpolarization)
Illumination modes	– Cross-polarized light (sliding clip) – Nonpolarized light (sliding spacer unit)	– Cross-polarized light – Nonpolarized light	– Cross-polarized light – Nonpolarized light
Magnification	10×	10×	Up to 20×
Supported smart devices	– iPhone 4/4S/5/5S/5C – iPad 3/4/Air/mini – Samsung Galaxy S3/S4	– iPhone 4/4S/5/5S/5C – iPad 3/4/Air/mini – Samsung Galaxy S3/S4	– iPhone 4/4S/5/5S – iPod Touch
Battery life	1 hour	5 hours	6–8 hours
Stand-alone usability	Yes	Yes	No

We tested five different combinations of the considered smartphones and dermoscopes: (1) Samsung Galaxy S4 with Dermlite DL1, (2) Samsung Galaxy S4 with Dermlite DL3, (3) iPhone 5 with Dermlite DL1, (4) iPhone 5 with Dermlite DL3, and (5) iPhone 5 with Handyscope. Regarding dermoscope comparison, the case reports and reviews available in the literature were pretty scarce for handheld dermoscopes [114, 115], and nonexistent if we only considered smartphone-adaptable dermoscopes. Therefore, we analyzed the five different combinations of smartphones and mobile-adaptable dermoscopes in terms of color reproduction, image area, image distortion, illumination, sharpness, and differential structure visibility.

12.5.1 COLOR REPRODUCTION

To test the color reproducibility of the combinations of the considered smart-phones and dermoscopes, we chose 12 different reference colors from the ColorChecker chart [116]: 6 grayscale colors, 3 primary colors, and 3 secondary colors. The reference colors were printed on standard office paper, and all the images were acquired using cross-polarized light with $10\times$ magnification. For comparison purposes, only a square of 1000×1000 pixels at the center of the acquired images was considered, since in dermoscopic images the best illumination conditions are usually achieved at the center of the image. The obtained results using all the combinations are depicted in Table 12.6.

From the analysis of Table 12.6, one can observe that the color reproducibility of the Handyscope with the iPhone 5 seems to be the most accurate, principally for the primary and secondary color patches. The Dermlite DL3 had a similar performance in terms of the primary and secondary colors; however, the images acquired with the Dermlite DL3 for the grayscale colors have a significant bluish tint. This clear tendency toward the blue color was present on both smartphones, which might indicate that it could be related to intrinsic characteristics of the Dermlite DL3. Comparatively, the images acquired with the Dermlite DL1 look considerably washed out and had subdued colors. These types of artifacts are commonly present in overexposed images, so in the case of the Dermlite DL1, probably more light than required was acquired by the camera.

12.5.2 IMAGE AREA AND DISTORTION

To compare the visible area and image distortion of the acquired images, we used millimeter paper, and images were acquired using cross-polarized illumination. The width and length of the visible area were calculated by counting the lines of the millimeter paper grid (see Table 12.7). Moreover, to analyze the image distortion of the captured images, a $10 \times 10 \, \text{mm}^2$ was centered in the image and the images were qualitatively compared (see Table 12.8).

In terms of visible area, the Dermlite DL3 dermoscope presents the biggest area, followed by the Handyscope, and finally the Dermlite DL1. Comparing the dermoscopes of the Dermlite line on both smartphones, it is worth noting that the iPhone 5 guarantees a wider visible area.

Regarding the image distortion, one can verify that all tested combinations produced pincushion distortion on the acquired images; that is, lines that did not pass through the center of the image were curved inward, toward the center of the image. The minimal pincushion distortion was obtained using iPhone 5 with Handyscope, followed by Dermlite DL1 with both smartphones. On the other hand, the images with the most pincushion distortion were acquired with Dermlite DL3 for both smartphones.

TABLE 12.6 (See color insert.)
Color Reproduction

Reference Color	Samsung Galaxy S4		iPhone 5		
	DL1	DL3	DL1	DL3	Handyscope

TABLE 12.7
Visible Area Comparison

Samsung Galaxy S4		iPhone 5		
DL1	DL3	DL1	DL3	Handyscope
$17 \times 13\,\mathrm{mm}^2$	$24 \times 15\,\mathrm{mm}^2$	$18 \times 18\,\mathrm{mm}^2$	$24 \times 18\,\mathrm{mm}^2$	$21 \times 18\,\mathrm{mm}^2$

TABLE 12.8
Image Distortion Comparison

Samsung Galaxy S4		iPhone 5		
DL1	DL3	DL1	DL3	Handyscope

12.5.3 ILLUMINATION

In order to compare possible differences in light spreading and brightness, images of the same skin mole were acquired using the five different considered combinations of smartphones and dermoscopes (Table 12.9).

The Dermlite DL1 appears to have the worst performance in terms of light spreading, with a brighter vertical area in the center of the image (more visible when using iPhone 5). Moreover, comparatively with the other dermoscopes, the Dermlite DL1 led to the biggest shadow area near the black border of the dermoscopic image.

Regarding the light spreading, the best performance was achieved by Dermlite DL3 and Handyscope using iPhone 5. Comparing the Dermlite line for both smartphones, the images acquired with iPhone 5 appeared to be brighter and with less shadow areas near the border of the dermoscopic images. However, color reproducibility seemed to be better for Samsung Galaxy S4, while being excessively white for Handyscope and Dermlite DL1 when using iPhone 5.

12.5.4 SHARPNESS AND DIFFERENTIAL STRUCTURES

To compare the sharpness and visibility of the differential structures, images of four different skin lesions were acquired using the five considered combinations of smartphones and dermoscopes. For each lesion, three different types of

TABLE 12.9
Light Spreading Comparison

Samsung Galaxy S4		iPhone 5		
DL1	DL3	DL1	DL3	Handyscope

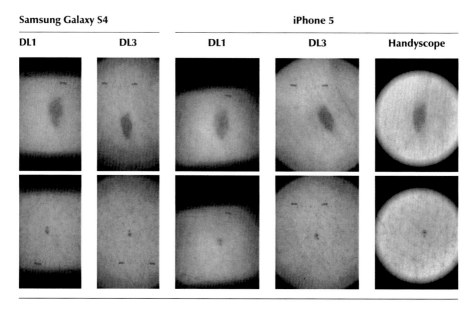

images were acquired: a dermoscopic image with cross-polarized light for each smartphone–dermoscope combination (see Table 12.10) and a nondermoscopic image using only the built-in smartphone camera, with and without flash (see Table 12.11).

Considering the dermoscopic images with cross-polarized light, the sharpest images seem to be obtained with Dermlite DL3 and iPhone 5, being simultaneously the images where the differential structures were most clearly visible. This combination also seemed to be the one that guarantees the best color reproducibility and contrast. Handyscope and Dermlite DL3 with Samsung Galaxy S4 closely followed the image quality delivered by Dermlite DL3 in terms of sharpness and visibility of differential structures. The worst results were with Dermlite DL1, with images that comparatively looked considerably washed out and with a lower contrast. Moreover, the borders of the skin lesions on Dermlite DL1 were less marked and the differential structures more difficult to see.

Finally, to analyze the impact of the flashlight in the mobile image acquisition process of skin lesions, images of the same skin moles were also acquired using both smartphones. As we can see in Table 12.11, the images acquired using the flashlight are sharper and the inner structures of the skin lesions are more visible. The acquisition process without the flashlight was significantly more difficult, being inclusively not possible to obtain focused images

TABLE 12.10

Dermoscopic Skin Lesion Images Acquired Using Cross-Polarized Light

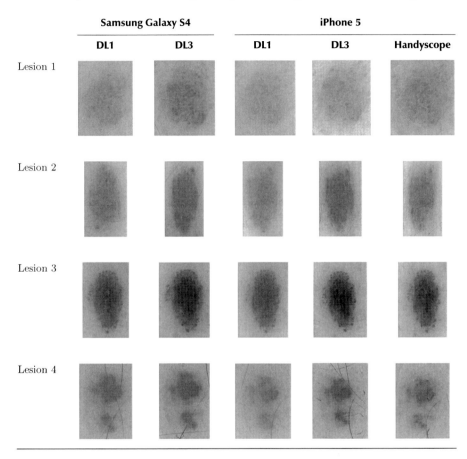

even after several attempts, as was the case for lesions 3 and 4 using the Samsung Galaxy S4. However, when using the flashlight, it should be taken into consideration that the likely appearance of highlight artifacts caused by the reflections of the skin might considerably reduce the skin lesion visibility.

12.6 FINAL REMARKS

Mobile teledermatology has indeed several potential applicabilities for both doctors and patients, being an important tool for skin cancer prevention. Statistics say that skin cancer is the most common malignancy in the Caucasian population, and the indicators show that each year this number

TABLE 12.11

Skin Lesion Images Acquired Using the Smartphones' Built-In Cameras

	Samsung Galaxy S4		iPhone 5	
	With Flash	**No Flash**	**With Flash**	**No Flash**
Lesion 1				
Lesion 2				
Lesion 3		N.A.		
Lesion 4		N.A.		

is alarmingly growing. Therefore, the development of prevention measures is essential, and MT can significantly add value in this case.

Here, a survey was presented on the new trends of MT, covering topics such as the available dermatological databases that can be used for developing robust detection methods and topics related to medical imaging, including image acquisition types, preprocessing challenges of the acquired images, and some solutions to overcome them. A new MT patient-oriented design approach was proposed, and finally, the existing smart device–adaptable dermoscopes were discussed.

Yet, being that this a recent area of investigation, several directions may be fruitful to explore in order to advance the MT field:

- **Preprocessing tasks**: It is important to develop robust methodologies focused on the normalization of images acquired using different mobile devices under uncontrolled conditions, in terms of both illumination and color calibration. Moreover, reliable image quality assessment should also be considered one of the key aspects for the successful deployment of these types of systems.

- **System design**: The patient-oriented approach opens up new possibilities for an active role of the patient in managing his or her skin health status, as well as simultaneously improving the patient–doctor relationship. Thus, the design of these types of systems should be rethought and improved in order to meet both personal and expert requirements.

- **Smart devices–adaptable dermoscopes**: The recent appearance of these devices on the market can bring significant advantages to dermatology specialists in terms of data acquisition, transmission, and storage. Taking into account the current global penetration of smart devices, if the price range of smart device–adaptable dermoscopes considerably decreases in the following years, it is expected that these devices will start spreading among the general population. Thus, it is important to start investigating the advantages and limitations of these devices in terms of image quality, so that the image processing and analysis techniques proposed to date for standard dermoscopic images can be improved accordingly.

ACKNOWLEDGMENTS

This work was done under the scope of the projects "SMARTSKINS: A Novel Framework for Supervised Mobile Assessment and Risk Triage of Skin Lesion via Non-invasive Screening," with reference PTDC/BBB-BMD/3088/2012 financially supported by Fundação para a Ciência e a Tecnologia in Portugal (sections 1 to 4), and "SAL: Service Assisted Living," with reference "Projecto n.º 30377-SAL" financially supported by Fundo Europeu de Desenvolvimento Regional (FEDER) through COMPETE—Programa Operacional Factores de Competitividade (POFC) (section 5).

REFERENCES

1. World Health Organization, http://www.who.int/, January 2014.
2. Portuguese Cancer League, http://www.ligacontracancro.pt/, January 2014.
3. SNS, Actuais e futuras necessidades previsionais de médicos, Tech. Rep., Unidade Operacional Planeamento e Investimentos, Unidade Funcional Estudos e Planeamento de Recursos Humanos, 2011.
4. Digital agenda for Europe: Research in eHealth, http://ec.europa.eu/digital-agenda/en/living-online/ehealth-and-ageing, January 2014.
5. J. P. Van der Heijden, N. F. De Keizer, J. D. Bos, P. I. Spuls, and L. Witkamp, Teledermatology applied following patient selection by general practitioners in daily practice improves efficiency and quality of care at lower cost, *British Journal of Dermatology*, vol. 165, no. 5, pp. 1058–1065, 2011.

6. G. R. Kanthraj, Newer insights in teledermatology practice, *Indian Journal of Dermatology, Venereology, and Leprology*, vol. 77, no. 3, p. 276, 2011.

7. E. A. Krupinski, B. LeSueur, L. Ellsworth, N. Levine, R. Hansen, N. Silvis, P. Sarantopoulos, P. Hite, J. Wurzel, R. S. Weinstein, and A. M. Lopez, Diagnostic accuracy and image quality using a digital camera for teledermatology, *Telemedicine Journal*, vol. 5, no. 3, pp. 257–263, 1999.

8. C. Massone, R. Hofmann-Wellenhof, V. Ahlgrimm-Siess, G. Gabler, C. Ebner, and H. P. Soyer, Melanoma screening with cellular phones, *PloS One*, vol. 2, no. 5, p. e483, 2007.

9. K. Tran, M. Ayad, J. Weinberg, A. Cherng, M. Chowdhury, S. Monir, M. El Hariri, and C. Kovarik, Mobile teledermatology in the developing world: Implications of a feasibility study on 30 Egyptian patients with common skin diseases, *Journal of the American Academy of Dermatology*, vol. 64, no. 2, pp. 302–309, 2011.

10. K. Korotkov and R. Garcia, Computerized analysis of pigmented skin lesions: A review, *Artificial Intelligence in Medicine*, vol. 56, no. 2, pp. 69–90, 2012.

11. M. E. Celebi, W. V. Stoecker, and R. H. Moss, Advances in skin cancer image analysis, *Computerized Medical Imaging and Graphics*, vol. 35, no. 2, pp. 83–84, 2011.

12. J. Scharcanski and M. E. Celebi, *Computer Vision Tecnhiques for the Diagnosis of Skin Cancer*, Springer, Berlin, 2013.

13. W. Stolz, A. Riemann, A. B. Cognetta, L. Pillet, W. Abmayr, D. Holzel, P. Bilek, F. Nachbar, and M. Landthaler, ABCD rule of dermatoscopy: A new practical method for early recognition of malignant-melanoma, *European Journal of Dermatology*, vol. 4, no. 7, pp. 521–527, 1994.

14. J. E. McWhirter and L. Hoffman-Goetz, Visual images for patient skin self-examination and melanoma detection: A systematic review of published studies, *Journal of the American Academy of Dermatology*, vol. 69, pp. 47–55, 2013.

15. Fraunhofer Portugal, Melanoma detection, http://www.fraunhofer.pt/en/fraunhofer_aicos/projects/internal_research/melanoma_detection.html, February 2014.

16. G. Argenziano, H. P. Soyer, V. De Giorgi, D. Piccolo, P. Carli, and M. Delfino, *Dermoscopy: A Tutorial*, EDRA Medical Publishing and New Media, Milan, 2002.

17. T. Mendonca, P. M. Ferreira, J. S. Marques, A. R. Marcal, and J. Rozeira, PH 2: A dermoscopic image database for research and benchmarking, in *2013 35th Annual International Conference of the IEEE Engineering in Medicine and Biology Society (EMBC)*, pp. 5437–5440, 2013.

18. S. W. Menzies, K. A. Crotty, C. Ingvar, and W. H. McCarthy, *An Atlas of Surface Microscopy of Pigmented Skin Lesions: Dermoscopy*, McGraw-Hill, Roseville, CA, 2003.

19. Dermnet, http://www.dermnet.com/, February 2014.

20. Atlas of dermatology, http://www.danderm-pdv.is.kkh.dk/atlas/index.html, January 2014.

21. Heenen, MED atlas de dermatologie, http://bib18.ulb.ac.be/cdm4/browse.php?CISOROOT=%2Fmed004&CISOSTART=31,601, January 2014.

22. S. Silva, Dermatology atlas, http://www.atlasdermatologico.com.br/, January 2014.

23. Interactive dermatology atlas, http://www.dermatlas.net/, January 2014.

24. Dermoscopy atlas, http://www.dermoscopyatlas.com/index.cfm, January 2014.
25. DermIS, http://www.dermis.net/dermisroot/en/home/index.htm, January 2014.
26. DermQuest, https://www.dermquest.com/, January 2014.
27. R. J. Friedman, D. S. Rigel, and A. W. Kopf, Early detection of malignant melanoma: The role of physician examination and self-examination of the skin, *CA: A Cancer Journal for Clinicians*, vol. 35, no. 3, pp. 130–151, 1985.
28. G. Argenziano and I. Zalaudek, Recent advances in dermoscopic diagnostic technologies, *European Oncological Disease*, vol. 1, no. 2, pp. 104–106, 2007.
29. H. Kittler, H. Pehamberger, K. Wolff, and M. Binder, Diagnostic accuracy of dermoscopy, *Lancet Oncology*, vol. 3, no. 3, pp. 159–165, 2002.
30. D. Piccolo, A. Ferrari, K. Peris, R. Diadone, B. Ruggeri, and S. Chimenti, Dermoscopic diagnosis by a trained clinician vs. a clinician with minimal dermoscopy training vs. computer-aided diagnosis of 341 pigmented skin lesions: A comparative study, *British Journal of Dermatology*, vol. 147, pp. 481–486, 2002. PMID: 12207587.
31. R. Asaid, G. Boyce, and G. Padmasekara, Use of a smartphone for monitoring dermatological lesions compared to clinical photography, *Journal of Mobile Technology in Medicine*, vol. 1, no. 1, pp. 16–18, 2012.
32. C. Poynton, A guided tour of color space, in *SMPTE Advanced Television and Electronic Imaging Conference*, pp. 167–180, 1995.
33. J. B. Park and A. C. Kak, A new color representation for non-white illumination conditions, *ECE Technical Reports*, p. 8, 2005.
34. F. Kristensen, P. Nilsson, and V. Öwall, Background segmentation beyond RGB, in *Computer Vision—ACCV 2006* (P. Narayanan, S. Nayar, and H.-Y. Shum, eds.), vol. 3852 of *Lecture Notes in Computer Science*, pp. 602–612, Springer, Berlin, 2006.
35. F. Vogt, D. Paulus, B. Heigl, C. Vogelgsang, H. Niemann, G. Greiner, and C. Schick, Making the invisible visible: Highlight substitution by color light fields, in *Conference on Colour in Graphics, Imaging, and Vision*, vol. 2002, pp. 352–357, Society for Imaging Science and Technology, 2002.
36. L. Zhang, X. Mao, C. Zhou, and P. Yu, Improved HIS model with application to edge detection for color image, *Journal of Computers*, vol. 7, no. 6, pp. 1400–1404, 2012.
37. T. Gevers and A. W. M. Smeulders, Color-based object recognition, *Pattern Recognition*, vol. 32, no. 3, pp. 453–464, 1999.
38. E. Todt and C. Torras, Detecting salient cues through illumination-invariant color ratios, *Robotics and Autonomous Systems*, vol. 48, no. 2, pp. 111–130, 2004.
39. B. Wang, X. Chang, and C. Liu, Skin detection and segmentation of human face in color images, *International Journal of Intelligent Engineering and Systems*, vol. 4, no. 1, pp. 10–17, 2011.
40. C. Lin, Face detection in complicated backgrounds and different illumination conditions by using YCbCr color space and neural network, *Pattern Recognition Letters*, vol. 28, no. 16, pp. 2190–2200, 2007.
41. H.-J. Lee and C.-C. Lee, *Human Skin Tone Detection in YCbCr Space*, Google Patents, 2008.
42. K. H. B. Ghazali, J. Ma, R. Xiao, and S. A. Lubis, An innovative face detection based on YCgCr color space, *Physics Procedia*, vol. 25, pp. 2116–2124, 2012.

43. S. V. Tathe and S. P. Narote, Face detection using color models, *World Journal of Science and Technology*, vol. 2, no. 4, 2012.

44. A. Kaur and B. V. Kranthi, Comparison between YCbCr color space and CIELab color space for skin color segmentation, *International Journal of Applied Information Systems (IJAIS)*, vol. 3, no. 4, pp. 30–33, 2012.

45. J. F. Alcn, C. Ciuhu, W. Ten Kate, A. Heinrich, N. Uzunbajakava, G. Krekels, D. Siem, and G. de Haan, Automatic imaging system with decision support for inspection of pigmented skin lesions and melanoma diagnosis, *IEEE Journal of Selected Topics in Signal Processing*, vol. 3, no. 1, pp. 14–25, 2009.

46. P. G. Cavalcanti, J. Scharcanski, and C. B. O. Lopes, Shading attenuation in human skin color images, in *Advances in Visual Computing* (G. Bebis, R. Boyle, B. Parvin, D. Koracin, R. Chung, R. Hammoud, M. Hussain et al., eds.), vol. 6453 of *Lecture Notes in Computer Science*, pp. 190–198, Springer, Berlin, 2010.

47. A. Madooei, M. S. Drew, M. Sadeghi, and M. S. Atkins, Automated preprocessing method for dermoscopic images and its application to pigmented skin lesion segmentation, in *Color and Imaging Conference*, vol. 2012, pp. 158–163, Society for Imaging Science and Technology, 2012.

48. M.-J. Seow and V. K. Asari, Ratio rule and homomorphic filter for enhancement of digital colour image, *Neurocomputing*, vol. 69, no. 7, pp. 954–958, 2006.

49. Q. Abbas, M. E. Celebi, and I. F. Garcia, Hair removal methods: A comparative study for dermoscopy images, *Biomedical Signal Processing and Control*, vol. 6, no. 4, pp. 395–404, 2011.

50. J. Glaister, R. Amelard, A. Wong, and D. Clausi, MSIM: Multi-stage illumination modeling of dermatological photographs for illumination-corrected skin lesion analysis, *IEEE Transactions on Biomedical Engineering*, vol. 60, no. 7, pp. 1873–1883, 2013.

51. N. V. Matveev and B. A. Kobrinsky, Automatic colour correction of digital skin images in teledermatology, *Journal of Telemedicine and Telecare*, vol. 12, suppl 3, pp. 62–63, 2006.

52. J. Marguier, N. Bhatti, H. Baker, M. Harville, and S. Ssstrunk, Assessing human skin color from uncalibrated images, *International Journal of Imaging Systems and Technology*, vol. 17, no. 3, pp. 143–151, 2007.

53. G. Schaefer, M. I. Rajab, M. E. Celebi, and H. Iyatomi, Skin lesion extraction in dermoscopic images based on colour enhancement and iterative segmentation, in *16th IEEE International Conference on Image Processing, 2009*, pp. 3361–3364, 2009.

54. H. Iyatomi, M. E. Celebi, G. Schaefer, and M. Tanaka, Automated color calibration method for dermoscopy images, *Computerized Medical Imaging and Graphics*, vol. 35, no. 2, pp. 89–98, 2011.

55. G. Schaefer, M. I. Rajab, M. E. Celebi, and H. Iyatomi, Colour and contrast enhancement for improved skin lesion segmentation, *Computerized Medical Imaging and Graphics*, vol. 35, no. 2, pp. 99–104, 2011.

56. H. Wannous, Y. Lucas, S. Treuillet, A. Mansouri, and Y. Voisin, Improving color correction across camera and illumination changes by contextual sample selection, *Journal of Electronic Imaging*, vol. 21, no. 2, pp. 23011–23015, 2012.

57. S. M. Pizer, E. P. Amburn, J. D. Austin, R. Cromartie, A. Geselowitz, T. Greer, B. ter Haar Romeny, J. B. Zimmerman, and K. Zuiderveld, Adaptive

histogram equalization and its variations, *Computer Vision, Graphics, and Image Processing*, vol. 39, no. 3, pp. 355–368, 1987.

58. K. Zuiderveld, Contrast limited adaptive histogram equalization, in *Graphics Gems IV*, pp. 474–485, Academic Press Professional, 1994.

59. M. J. Carlotto, Histogram analysis using a scale-space approach, *IEEE Transactions on Pattern Analysis and Machine Intelligence*, no. 1, pp. 121–129, 1987.

60. M. Abdullah-Al-Wadud, M. H. Kabir, M. A. A. Dewan, and O. Chae, A dynamic histogram equalization for image contrast enhancement, *IEEE Transactions on Consumer Electronics*, vol. 53, no. 2, pp. 593–600, 2007.

61. D. D. Gmez, C. Butakoff, B. K. Ersboll, and W. Stoecker, Independent histogram pursuit for segmentation of skin lesions, *IEEE Transactions on Biomedical Engineering*, vol. 55, no. 1, pp. 157–161, 2008.

62. N. Otsu, A threshold selection method from gray-level histograms, *IEEE Transactions on Systems, Man and Cybernetics*, vol. 9, no. 1, pp. 62–66, 1979.

63. M. E. Celebi, H. Iyatomi, and G. Schaefer, Contrast enhancement in dermoscopy images by maximizing a histogram bimodality measure, in *16th IEEE International Conference on Image Processing, 2009*, pp. 2601–2604, 2009.

64. A. Sultana, M. Ciuc, T. Radulescu, L. Wanyu, and D. Petrache, Preliminary work on dermatoscopic lesion segmentation, in *Proceedings of the 20th European Signal Processing Conference (EUSIPCO), 2012*, pp. 2273–2277, 2012.

65. M. E. Celebi, H. Iyatomi, G. Schaefer, and W. V. Stoecker, Lesion border detection in dermoscopy images, *Computerized Medical Imaging and Graphics*, vol. 33, no. 2, pp. 148–153, 2009.

66. I. Fondn, Q. Abbas, M. E. Celebi, W. Ahmad, and Q. Mushtaq, Software tool for contrast enhancement and segmentation of melanoma images based on human perception, *Imagen-A*, vol. 3, no. 5, pp. 45–47, 2013.

67. S. Fischer, P. Schmid, and J. Guillod, Analysis of skin lesions with pigmented networks, in *Proceedings of the 1996 International Conference on Image Processing*, vol. 1, pp. 323–326, 1996.

68. E. Zagrouba and W. Barhoumi, A preliminary approach for the automated recognition of malignant melanoma, *Image Analysis and Stereology Journal*, vol. 23, no. 2, pp. 121–135, 2004.

69. M. K. A. Mahmoud, A. Al-Jumaily, and M. Takruri, Wavelet and curvelet analysis for automatic identification of melanoma based on neural network classification, in *International Journal of Computer Information Systems and Industrial Management*, vol. 5, pp. 600–614, 2013.

70. T. Lee, V. Ng, R. Gallagher, A. Coldman, and D. McLean, Dullrazor: A software approach to hair removal from images, *Computers in Biology and Medicine*, vol. 27, no. 6, pp. 533–543, 1997.

71. P. Schmid, Segmentation of digitized dermatoscopic images by two-dimensional color clustering, *IEEE Transactions on Medical Imaging*, vol. 18, no. 2, pp. 164–171, 1999.

72. M. E. Celebi, A. Aslandogan, and W. V. Stoecker, Unsupervised border detection in dermoscopy images, *Skin Research and Technology*, vol. 13, no. 4, pp. 454–462, 2007.

73. P. Schmid-Saugeon, J. Guillod, and J.-P. Thiran, Towards a computer-aided diagnosis system for pigmented skin lesions, *Computerized Medical Imaging and Graphics*, vol. 27, no. 1, pp. 65–78, 2003.

74. M. G. Fleming, C. Steger, J. Zhang, J. Gao, A. B. Cognetta, I. Pollak, and C. R. Dyer, Techniques for a structural analysis of dermatoscopic imagery, *Computerized Medical Imaging and Graphics*, vol. 22, no. 5, pp. 375–389, 1998.

75. Z. She, P. J. Fish, and A. W. Duller, Improved approaches to hair removal from skin image, in *Proceedings of SPIE*, vol. 4322, p. 492, 2001.

76. M. Bertalmio, G. Sapiro, V. Caselles, and C. Ballester, Image inpainting, in *Proceedings of the 27th Annual Conference on Computer Graphics and Interactive Techniques*, pp. 417–424, ACM Press/Addison-Wesley Publishing Co., 2000.

77. P. Wighton, T. K. Lee, and M. S. Atkins, Dermascopic hair disocclusion using inpainting, in *Proceedings of SPIE*, vol. 6914, pp. 691427V1–691427V8, 2008.

78. F.-Y. Xie, S.-Y. Qin, Z.-G. Jiang, and R.-S. Meng, PDE-based unsupervised repair of hair-occluded information in dermoscopy images of melanoma, *Computerized Medical Imaging and Graphics*, vol. 33, no. 4, pp. 275–282, 2009.

79. N. H. Nguyen, T. K. Lee, and M. S. Atkins, Segmentation of light and dark hair in dermoscopic images: A hybrid approach using a universal kernel, in *Proceedings of SPIE*, vol. 7623, pp. 76234N–76234N8, 2010.

80. G. Capdehourat, A. Corez, A. Bazzano, R. Alonso, and P. Musé, Toward a combined tool to assist dermatologists in melanoma detection from dermoscopic images of pigmented skin lesions, *Pattern Recognition Letters*, vol. 32, no. 16, pp. 2187–2196, 2011.

81. A. Criminisi, P. Perez, and K. Toyama, Object removal by exemplar-based inpainting, in *Proceedings of the 2003 IEEE Computer Society Conference on Computer Vision and Pattern Recognition*, vol. 2, pp. II721–II728, 2003.

82. M. Fiorese, E. Peserico, and A. Silletti, VirtualShave: Automated hair removal from digital dermatoscopic images, in *2011 Annual International Conference of the IEEE Engineering in Medicine and Biology Society EMBC*, pp. 5145–5148, 2011.

83. K. Kiani and A. R. Sharafat, E-shaver: An improved DullRazor for digitally removing dark and light-colored hairs in dermoscopic images, *Computers in Biology and Medicine*, vol. 41, no. 3, pp. 139–145, 2011.

84. R. Nathan, Digital video-data handling, Tech. Rep. 32-877, Jet Propulsion Laboratory, Pasadena, CA, 1966.

85. B. R. Hunt, The application of constrained least squares estimation to image restoration by digital computer, *IEEE Transactions on Computers*, vol. 100, no. 9, pp. 805–812, 1973.

86. B. Caputo, V. Panichelli, and G. E. Gigante, Toward a quantitative analysis of skin lesion images, *Studies in Health Technology and Informatics*, pp. 509–513, 2002.

87. M. K. A. Mahmoud and A. Al-Jumaily, Segmentation of skin cancer images based on gradient vector flow (GVF) snake, in *2011 International Conference on Mechatronics and Automation (ICMA)*, pp. 216–220, 2011.

88. M. Jiang and G. Wang, Development of blind image deconvolution and its applications, *Journal of X-Ray Science and Technology*, vol. 11, no. 1, pp. 13–19, 2003.

89. P. Campisi and K. Egiazarian, *Blind Image Deconvolution: Theory and Applications*, CRC Press, Boca Raton, FL, 2007.

90. P. A. Patil and R. B. Wagh, Review of blind image restoration methods, *World Journal of Science and Technology*, vol. 2, no. 3, pp. 168–170, 2012.

91. R. Nakagaki and A. K. Katsaggelos, A VQ-based blind image restoration algorithm, *IEEE Transactions on Image Processing*, vol. 12, no. 9, pp. 1044–1053, 2003.

92. A. C. Likas and N. P. Galatsanos, A variational approach for Bayesian blind image deconvolution, *IEEE Transactions on Signal Processing*, vol. 52, no. 8, pp. 2222–2233, 2004.

93. S. D. Babacan, R. Molina, and A. K. Katsaggelos, Variational Bayesian blind deconvolution using a total variation prior, *IEEE Transactions on Image Processing*, vol. 18, no. 1, pp. 12–26, 2009.

94. B. Amizic, R. Molina, and A. K. Katsaggelos, Sparse Bayesian blind image deconvolution with parameter estimation, *EURASIP Journal on Image and Video Processing*, vol. 2012, no. 1, pp. 1–15, 2012.

95. M. J. M. Vasconcelos and L. Rosado, No-reference blur assessment of dermatological images acquired via mobile devices, in *International Conference on Image and Signal Processing 2014*, Cherbourg, France, pp. 350–357, 2014.

96. M. J. M. Vasconcelos and L. Rosado, Automatic reflection detection algorithm of dermatological images acquired via mobile devices, in *18th Annual Conference in Medical Image Understanding and Analysis 2014*, Egham, UK, pp. 85–90, 2014.

97. H.-H. Tsai, Y.-P. Pong, C.-C. Liang, P.-Y. Lin, and C.-H. Hsieh, Teleconsultation by using the mobile camera phone for remote management of the extremity wound: A pilot study, *Annals of Plastic Surgery*, vol. 53, no. 6, pp. 584–587, 2004.

98. C.-H. Hsieh, S.-F. Jeng, C.-Y. Chen, J.-W. Yin, J. C.-S. Yang, H.-H. Tsai, and M.-C. Yeh, Teleconsultation with mobile camera-phone in remote evaluation of replantation potential, *Journal of Trauma and Acute Care Surgery*, vol. 58, no. 6, pp. 1208–1212, 2005.

99. R. P. Braun, J. L. Vecchietti, L. Thomas, C. Prins, L. E. French, A. J. Gewirtzman, J.-H. Saurat, and D. Salomon, Telemedical wound care using a new generation of mobile telephones: a feasibility study, *Archives of Dermatology*, vol. 141, no. 2, p. 254, 2005.

100. P. Chung, T. Yu, and N. Scheinfeld, Using cellphones for teledermatology, a preliminary study, *Dermatology Online Journal*, vol. 13, no. 3, p. 2, 2007.

101. C. May, L. Giles, and G. Gupta, Prospective observational comparative study assessing the role of store and forward teledermatology triage in skin cancer, *Clinical and Experimental Dermatology*, vol. 33, no. 6, pp. 736–739, 2008.

102. C. Massone, A. Di Stefani, and H. P. Soyer, Dermoscopy for skin cancer detection, *Current Opinion in Oncology*, vol. 17, no. 2, pp. 147–153, 2005.

103. C. Massone, A. M. G. Brunasso, T. M. Campbell, and H. P. Soyer, Mobile teledermoscopy: Melanoma diagnosis by one click? in *Seminars in Cutaneous Medicine and Surgery*, vol. 28, pp. 203–205, 2009.

104. J. D. Whited, Economic analysis of telemedicine and the teledermatology paradigm, *Telemedicine and e-Health*, vol. 16, no. 2, pp. 223–228, 2010.

105. E. M. Warshaw, Y. J. Hillman, N. L. Greer, E. M. Hagel, R. MacDonald, I. R. Rutks, and T. J. Wilt, Teledermatology for diagnosis and management of skin conditions: A systematic review, *Journal of the American Academy of Dermatology*, vol. 64, no. 4, pp. 759–772, 2011.

106. C. A. Morton, F. Downie, S. Auld, B. Smith, M. Van Der Pol, P. Baughan, J. Wells, and R. Wootton, Community photo-triage for skin cancer referrals: An aid to service delivery, *Clinical and Experimental Dermatology*, vol. 36, no. 3, pp. 248–254, 2011.

107. C. M. Grin, A. W. Kopf, B. Welkovich, R. S. Bart, and M. J. Levenstein, Accuracy in the clinical diagnosis of malignant melanoma, *Archives of Dermatology*, vol. 126, no. 6, p. 763, 1990.

108. M. Gray and A. Bowling, Considerations for a successful teledermatology application, *Health Informatics New Zealand*, 2010.

109. L. Rosado, M. J. Vasconcelos, and M. Ferreira, A mobile-based prototype for skin lesion analysis: Towards a patient-oriented design approach, *International Journal of Online Engineering (iJOE)*, vol. 9, pp. 27–29, 2013.

110. Jersey, The open source JAX-RS reference implementation for building RESTful web services, https://jersey.java.net/, 2014.

111. G. Bradski and A. Kaehler, *Learning OpenCV: Computer Vision with the OpenCV Library*, O'Reilly Media, 2008.

112. 3Gen, Dermlite, http://dermlite.com/collections/pocket-dermoscopy-devices, 2014.

113. FotoFinder, Handyscope, http://www.handyscope.net/, 2014.

114. A. Blum and S. Jaworski, Clear differences in hand-held dermoscopes, *Journal der Deutschen Dermatologischen Gesellschaft JDDG*, vol. 4, pp. 1054–1057, 2006. PMID: 17176414.

115. A. Blum, S. Jaworski, H. Ludtke, and U. Ellwanger, Systematic comparison of five hand-held dermoscopes reveals clear differences, *Aktuelle Dermatologie*, vol. 34, no. 1–2, pp. 9–15, 2008.

116. ColorChecker, http://en.wikipedia.org/w/index.php?title=ColorChecker&oldid =565716177, February 2014.

13 PH²
A Public Database for the Analysis of Dermoscopic Images

Teresa F. Mendonça
Universidade do Porto
Porto, Portugal

Pedro M. Ferreira
Universidade do Porto
Porto, Portugal

André R. S. Marçal
Universidade do Porto
Porto, Portugal

Catarina Barata
Instituto Superior Técnico
Lisbon, Portugal

Jorge S. Marques
Instituto Superior Técnico
Lisbon, Portugal

Joana Rocha
Hospital Pedro Hispano
Matosinhos, Portugal

Jorge Rozeira
Hospital Pedro Hispano
Matosinhos, Portugal

CONTENTS

13.1 INTRODUCTION

Skin cancer represents a serious public health problem because of its increasing incidence and subsequent mortality. Among skin cancers, malignant melanoma is by far the most deadly form. Because the early detection of melanoma significantly increases the survival rate of the patient, several noninvasive imaging techniques, such as dermoscopy, have been developed to aid the screening process [1]. Dermoscopy involves the use of an optical instrument paired with a powerful lighting system, allowing the examination of skin lesions in a higher magnification. Therefore, dermoscopic images provide a more detailed view of the morphological structures and patterns than normally magnified images of the skin lesions [1, 2]. However, the visual interpretation and examination of dermoscopic images can be a time-consuming task and, as shown by Kittler et al. [3], the diagnosis accuracy of dermoscopy significantly depends on the experience of the dermatologists. Several medical diagnosis procedures have been introduced in order to guide dermatologists and other health care professionals, for example, pattern analysis, the ABCD rule, the 7-point checklist, and the Menzies method. A number of dermoscopic criteria (i.e., asymmetry, border, colors, differential structures) have to be assessed in these methods to produce the final clinical diagnosis. However, the diagnosis of skin lesions is still a challenging task, even using these medical procedures, mainly due to the subjectivity of clinical interpretation and lack of reproducibility [1, 2].

Several computer-aided diagnosis (CAD) systems for digital dermoscopic images have been proposed to assist the clinical evaluation of skin lesions. Such CAD systems are usually based on three stages: image segmentation, feature extraction/selection, and lesion classification. Each of these stages has challenges and therefore needs to have a proper evaluation and validation, which requires reliable reference (or ground truth) data. The reference data have to be prepared and validated by expert dermatologists. The process is, however, time-consuming, particularly in what is referred to as the manual segmentation of the lesion in each dermoscopic image. For this reason, there is currently a lack of ground truth dermoscopy image databases available for public use (possibility limited to research and educational purposes). This was recognized in the Automatic Computer-Based Diagnosis System for Dermoscopy Images (ADDI) project [4], and thus one of its main objectives was to prepare and make available a dermoscopic reference database.

In this chapter, a dermoscopic image database is presented: PH^2. This database can be used as ground truth in the evaluation and validation of both segmentation and classification algorithms. The PH^2 database contains a total of 200 melanocytic lesions, including 80 common nevi, 80 atypical nevi, and 40 melanomas. The rather small number of melanomas, compared with the other two types of melanocytic lesions, can be explained by two main reasons. First of all, the number of real cases of melanomas is actually much smaller than the number of other ones. In addition, as melanomas are usually not completely contained within the image frame and present many image artifacts, they are not always suitable to be used as ground truth in the evaluation of CAD systems.

For each image in the database, the manual segmentation and the clinical diagnosis of the skin lesion, as well as the identification of other important dermoscopic criteria, are available. These dermoscopic criteria include the assessment of the lesion asymmetry and also the identification of colors and several differential structures, such as pigment network, dots, globules, streaks, regression areas, and blue–white veil. The PH^2 database is freely available for research and educational purposes, following a brief registration process at the website [4].

The size of the PH^2 database (200 images) might seem small, particularly when compared with traditional machine learning ground truth databases, which may have hundreds or thousands of annotated images. However, it is important to highlight that the annotation of dermoscopic images is not just a binary issue (benign or malign). The annotation of each image requires a large amount of time and effort, since several dermoscopic features have to be assessed to perform the lesion diagnosis. Moreover, the skin lesion and the color classes present in each image have to be manually segmented by expert clinicians. The PH^2 database can also be used for medical training. For instance, dermatologist trainees can test their skills by comparing their own diagnosis and evaluation with the ground truth available in the PH^2 database.

13.2 PH^2 DATABASE

The creation of the PH^2 database was made possible by a joint collaboration between the Universidade do Porto and Universidade de Lisboa in conjunction with the dermatology service of Hospital Pedro Hispano in Matosinhos,

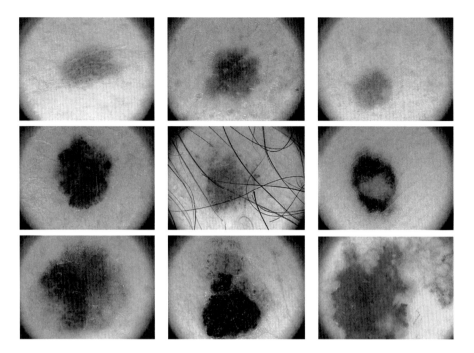

FIGURE 13.1 A sample of images from the PH^2 database, including common nevi (first row), atypical nevi (second row), and melanomas (third row).

Portugal. The PH^2 database was mainly created to make available a common dataset that may be used for the performance evaluation of different computer-aided diagnosis systems of dermoscopic images.

The database currently consists of 200 dermoscopic images along with the corresponding medical annotations, comprising 80 common nevi, 80 atypical nevi, and 40 malignant melanomas. The dermoscopic images were carefully acquired using a magnification of 20× under unchanged conditions. They are 8-bit red, green, blue (RGB) color images with a resolution of 768 × 560 pixels. The set of images available in the PH^2 database was selected with some constraints, regarding their quality, resolution, and dermoscopic features, so that they are suitable enough to be used in a dermoscopic reference database. An illustrative collection of the images that can be found in the PH^2 database is presented in Figure 13.1.

Each image of the database was visually inspected and manually annotated by an expert dermatologist with regard to three main parameters:

1. Manual segmentation of both lesion and colors (although the segmentation of the lesion is available for the entire PH^2 dataset, the segmentation of the colors is only available for a subset of 29 images)
2. Clinical and histological diagnosis

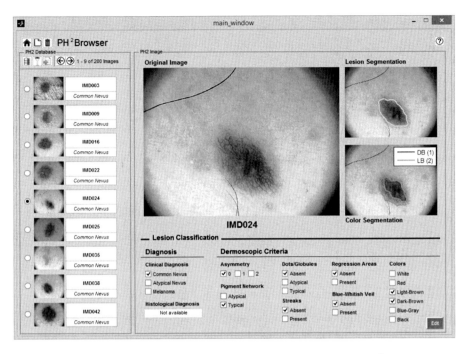

FIGURE 13.2 (**See color insert.**) Graphical user interface of the PH^2 Browser.

3. Dermoscopic criteria, which include the assessment of the following features: asymmetry, colors, pigment network, dots/globules, streaks, regression areas, and blue–white veil

The PH^2 dataset is available in [4], together with an interactive image tool called PH^2 Browser. This tool allows the visualization of the medical segmentations and classifications of each image of the database. Furthermore, it allows searching dermoscopic images according to the desired criteria, as well as the exportation of the images, along with their corresponding segmentation and classification, into several formats. Figure 13.2 shows the graphical user interface of the PH^2 Browser.

13.2.1 MANUAL SEGMENTATION OF THE SKIN LESION

The availability of manually segmented skin lesions, performed by expert dermatologists, is of crucial importance since they give essential information for the evaluation of the segmentation step of a CAD system.

The manual segmentation of each image of the database is available in a binary format, more concretely as a binary mask with the same size as the original image. The pixels of the skin lesion are labeled with the intensity value of 1, whereas all pixels of the background region have values of 0. This output format was chosen because it can be easily used to extract

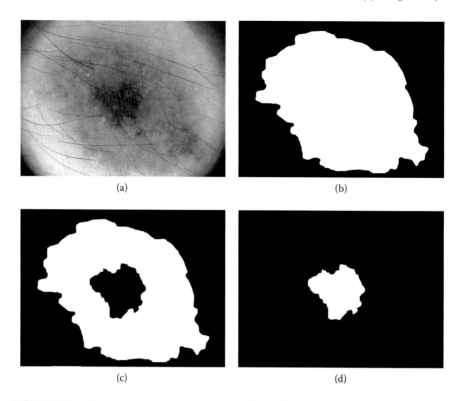

(a)   (b)

(c)   (d)

FIGURE 13.3 Manual segmentation of both skin lesion and color classes of a dermo-scopic image: (a) original image, (b) manual segmentation of the skin lesion, (c) manual segmentation of the light-brown color class, and (d) manual segmentation of the dark-brown color class.

the boundary position of the skin lesion. An example of a dermoscopic image and the corresponding manual segmentation is presented in Figure 13.3.

13.2.2 CLINICAL DIAGNOSIS

Regarding the nature of melanocytic lesions, they can be broadly classified into benign nevi and malignant melanomas. Benign nevi can be further classified into common and atypical nevi, concerning their atypia degree. This classification procedure was adopted and followed during the assessment of the PH^2 images, and hence each image of the database is classified into common nevus, atypical nevus, or melanoma. Although the clinical diagnosis is available for all images of the database, the histological diagnosis is only available for a subset of them, since the histological test is only performed for those lesions considered highly suspicious by dermatologists. Examples of each type of skin lesion are shown in Figure 13.1.

13.2.3 DERMOSCOPIC CRITERIA

The dermoscopic features available in the PH^2 database are asymmetry, colors, pigment network, dots, globules, streaks, regression areas, and blue–white veil. These dermoscopic features were selected for two main reasons. First, this set of dermoscopic criteria corresponds to those features that are commonly used by dermatologists to perform a clinical diagnosis. In addition, this set of features comprises the majority of the dermoscopic features that have to be assessed in the most widely used medical diagnosis procedures, such as the ABCD rule [5], the 7-point checklist [6], and the Menzies method [7]. The definitions of each of these features, along with the descriptions of their assessment processes, are described in the following.

13.2.3.1 Asymmetry

Asymmetry plays an important role in the diagnosis of a melanocytic lesion. For instance, it has the largest weight factor in the ABCD rule of dermoscopy.

In the PH^2 database, the lesion asymmetry was evaluated by the dermatologist according to the ABCD rule. Therefore, the asymmetry of a lesion is assessed regarding its contour, colors, and structure distribution simultaneously. Moreover, there are three possible labels for this parameter: 0 for fully symmetric lesions, 1 for asymmetric lesions with respect to one axis, and 2 for asymmetric lesions with respect to two axes.

13.2.3.2 Colors

Overall, six different colors are taken into account during the diagnosis of a melanocytic lesion. The set of color classes comprises white, red, light brown, dark brown, blue–gray, and black [1].

Each image of the database was evaluated by a dermatologist in order to identify the presence of the six color classes. Moreover, the manual segmentation of the color classes was performed by a dermatolgist for a subset of 29 images of the PH^2 database. The location (manual segmentation) of each color in an image was recorded as a binary mask, manually segmented by the dermatologist. An example is presented in Figure 13.3, where two color classes were identified.

13.2.3.3 Pigment Network

The pigment network appears in melanocytic lesions as a grid-like network consisting of thin pigmented lines and hypopigmented holes, creating a shape similar to that of a honeycomb [1]. The pigment network is one of the most important structures in dermoscopy, since its presence allows the distinction between different skin lesion classes, as well as the identification of the lesion diagnosis. Since the presence of an atypical network is usually a sign of a malignant lesion, this structure was visually evaluated by dermatologists and

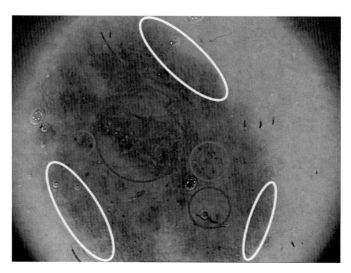

FIGURE 13.4 (See color insert.) Dermoscopic feature identification: atypical pigment network (yellow ellipses), atypical dots/globules (red circles), and blue–white veil (blue circles).

classified as typical or atypical. The presence of an atypical pigmented network in a skin lesion is illustrated in Figure 13.4.

13.2.3.4 Dots/Globules

As illustrated in Figure 13.4, dots/globules are spherical or oval, variously sized, black, brown, or gray structures (dots are usually smaller than globules). The presence of these dermoscopic structures also has an important role in the distinction among skin lesion types [1].

These structures were visually evaluated by dermatologists and categorically classified as present or absent in each image of the PH² database. When dots/globules are present in a given lesion, these structures are further classified as regular or irregular concerning their distribution in the lesion.

13.2.3.5 Streaks

Streaks are finger-like projections of the pigment network from the periphery of the lesion. Instead of both pigment network and dots/globules, the presence of streaks in a skin lesion is by itself a sign of malignancy [1]. Therefore, these structures are only classified as present or absent in each image of the database.

13.2.3.6 Regression Areas

Regression areas are defined as white, scarlike depigmentation often combined with pepperlike regions (speckled blue–gray granules) [1]. In the PH² database, this parameter is classified in two main groups (present or absent) concerning its presence in the skin lesion.

13.2.3.7 Blue–White Veil

The blue–white veil can be defined as a confluent, opaque, irregular blue pigmentation with an overlying, white, ground-glass haze. Its presence is a strong malignancy indicator [1]. This dermoscopic structure is categorically labeled as present or absent, in each image of the database. The presence of the blue–white veil in a melanocytic lesion is illustrated in Figure 13.4.

13.3 DERMOSCOPY IMAGE ANALYSIS

This section presents three image analysis techniques developed and tested using the PH^2 database.

13.3.1 IMAGE SEGMENTATION

Image segmentation is one of the most important tasks in image processing, since its accuracy determines the eventual success or failure of computerized analysis procedures. In the dermoscopy image analysis field, segmentation is used in order to automatically extract the pigmented skin lesion from the surrounding skin. However, dermoscopic images are a great challenge for segmentation algorithms, because there is a great diversity of lesion shapes, boundaries, and colors, along with several skin types and textures. Moreover, dermoscopic images usually contain some intrinsic skin features such as hairs, blood vessels, and air bubbles. Therefore, several segmentation algorithms have been suggested to overcome these difficulties. A comprehensive survey of the methods applied to the segmentation of skin lesions in dermoscopic images is provided in [8].

Herein, the segmentation problem is addressed using gradient vector flow (GVF) snakes [9]. Snakes (or active contours) are deformable curves that are pushed toward nearby edges under the influence of external and internal forces computed from the curve itself and the image data, respectively. Active contour algorithms are often very sensitive to initialization. The initial snake points can be manually defined by an operator or automatically determined. In this work, an automatic snake initialization method is proposed, in order to make the segmentation process fully automated.

Before performing segmentation itself, a preprocessing procedure is applied to dermoscopic images (Figure 13.5). First, the RGB dermoscopic image is converted into a grayscale image through the selection of the blue color channel, since this is the one that provides the best discrimination between the lesion and the skin. Afterwards, dermoscopic images are filtered with a hair removal filter [10], followed by a median filter for image smoothing. Finally, a binary mask of the dark regions in the four corners of the image is created to remove the influence of these regions on the segmentation results.

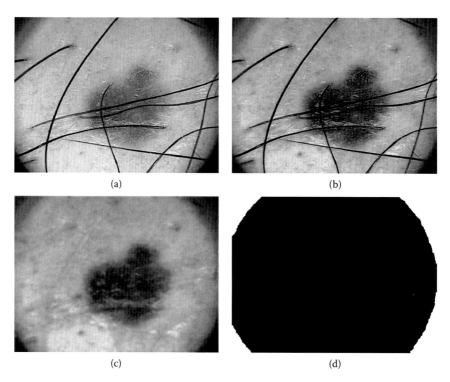

(a)   (b)

(c)   (d)

FIGURE 13.5 Preprocessing: (a) original image, (b) grayscale image, (c) filtered image, and (d) binary mask of the dark regions.

13.3.1.1 Gradient Vector Flow (GVF) Background

The gradient vector flow (GVF) snake method is an extension of the classic snake algorithm [11]. The snake is defined by a parametric curve $\mathbf{x}(s) = (x(s), y(s))$, where x and y are the 2D coordinates of the contour points, and $s \in [0, 1]$ is the parameter. The evolution of the snake from an initial position to the object boundary is performed according to a differential equation

$$\mathbf{x}_t(s, t) = \alpha \mathbf{x}''(s, t) - \beta \mathbf{x}''''(s, t) + \mathbf{v}(x, y), \qquad (13.1)$$

where $\mathbf{x}_t(x, y)$ denotes the partial derivative with respect to t, $\mathbf{x}''$, $\mathbf{x}''''$ denote partial derivatives with respect to s, and $\mathbf{v}(x, y) = (\mathrm{u}(x, y), \mathrm{v}(x, y))$ is the GVF field. The GVF field is computed as a diffusion of the gradient of an edge map f, derived from the image. This is achieved by minimizing an energy function:

$$\epsilon = \iint \mu (u_x^2 + u_y^2 + v_x^2 + v_y^2) + |\nabla f|^2 |\mathbf{v} - \nabla f|^2 dx dy, \qquad (13.2)$$

where µ is a regularization parameter that controls the degree of smoothness of the GVF field, and hence should be defined according to the amount of noise present in the image [9].

13.3.1.2 Automatic Snake Initialization

The proposed automatic snake initialization method is mainly based on the information obtained from the Canny edge detector [12] and can be described by three main steps: (1) edge detection, (2) edge validation, and (3) initial curve determination.

13.3.1.2.1 Edge Detection

The aim of this step is to create a binary edge map from the gray-level image. To accomplish this purpose, the Canny edge detector algorithm is used. The binary edge map obtained through the Canny edge detector is shown in Figure 13.6b, in which each pixel is labeled as either an edge point (value 1) or a nonedge point (value 0).

13.3.1.2.2 Edge Validation

At this stage the edge map includes a large number of false positive edge segments. These false positives are usually a result of the presence of the dark regions in the four corners of the image, and also pigment network segments, skin lines, and even hairs when these artifacts have not been completely removed in the preprocessing step. Therefore, the edge segments corresponding to the dark corners are first eliminated. Then, since edges of the skin lesions are larger than most of noisy edges, the length is used as a criterion to eliminate the edges whose length is less than a predefined threshold. The effect of this step is illustrated in Figure 13.6c.

The next step aims to quantify the relative importance of each edge. To accomplish this purpose, the peripheral regions of each edge are identified (Figure 13.6d). These two regions on both sides of the edges are obtained with the application of morphological dilation to each edge individually, using a flat disk-shaped structuring element with a kernel size defined based on the skin lesions available in the PH^2 dataset. It is important to note that the pixels immediately adjacent to the edges are not considered in the peripheral regions in order to reduce the relative importance of the edges created by small transitions (i.e., skin lines, hairs, etc.).

The difference between the mean intensities of the peripheral regions is computed as a measure of the relative importance of each edge. The underlying assumption is that this difference is larger in the edges of the skin lesion. Given n edge segments E_i, $i = 1, \ldots, n$, the measure of the importance of each edge is given by

$$I_{E_i} = \left| P_{E_{i_1}} - P_{E_{i_2}} \right| \tag{13.3}$$

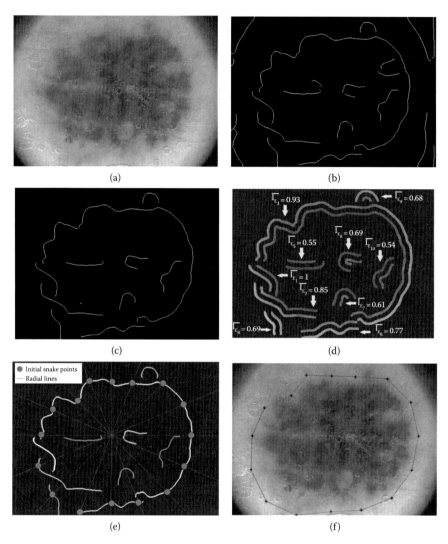

FIGURE 13.6 (**See color insert.**) Automatic snake initialization method: (a) original RGB image, (b) edge map obtained through the Canny edge detector, (c) edge map after removing some false positive edge segments, (d) determination of the normalized mean intensity difference between the peripheral regions, (e) initial snake point finding process, and (f) initial snake curve.

where $P_{E_{i_1}}$ and $P_{E_{i_2}}$ are the mean intensities of the peripheral regions. The maximal mean intensity difference is used to normalize I_{E_i}, thus yielding

$$\overline{I_{E_i}} = \frac{I_{E_i}}{\max_i I_{E_i}} \tag{13.4}$$

Then, every pixel of a given edge E_i is assigned with the value of the respective normalized mean intensity difference between the peripheral regions $\overline{I_{E_i}}$. $\overline{I_{E_i}}$ values range from 0 to 1, and as expected, the edges of the skin lesion have the highest $\overline{I_{E_i}}$ values (Figure 13.6d).

13.3.1.2.3 Initial Curve Determination

In this step the initial curve to be used in the initialization of the GVF method is automatically defined, by first determining a set of initial points that are then connected to form a closed curve. To accomplish this purpose, a number of radial lines R_{θ_j} are drawn from a point within the lesion to the exterior, each of them with a particular orientation $\theta_j \in [0, \ldots, 2\pi]$, $j = 1, \ldots, 16$. The center point, $C(x_c, y_c)$, is automatically computed based on the vertical and horizontal projections of the image. As skin lesions are darker than the surrounding skin, the global minimizers of the image projections are used to provide the coordinates of C.

Then, an initial snake point is defined on each radial line R_{θ_j} as follows. First, take the intersection of this line with the edges E_i, $i = 1, \ldots, n$. Let P_{θ_j} be the set of all edge points detected along the radial line R_{θ_j}, that is, $P_{\theta_j} = \left\{ p_j^1, \ldots, p_j^{N_j} \right\}$, and let $Q_{\theta_j} = \left\{ q_j^1, \ldots, q_j^{N_j} \right\}$ be the set of values of the mean intensity difference between peripheral regions, $\overline{I_E}$, associated with each edge point p_j^k, $k = 1, \ldots, N_j$. Then a subset S_{θ_j} of P_{θ_j} containing the edge points with the highest Q_{θ_j} values is defined as

$$S_{\theta_j} = \left\{ p_j^k \mid q_j^* - q_j^k \leq T_E \right\} \tag{13.5}$$

where

$$q_j^* = \max_{k=1,\ldots,Nj} q_j^k \tag{13.6}$$

and T_E is a predefined threshold value. If S_{θ_j} only has one element, then this point is defined as the initial snake point, s_j, along the radial line R_{θ_j}. In case there is more than one point in the subset S_{θ_j}, the initial snake point is the point s_j^* whose distance to the inner point C is larger, provided that the distance between s_j^* and the point p_j^*, corresponding to the maximum value q_j^*, is not larger than a certain threshold T_d. Figure 13.6e illustrates the detection process of the initial snake point positions. It is important to note that when a given radial line R_{θ_j} does not intersect any edge ($P_{\theta_j} = \emptyset$), no initial snake point is defined in that line.

After detecting the initial snake point s_j, a curve is obtained using a linear interpolation of these points. Finally, in order to obtain the initial snake curve, this curve is uniformly expanded in all outward directions by 20 pixels to ensure that it contains the skin lesion (Figure 13.6f).

Figure 13.7 illustrates the robustness of the automatic snake initialization method, since it works well even in dermoscopic images with a large amount of hair, in images with fragmented skin lesions, and in images with skin lesions

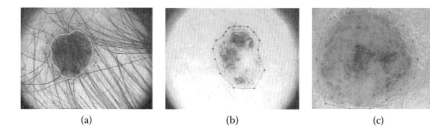

(a)   (b)   (c)

FIGURE 13.7 (**See color insert.**) GVF snake segmentation in difficult dermoscopic images: (a) presence of hairs, (b) fragmented skin lesion, and (c) skin lesion with multiple colors. In these images the dotted red contour represents the initial snake curve, whereas the green contour corresponds to the final segmentation.

with different colors and textures. Furthermore, the final segmentation result is achieved after few iterations, since the initial snake curves are in general placed very close to the skin lesion boundaries.

13.3.1.3 Segmentation Results

In this section, the experimental results of the implemented segmentation method are presented. As the proposed automatic initialization method is mainly based on the gradient information, it is not suitable enough to produce good results when the skin lesions are not completely contained in the image. Therefore, the segmentation algorithm was not tested on the entire PH^2 database, but only in the images of the database in which the skin lesion is contained in the image frame. This results in a subset of 174 images for test.

Three performance metrics were used to quantify the boundary differences: the border error rate (Err), the false negative rate (FNR), and the false positive rate (FPR). Err is given by $\#FP + \#FN/\#GT$, where GT represents the manually segmented area.

Table 13.1 shows the mean, the median, and the standard deviation (Std) of the performance metrics obtained by the implemented segmentation method. The segmentation method achieved an average Err, FPR, and FNR of 11.9%,

TABLE 13.1

Performance of the Implemented Segmentation Algorithm

	Err (%)	FPR (%)	FNR (%)
Mean	11.9%	5.15%	2.05%
Median	9.2%	3.48%	1.00%
Std	7.1%	5.46%	3.30%

5.15%, and 2.05%, respectively. These results demonstrate that the implemented segmentation algorithm provides good results for the majority of the tested images. However, there are three main groups of images in which the algorithm may demonstrate limitations: (1) images in which the lesion is fragmented, (2) lesions presenting a great variety of colors and textures, and (3) images with a very low contrast between the lesion and the skin.

13.3.2 COLOR LABELING

Color plays a major role in the analysis of dermoscopy images [1]. For example, the ABCD rule of dermoscopy considers six clinically significant colors (blue–gray, black, white, dark and light brown, red) that medical doctors try to detect in melanocytic lesions. The number of colors observed in an image is a malignancy measure that is combined with other criteria (border, symmetry, differential structures) [5].

The detection of colors is a subjective task that requires considerable training. Nonetheless, the development of computational methods for this task is a desired goal. This problem is addressed in [13], assuming that the feature vector $\mathbf{y}$, associated with a small patch of size 12×12 and a color c, is a random variable described by a mixture of Gaussians

$$p(\mathbf{y}|c, \theta^c) = \sum_{m=1}^{k_c} \alpha_m^c \, p(\mathbf{y}|c, \theta_m^c) \qquad (13.7)$$

where k_c is the number of Gaussians in the mixture and $\theta_m^c = (\alpha_m^c, \boldsymbol{\mu}_m^c, \boldsymbol{R}_m^c)$ denotes the set of parameters (weight, mean, covariance matrix) of the mth Gaussian mode.

The number of Gaussians, k_c, and their parameters, θ_m^c, should be estimated from a set of dermoscopy images annotated by an expert. This problem can be solved since the PH^2 database contains 29 images with color segmentations performed by an experienced dermatologist. The estimation of the mixture order and parameters was carried out using the algorithm proposed in [14]. This procedure is repeated for each of the five colors considered in this chapter (blue–gray, black, white, dark and light brown). The red color was excluded due to the lack of examples associated with this color in the annotated images.

After estimating the five mixtures, each pixel is then classified into the most probable color. This is achieved by the Bayes' law

$$p(c|\mathbf{y}) = \frac{p(\mathbf{y}|c, \widehat{\theta}^c)p(c)}{p(\mathbf{y}|\widehat{\theta})} \qquad c = 1, \ldots, 5 \qquad (13.8)$$

where $\widehat{\theta}^c = (\widehat{\theta}_1^c, \ldots, \widehat{\theta}_{k_c}^c)$, $\widehat{\theta} = (\widehat{\theta}^1, \ldots, \widehat{\theta}^5)$ are the estimates of the mixture parameters. A label c is assigned to the pixel $\mathbf{y}$ using the following decision rule. First, the degrees of membership to each of the five colors are sorted.

The highest and second-highest values are denoted as c_1 and c_2, respectively. Then, this information is used to either label the patch or reject it, as follows:

1. If $p(c_1|\mathbf{y}) \geq \delta$ and $p(c_1|\mathbf{y}) - p(c_2|\mathbf{y}) > \epsilon$, where δ and ϵ are empirically determined thresholds, the patch is labeled according to color c_1.
2. If $p(c_1|\mathbf{y}) \geq \delta$ and $p(c_1|\mathbf{y}) - p(c_2|\mathbf{y}) \leq \epsilon$, the patch receives a label that expresses doubt between c_1 and c_2.
3. If $p(c_1|\mathbf{y}) < \delta$, the patch is rejected.

Finally, we assign color labels to the test images. This task is performed using the patches previously labeled with one of the five colors. We do not consider the patches that have doubt labels in this process. For each color, we compute the area of the patches with its label (i.e., the number of pixels) and compare it with an empirically determined area ratio threshold. Each color is validated only if its area ratio is above a specific threshold, where the area ratio (λ_c) for color c is defined as

$$\lambda_c = \frac{A_{patches^c}}{A_{lesion}} \qquad (13.9)$$

For each color we have a different area ratio threshold, which was empirically determined.

We will now present experimental results obtained on the PH^2 database. The five mixture models were estimated using 29 annotated images from the PH^2 database (see Section 13.2). Each of these images is associated with five binary masks defining examples of each color. Then, we selected another 123 images (test set) to evaluate the performance of the algorithm. The test images were classified according to the learned models, and a set of labels was automatically computed for each image and compared with the colors annotated by a medical specialist. Table 13.2 compares the performance of the proposed system with the labeling performed by a specialist. We used the following

---

TABLE 13.2

Evaluation of Color Labeling Algorithm in the PH^2 Database

	CD	DF	CND	FA	SE	SP	ACC
Blue–gray	24	2	62	15	92.3%	80.5%	86.4%
Dark brown	74	4	16	9	94.9%	64.0%	79.4%
Light brown	71	7	19	6	91.0%	76.0%	83.5%
Black	24	4	54	21	85.7%	72.0%	78.9%
White	6	1	71	25	85.7%	74.0%	79.8%
Total	199	18	222	76	91.7%	74.5%	81.7%

Note: CD, correct detections; DF, detection failures; CND, correct non detections; FA, false alarms; SE, sensitivity, SP, specificity, and ACC, accuracy.

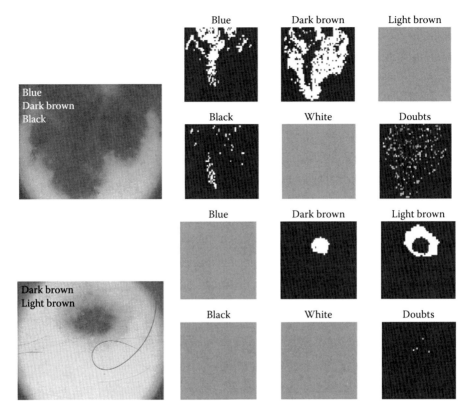

FIGURE 13.8 Examples of color detection in melanoma (top) and benign lesions (bottom).

metrics to evaluate the algorithm. Each color correctly identified in an image is considered a *correct detection* (CD), a missed color is a *detection failure* (DF), a detected color that has no corresponding label is a *false alarm* (FA), and each color that is correctly nondetected is a *correct nondetection* (CND). Additionally, we also compute three different statistics: sensitivity (SE), specificity (SP), and accuracy (ACC). It is possible to see that a good match was obtained in this dataset. Figure 13.8 shows two examples of color detection.

13.3.3 MELANOMA DETECTION

Melanoma is the most aggressive type of skin cancer. The early detection of melanomas is therefore a major goal in dermoscopy analysis. Several methods have been proposed in the literature to perform this task [15–19]. Most of them fit into a three-step structure: (1) lesion segmentation, (2) feature extraction, and (3) feature classification. First, the lesion boundary is estimated in the input images. Then, a set of features (color, texture, shape, symmetry) is extracted from each lesion. Finally, a classifier (e.g., support vector machine (SVM)) is trained to distinguish benign lesions from malign ones.

We developed computer diagnosis systems for the detection of melanomas, based on two classification strategies: (1) global classification strategy, using global features extracted from the lesion [19] and (2) local strategy, representing the lesion by a set of local patches, each of them described by local features; the decision is obtained using a bag-of-features (BoF) approach [19, 20].

Several types of features were considered in the global approach: color features, texture features, shape, and symmetry features. The BoF approach also considered color and texture features associated with lesion patches. See the different descriptors in Table 13.3. In each approach, the color features were computed using multiple color spaces (RGB, HSV, CIE L*a*b*, and opponent).

The global system used a k-nearest neighbor (kNN) classifier with $k \in \{3, 5, \ldots, 25\}$ neighbors. The BoF system used a dictionary of $\{100, 200, 300\}$ words; the decision is made by a kNN classifier as well, with $k \in \{3, 5, \ldots, 25\}$. Details can be found in [19, 20].

The algorithms were evaluated by 10-fold cross-validation. The set of 200 images is split into 10 subsets (folds) of 20 images each; 9 folds are used for training and 1 fold for testing. This procedure is repeated 10 times with different test folds. The results are shown in Table 13.4 for both classification strategies and different types of features. Very good performance is achieved by several configurations. The best types of features are color and color symmetry features. Both strategies (global and local) lead to very good results. We prefer local classifiers since they take into account local properties of the dermoscopy image, as the examination is performed by medical experts. The global methods, however, are much faster during the training phase.

TABLE 13.3
Considered Features

Features	Global	Local
Color	Color histograms	Color histograms
	Mean color vectors	Mean color vectors
Texture	Gradient histograms	Gradient histograms
	Gray Level Co-occurence Matrix (GLCM)	GLCM
	Laws' masks	Laws' masks
	Gabor filters	Gabor filters
Shape	Simple shape descriptors	—
	Fourier descriptors	—
	Wavelet descriptors	—
	Moment invariants	—
Symmetry	Shape symmetry	—
	Color symmetry (histograms and mean color vector)	—

TABLE 13.4

Performance of Melanoma Detection Algorithms for Different Types of Features and Classification Strategies

Features	Global			Local		
	Sensitivity	**Specificity**	**Descriptor**	**Sensitivity**	**Specificity**	**Descriptor**
Color	90%	89%	HSV histogram	93%	84%	L*a*b* histogram
Texture	93%	78%	Gradient histogram	88%	76%	Laws' masks
Shape	81%	88%	Wavelets	—	—	—
Symmetry	92%	85%	HSV mean color	—	—	—

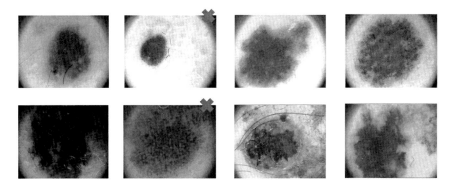

FIGURE 13.9 Examples of benign (top) and malign (bottom) lesions classified by global system (the symbol × denotes a misclassification).

Figures 13.9 and 13.10 show examples of melanocytic lesions extracted from the PH^2 database, together with the decision provided by the two systems described in this section. Color features were used in both cases to characterize the lesion or its patches. We observe that the systems provide correct decisions in most cases and solve some difficult examples in which the classification of the skin lesions is not simple.

13.4 CONCLUSIONS

This chapter presents a dataset of 200 dermoscopic images with medical annotations, publicly available at www.fc.up.pt/addi. The images and medical annotations were provided by the dermatology service of Hospital Pedro Hispano, Matosinhos, Portugal, and comprise both benign nevi (160) and malign melanomas (40).

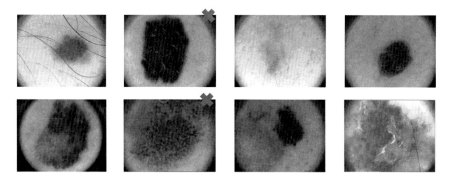

FIGURE 13.10 Examples of benign (top) and malign (bottom) lesions classified by the local system (the symbol × denotes a misclassification).

The PH^2 dataset aims to provide a benchmarking tool for the comparison of computer-aided diagnosis systems for the analysis of dermoscopic images. This chapter includes examples of such systems trained with the PH^2 database and tested using 10-fold cross-validation. The results presented in this chapter for illustrative purposes allow a direct comparison with other systems.

The PH^2 database was made available online in September 2013. Since its release, the PH^2 database has been downloaded 51 times by research groups from 21 countries. These download statistics are a strong indicator of the impact of the PH^2 database in the research community due to the lack of public ground truth databases of dermoscopic images.

ACKNOWLEDGMENTS

This work was partially funded with grant SFRH/ BD/84658/2012 and by the FCT Fundação para a Ciência e Tecnologia projects PTDC/SAU-BEB/103471/2008 and [UID/EEA/50009/2013].

REFERENCES

1. G. Argenziano, H. P. Soyer, V. De Giorgi, D. Piccolo, P. Carli, M. Delfino, A. Ferrari et al., *Interactive Atlas of Dermoscopy*, EDRA Medical Publishing and New Media, 2000.
2. G. C. do Carmo and M. R. e Silva, Dermoscopy: Basic concepts, *International Journal of Dermatology*, vol. 47, pp. 712–719, 2008.
3. H. Kittler, H. Pehamberger, K. Wolff, and M. Binder, Diagnostic accuracy of dermoscopy, *Lancet Oncology*, vol. 3, pp. 159–165, 2002.
4. ADDI project: Automatic computer-based diagnosis system for dermoscopy images, http://www.fc.up.pt/addi.
5. W. Stolz, A. Riemann, and A. B. Cognetta, ABCD rule of dermatoscopy: A new practical method for early recognition of malignant melanoma, *European Journal of Dermatology*, vol. 4, pp. 521–527, 1994.

6. G. Argenziano, G. Fabbrocini, P. Carli, V. D. Giorgi, E. Sammarco, and M. Delfino, Epiluminescence microscopy for the diagnosis of doubtful melanocytic skin lesions: Comparison of the ABCD rule of dermatoscopy and a new 7-point checklist based on pattern analysis, *Archives of Dermatology*, vol. 12, no. 134, pp. 1563–1570, 1998.

7. S. Menzies, C. Ingvar, K. Crotty, and W. H. McCarthy, Frequency and morphologic characteristics of invasive melanomas lacking specific surface microscopic features, *Archives of Dermatology*, vol. 132, pp. 1178–1182, 1996.

8. M. E. Celebi, G. Schaefer, H. Iyatomi, and W. V. Stoecker, Lesion border detection in dermoscopy images, *Computerized Medical Imaging and Graphics*, vol. 33, pp. 148–153, 2009.

9. C. Xu and J. L. Prince, Snakes, shapes, and gradient vector flow, *IEEE Transactions on Image Processing*, vol. 17, no. 3, 1998.

10. C. Barata, J. S. Marques, and J. Rozeira, A system for the detection of pigment network in dermoscopy images using directional filters, *IEEE Transactions on Biomedical Engineering*, vol. 10, pp. 2744–2754, 2012.

11. M. Kass, A. Witkin, and D. Terzopoulos, Snakes: Active contour models, *International Journal of Computer Vision*, pp. 321–331, 1988.

12. J. Canny, A computational approach to edge detection, *IEEE Transactions on Pattern Analysis and Machine Intelligence*, vol. 8, no. 6, pp. 679–714, 1986.

13. C. Barata, M. A. T. Figueiredo, M. E. Celebi, and J. S. Marques, Color identification in dermoscopy images using Gaussian mixture models, in *IEEE International Conference on Acoustics, Speech, and Signal Processing*, pp. 3611–3615, Florence, Itlay, 2014.

14. M. A. T. Figueiredo and A. K. Jain, Unsupervised learning of finite mixture models, *IEEE Transactions on Pattern Analysis and Machine Intelligence*, vol. 24, no. 3, pp. 381–396, 2002.

15. H. Ganster, P. Pinz, R. Rohrer, E. Wildling, M. Binder, and H. Kittler, Automated melanoma recognition, *IEEE Transactions on Medical Imaging*, vol. 20, no. 3, pp. 233–239, 2001.

16. M. E. Celebi, H. Kingravi, B. Uddin, H. Iyatomi, Y. Aslandogan, W. Stoecker, and R. Moss, A methodological approach to the classification of dermoscopy images, *Computerized Medical Imaging and Graphics*, vol. 31, pp. 362–373, 2007.

17. H. Iyatomi, H. Oka, M. E. Celebi, M. Hashimoto, M. Hagiwara, M. Tanaka, and K. Ogawa, An improved Internet-based melanoma screening system with dermatologist-like tumor area extraction algorithm, *Computerized Medical Imaging and Graphics*, vol. 32, pp. 566–579, 2008.

18. Q. Abbas, M. E. Celebi, I. F. Garcia, and W. Ahmad, Melanoma recognition framework based on expert definition of ABCD for dermoscopic images, *Skin Research and Technology*, vol. 19, pp. e93–e102, 2013.

19. C. Barata, M. Ruela, M. Francisco, T. Mendonça, and J. S. Marques, Two systems for the detection of melanomas in dermoscopy images using texture and color features, *IEEE Systems Journal*, vol. 8, no. 3, pp. 965–979, 2014.

20. C. Barata, M. Ruela, T. Mendonça, and J. S. Marques, A bag-of-features approach for the classification of melanomas in dermoscopy images: The role of color and texture descriptors, in *Computer Vision Techniques for the Diagnosis of Skin Cancer* (J. Scharcanski and M. E. Celebi, eds.), pp. 49–69, Springer, Berlin, 2014.

Index

Abbas methods
  global pattern classification,
    193–194
  numerical results, 172–173
  reticular pattern recognition,
    135, 153–159
  techniques used, 167–168
ABCDE rule, 252, 258
ABCD rule
  Abbas methods, 156
  asymmetry, 303, 423
  basic concepts, 250–251, 420
  border blurriness, 306
  color, 308
  color detection, 13
  color information, 232–233
  color labeling, 433
  color/texture features, 51
  computer-aided diagnostics, 253
  databases, 388
  dermoscopic criteria, 423
  feature extraction, 303
  feature selection, 313
  global pattern classification, 184
  Gola methods, 148
  image acquisition, 389
  image features, 257
  learning color mixture
    models, 13
  melanoma diagnosis, 295
  reticular patterns, 132
  streak detection, 212
ABC features, 296
Absence of streaks, 223, 224
Accuracy (ACC)
  artificial neural networks, 296
  color assessment, 240, 243
  color identification, 16
  color labeling, 435
  computer system *vs.* humans,
    253–254
  dermatoscopy, 250

DMB system, 240
ensemble classifiers, 315
evaluation, 107
hair detection, 364
lesion classification results, 10
lesion segmentation, 367–368
perceptible grade, 243
support vector machine, 373
Accurate and scalable system,
    melanoma automatic
    detection
  artificial neural networks, 314
  asymmetry, 303–306
  background, 297
  basic concepts, 294–297
  blurriness, 306–307
  borders, 306–308
  classification, 313–317
  color, 305–306, 308–309
  comparisons, 316–317
  datasets, 323
  decision trees, 315
  differential structures, 310–311
  discriminant analysis, 313–314
  disease classification, 324–328
  ensemble classifiers and
    modeling, 315, 320–321,
    326–328
  experimental results, 322–328
  feature extraction, 303–311
  feature selection, 311–313
  high-level intuitive
    features, 311
  image acquisition, 297–298
  irregularity, borders, 307–308
  k-nearest neighborhood, 314
  large-scale training, 322
  low-level features, 318–320,
    324–325
  machine learning method
    comparisons, 316–317
  palette, color, 308

441

Printed and bound by CPI Group (UK) Ltd, Croydon, CR0 4YY

28/10/2024

01779788-0001